Handbook of Intensive Care
Organization and Management

Handbook of Intensive Care

Organization and Management

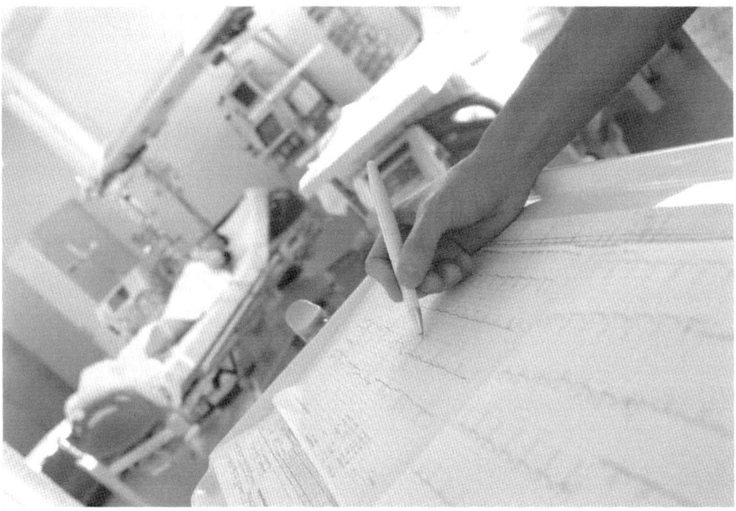

Editor

Andrew Webb

Clinical Professor, Division of Critical Care, Department of Medicine,
University of British Columbia

Imperial College Press

ICP

Published by

Imperial College Press
57 Shelton Street
Covent Garden
London WC2H 9HE

Distributed by

World Scientific Publishing Co. Pte. Ltd.
5 Toh Tuck Link, Singapore 596224
USA office: 27 Warren Street, Suite 401-402, Hackensack, NJ 07601
UK office: 57 Shelton Street, Covent Garden, London WC2H 9HE

Library of Congress Cataloging-in-Publication Data
Names: Webb, Andrew R. (Andrew Roy), editor.
Title: Handbook of intensive care organization and management / [edited by] Andrew Webb.
Description: New Jersey : Imperial College Press, [2016]
Identifiers: LCCN 2015049357 | ISBN 9781783269501 (hc : alk. paper)
Subjects: | MESH: Critical Care--organization & administration | Intensive Care Units--
organization & administration
Classification: LCC RC86.7 | NLM WX 218 | DDC 616.02/8--dc23
LC record available at http://lccn.loc.gov/2015049357

British Library Cataloguing-in-Publication Data
A catalogue record for this book is available from the British Library.

Desk Editors: Anthony Alexander/Mary Simpson

Typeset by Stallion Press
Email: enquiries@stallionpress.com

Printed in Singapore

Contents

About the Editor

Dr. Webb has 25 years of healthcare leadership experience. He has held executive roles as Vice President, Medicine at Fraser Health Authority, the second largest health authority in Canada, and Medical Director for UCL Hospitals NHS Foundation Trust in London, UK. He is a clinical professor in the Faculty of Medicine at the University of British Columbia. He has held expert medical advisory roles with the British Columbia, Irish and Welsh governments, supporting health system reform and critical care development. As Director of Critical Care at UCL Hospitals Dr. Webb was instrumental in building academic critical care through key appointments, as a clinical researcher, educator and consultant physician. He was awarded Honorary Membership of the Intensive Care Society in 2010.

Dr. Webb is co-editor of the *Oxford Handbook of Critical Care* and the *Oxford Textbook of Critical Care*, both in multiple editions.

Preface

The specialty of Critical Care Medicine is complex. In addition to required knowledge of physiology, pathophysiology, biochemistry, technology and pharmacology, practitioners need to act and react decisively. Clear communication with colleagues, patients and relatives, often in stressful situations, the importance of working cohesively within an expanded team drawn from different backgrounds, and the regular occurrence of ethical and life-and-death dilemmas all place heavy demands on critical care staff.

As the demand for critical care resources increases in our aging society, there is an increasing need for books on management and administration in clinical critical care medicine.

This book describes the principles of critical care organization and management. While some of the principles of organization and management cross international borders, many of the details do not. The divide between North America and Europe is significant in this respect with physicians providing independent services to hospitals rather than being salaried employees. There are also considerable differences in funding systems from 'for profit' insurance based services to single payer–multiple provider and single payer–single provider. There are significant differences in management in heavily unionized labor forces versus the more liberal workforces. Regulation and governance standards also vary from country to country. Even the mode of delivery of critical care varies with the closed unit still being relatively uncommon in North America yet the standard in much of Europe.

Organized in seven parts, the handbook covers organization, structure and governance of critical care, staffing and staff development, decision making and communication, performance, quality and safety, financial management, and emergency preparedness. The 20 chapters are written by international experts.

This book will serve academics, students and professionals in medicine, health and business, as a key reference for service providers, their employees, trainees/practitioners in medicine and management and those responsible for practice and administration in critical care.

Part I

Organization, Structure, and Governance

Leadership and Management

Pascale Gruber
Clinical Lead
Consultant in Anaesthesia and Intensive Care Medicine
The Royal Marsden NHS Foundation Trust
SW3 6JJ, Fulham Road, London

Timothy Wigmore
Divisional Medical Director
Consultant in Anaesthesia and Intensive Care Medicine
The Royal Marsden NHS Foundation Trust
SW3 6JJ, Fulham Road, London

Key Points

1. Nowadays clinicians are expected to be skilled in management and leadership as well as being clinically astute.
2. Key to good leadership is self-knowledge, excellent communication skills, emotional intelligence, and expertise in persuasion and negotiation.
3. Good leadership has been shown to improve patient safety, staff satisfaction and outcome in critical care.
4. Management and leadership roles in most well-functioning intensive care units (ICUs) are dispersed with distribution of responsibilities to a number of selective individuals.
5. Effective delegation is a key skill for a good leader and the art lies in knowing which tasks should be delegated and to who.

Introduction

In the past, the role of hospital management was predominantly restricted to non-clinical hospital managers but there has been an increasing recognition over the last 20 years that the involvement of clinicians has much to add. Management roles in hospitals are now more widely distributed with a significant proportion of management duties distributed to hybrid clinician-managers. Clinicians are increasingly required to play two roles — one that relies on their clinical skills and the other on their managerial and leadership capabilities.[1] This hybrid role enables doctors to influence care for individual patients by the bedside, pathways of patient care within their service and healthcare delivery at an organizational level. Service improvements are more likely to be sustain and succeed if clinically led. However, in the past, the clinician-manager role has received little recognition or remuneration with doctor-managers regarding the managerial aspects of their role as part-time and temporary with little authority over their peers.

Historically clinicians have been identified and promoted to leadership positions based on academic and career success rather than on their management skills and experience.[2] This has sometimes left clinicians poorly equipped for the requirements of management and leadership. The climate is now changing with under- and post-graduate training programs including management and leadership competences as an integral part of medical education.[2] Responsibilities of clinician-managers/leaders encompass a multitude of areas outside traditional bedside clinical care including strategy, service development, human resources, finance and business planning. As a consequence clinician-managers rely on broad knowledge and skills and require the ability to transition seamlessly between clinical, managerial and leadership roles depending on the context.[1]

What is Leadership?

To define leadership precisely is difficult. For many the definition of a leader is synonymous with a job title or role but leadership is not just a job description. It is about the specific skills and behaviour of the leader. Stogdill stated in an early definition of leadership that "leadership may be considered as the process (act) of influencing the activities of an organized group in its efforts towards goal setting and goal achievements". This definition views leadership as a process of influencing a group with the purpose of goal attainment and achievement.[3] In this, the work that the group does together is central to the definition, i.e. leadership in this context is a social rather than an individually focused activity. In contrast, in Warren Bennis' definition of leadership he focuses on a leader's qualities: "Leadership is a function of knowing yourself, having a vision that is well communicated, building trust among colleagues, and taking effective action to realize your own leadership potential".[4,5] Melissa Fitzpatrick, past president of the American Association of Critical Care Nurses, once stated, "Leadership is about influencing and making decisions. It is about taking appropriate actions at appropriate times. Leadership is about projecting ourselves and those around us into a future that is better. Effective leaders influence. They teach. They are role models. They evoke confidence in others".[6]

Leadership qualities

Surviving and succeeding in the healthcare environment of today requires leadership at all levels of the organization, not just at the top. There has been a drive towards leadership development amongst healthcare professionals.[1,7] The concept that individuals are "born to lead" is outdated and has been replaced by a focus on the development of leadership competencies.[7] Key leadership skills include self-knowledge, emotional intelligence, an ability to tolerate debate and disagreement, a capacity to understand the values and beliefs of others, excellent communication skills, and powers of persuasion and negotiation. These are crucial skills for leaders to empower and motivate individuals, to drive change and to communicate and collaborate across multi-organizational, multi-disciplinary and multi-functional boundaries in the modern healthcare system.[1] Today's leaders are not only required to have role related knowledge, clinical expertise and vision, but the emotional intelligence that encompasses so-called "people skills".[8] Emotional intelligence is most often cited as the quality most admired of leaders.[8] It is the ability to manage oneself and one's relationships effectively. Personal qualities such as self-awareness, self-management, resilience, personal reflection, social awareness, and social skill form the foundations of emotional intelligence.[8] Awareness of one's strengths and limitations in these areas has a direct impact on how one behaves and interacts with others. This in turn will impact on one's colleagues, overall culture and climate within the team and organization.[7]

Another commonly cited important quality of leaders is organizational orientation and political astuteness. In addition to knowing about the organizational structure and function, organizational orientation includes a commitment to improving the organization, even if it is at variance with personal or department goals. One cited example is "it's really about an organization that makes patient care better. So having an attitude that you know this is how I make things better in the organization, I'm not interested in people who work just for power, I'm interested in people interested in making things better and that involves changes, changes in management".[8] Political awareness is also an important skill, as leaders need to be able to work with diverse stakeholders inside and outside the organization, both locally and nationally.

Competency frameworks have become a widely used approach to thinking about leadership skill development.[7] The National Health Service (NHS) Leadership Qualities Framework has been used in healthcare in United Kingdom.[7] The competency frameworks cover a range of personal (self-awareness, confidence, integrity, and resilience), social (empathy, communication, maintaining cooperative relationships), and cognitive, or conceptual skills (analytical ability, creativity, foresight).

Leadership Styles and Theories

There is a wealth of published literature discussing styles of leadership.[9–15] Effective leaders tend to not rely on only one leadership style; they use most of them, seamlessly adapting and transitioning from one style to another depending on context. Summarized below are some commonly described leadership styles.

Behaviour or style theory

Psychologist Kurt Lewin described three major leadership styles: democratic, autocratic, and laissez-faire.[9] Democratic leadership is characterized by high staff engagement in decision-making; autocratic leadership where the decision-making is primarily directed by the leader; laissez-faire leadership is a more devolved style with a high level of autonomy given to team members. Autocratic leadership is useful when a quick decision needs to be made but can lead to poor staff engagement and high staff turnover. In contrast democratic and laissez-faire leadership styles often result in high levels of job satisfaction and productivity amongst the team but may not be effective when a decision needs to be expedited or staff are inexperienced.

Blake–Mouton managerial model

The Blake–Mouton managerial model adapts the style of leadership based on two axes — concern for people (accommodating people's needs) and concern for production/task (focus on getting the job done).[10] The end result are five key leadership styles: impoverished (the leader has not only little concern for employee satisfaction but also work deadlines), task (the leader is more concerned about the task/production and less about the people), middle of the road (the leader has a compromising style where they aim to maintain a balance between needs of the task and people), country club (the leader is characterized by low task but high people orientation) and team management (with the leader exhibiting high people and task focus).

Situational theory

The Hersey–Blanchard situational leadership theory relies on the maturity of the team members to determine the leadership style used.[11] Based on the maturity of the individual or group, the leader chooses to be more supportive or directive in their behaviour. Four key leadership behaviours are characterized: telling (the leader is very directive), selling (the leader provides information and direction), participating (the leader shares decision-making and ideas, working with the team to achieve the goal), and delegating (the leader passes responsibility to the group). Depending on the knowledge, skills and confidence of the individual or group the leader may choose different leadership styles. For example, the Lead Clinician in critical care may choose to use the telling/directing approach when guiding a new doctor through their first central line insertion, selling approach when writing a book chapter on ventilation with a senior trainee and delegating approach when handing over role of Educational Lead to their colleague.

Primal leadership

In primal leadership, Daniel Goleman, described six styles of leadership that effective leaders utilize depending on the context: visionary, coaching, affiliative, democratic, pacesetting, commanding.[12] In the visionary style the leader articulates the goal but leaves individuals to be free and creative in how they achieve that goal. When using the coaching style the leader focuses on helping individuals and teams develop and improve their performance. In the affiliative style, the leader focuses on creating harmony and increasing communication within the group; this has been demonstrated to be particularly useful when there has been mistrust within an organization. In the democratic style, the leader draws on the knowledge and skills within the group and uses the group's knowledge and experience to guide the direction of the service. In the pace-setting style, the leader sets high standards for performance. This style should be used cautiously, as setting overly high goals can demoralize groups if they are serially unable to achieve them. Finally, there is the commanding or 'military' style that is most effective in crises situations or when urgent turnaround is needed.

Transactional and transformational leadership

In transactional leadership the leader uses rewards or punishment to gain team compliance and to achieve goals.[13] In contrast, transformational leadership is about engaging, motivating and inspiring individuals to achieve goals. The focus of transformational leadership is on empowering others through intellectual simulation where "leaders and their followers raise one another to higher levels of morality and motivation".[13] This purportedly leads to high levels of productivity and engagement.

Collective leadership approach

More recently there has been a growing interest in a collective approach to leadership.[14,15] Experts argue that it is difficult for one individual to embody all the different traits required for good leadership.[14] This is a complete contrast to the previously discussed descriptions of leadership that are individually focused. The concept of collective leadership relies on it being a shared, team phenomenon where behaviours are enacted by multiple individuals rather than those solely in formal leadership roles.[14,15] This approach envisages collaborative working between individuals who trust and respect each other's contribution and have 'shared values' and is a move away from the traditional concept of the individual leader at the top of the organization (vertical hierarchy) to a shared and distributed leadership across the organization (horizontal hierarchy). Shared decision-making does not equate to shared accountability and in collective leadership clear lines of accountability remain. Opponents of this approach argue that while groups may make better decisions because of their ability to draw from the breadth and variety of team expertise, there remains a risk of gravitating towards 'group thinking' if members do not embrace individual differences. This radical approach to leadership requires a change in mindset with a shift away from 'command and control structures', silo working and hierarchy towards a collaborative process whereby influence is distributed amongst several individuals for the purpose of achieving favorable outcomes for the organization.

Management versus leadership

Management is often described as using resources effectively and efficiently to achieve the best outcome. Leadership has been described as about guiding, influencing, directing the team towards a specific goal or vision (Figure 1). Bennis eloquently stated: "Managers are people who do things right, and leaders are people who do the right thing".[5]

Leadership and management also tend to differ in their legitimacy, power, type of action, and position in the organization hierarchy (Table 1).[17]

Leaders and managers can influence and change behaviour by using power. A leader's or manager's power is proportional to their ability to create opportunities, control resources, and successfully deal with challenges. Leaders rarely use formal ways of exerting power. There are different types of power described by Yukl: legitimate power (formal; derived from the individual's administrative position), reward-based (formal; derived from the leader's or manager's ability to reward desirable

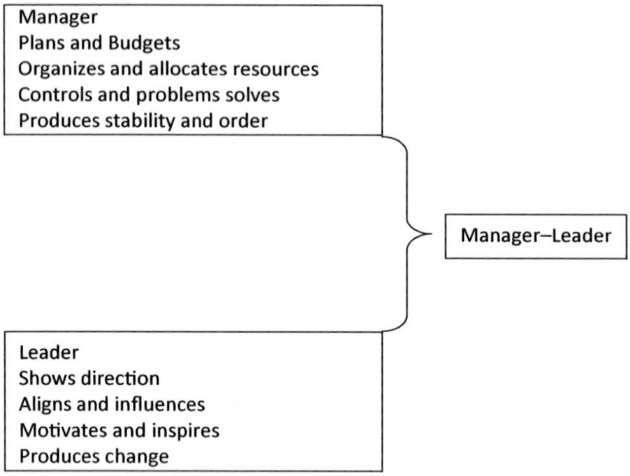

Figure 1. Differences between leaders and managers.[16]

Table 1. Differences in legitimacy, power, type of action, and hierarchy between leaders and managers.

	Manager	Leader
Legitimacy	Result-based	Ambiguous
Power	Formal	Informal
Type of action	Maintaining *status quo*	Change
Organization hierarchy	Middle-level positions	High-level positions

behaviours), coercive (formal; derived from the leader's or manager's ability to prevent an individual from achieving rewards), expert (informal; based on knowledge) and referent (informal; derived from the ability of the leader to create loyalty from others).[17]

Leadership and management are closely interlinked. Without good management, the vision set by a leader will rarely be achieved. Similarly, management without effective leadership will result in stagnation with no change, little adaptation to meet strategic goals and lack of optimal team performance. Most senior roles in hospital management demand expertise in both areas. The real challenge is to combine good leadership and management and use both to balance the other.[16]

The role of the manager

Typical managerial responsibilities include planning, organizing, controlling, budgeting, staffing, and auditing to ensure organizational objectives are met using available resources. A manager's focus is to ensure resources are used effectively, to the maximum benefit for patients, staff and the organization while maintaining the budget. For this managers must have good understanding of the technical aspect of the service being delivered and need to review regularly data/information about the service and use this to make informed choices.

Simplistically, the role clinician-manager can be divided into *three* categories:

1. Interpersonal: nominally in charge of the service.
2. Informational: takes responsibility for dissemination and communication of information to the team.
3. Decisional: takes responsibility for negotiating and allocating resources to help achieve the service's objectives.

To a degree, the role and responsibilities of a manager will depend on the type of services being delivered, resources available and people (staff, patients, partners, stakeholders). Examples of key functions of clinician-managers in the ICU are outlined in Table 2.

The management role involves skills and competencies such as motivating staff, managing poor performance and conflict, communicating and negotiating with stakeholders, maintaining attitudes and behaviours that maximize staff performance and satisfaction, and facilitate high quality service provision.

The role of the leader

Leadership is a group phenomenon; there is no leader without followers. Leadership is about aligning people to the vision, empowerment but also about change. This requires skills in communication, listening, influencing, and persuasion to get buy-in.[4]

Examples of key functions of clinician-leader in the ICU are outlined in Table 3.

Table 2. Examples of key functions of clinician-manager in the ICU.

	Functions of clinician-managers in the ICU					
	Planning	Organizing	Staffing	Controlling	Decision-making	Problem solving
Explanations	Providing the team guidance and direction and how to achieve the goals for the service	Delegation and task allocation of activities and roles on the ICU	Appointing and managing staff	Performance review and evaluation	Analysis of situations that require decisions	Identify and evaluate different solutions to address a problem, implement and review of results
Practical examples	Service reconfiguration, expansion	Allocating roles for individuals in the unit e.g. medical and nursing leads for patient safety, research, education, etc.	Job plans, appraisal, recruitment, coaching, mentorship	Service improvement, budgeting, clinical governance activities	Review of pathways for patient referral to the ICU	Introduction of electronic prescribing to reduce medication errors

Table 3. Examples of key functions of clinician-leader in the ICU.

	Functions of clinician-leaders in the ICU					
	Visionary	Motivate and inspire	Persuasion	Build relationships and teamwork	Mentorship, counselling, and coaching	Change
Explanation	A focus on long-term visions and goals	Motivate, empower and challenge the team	Bringing people willingly towards the right path	Build relationships and networks internally and externally with key stakeholders	Supporting, encouraging individuals to have the freedom to develop themselves	Bringing about positive change to the service
Practical examples	Articulate clear vision for the future of ICU, creating priorities and direction for the unit	Delegate suitable tasks (not just the routine ones) to team members	Engage individuals in the change management process, allowing them to own it	Devote time to attending both clinical and non-clinical meetings and take up opportunities for involvement beyond the hospital boundaries	Allocate mentors to new arrivals, and create an educational trust to fund educational endeavors	Develop a short, medium and long-term strategic plan and set about planning how each item can be enacted

To be successful, the clinician-leader should have a clear vision for the future of the service, be able to motivate staff to focus on activities (clinical, education, and academic) towards achieving the vision, to inspire change, to encourage staff development and growth, all while balancing the interests of the key stakeholders.[4,5]

Leadership and Management Roles in the ICU

The management roles within the ICU are usually not limited to the ICU Clinical Director or Lead Nurse (Figure 2). In fact management and

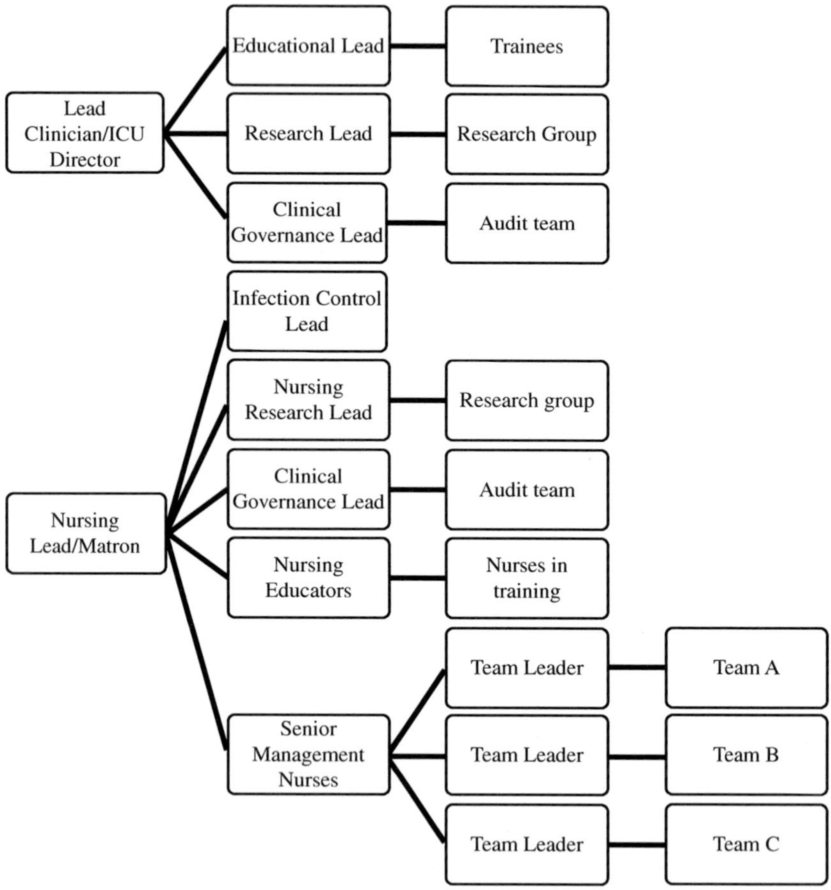

Figure 2. An example of different leadership roles in the ICU.

leadership roles in most well-functioning ICUs are often more widely distributed with dispersion of responsibilities to a number of selective individuals. One key skill required of the ICU Clinical Director is the ability to identify individual's strengths within the team and delegate tasks to the appropriate individual. For example, within the medical team in addition to the ICU Clinical Director whose primary responsibility is the operational and management activities of the unit, there will commonly be separate leads for research, education, and quality improvement/patient safety. Similarly, within the nursing hierarchy they may be separate leads for management, infection control, recruitment, education, audit, and clinical governance. Ultimately these roles should feedback to clinical medical and nursing leads that have responsibility and accountability for the overall service.

Role of the ICU Clinical Director

The ICU Clinical Director is typically considered a 'middle manager' within the hospital hierarchy. The ICU Clinical Director usually reports to the Divisional Medical Director, Medical Director and ultimately to the hospital Chief Executive Officer. These vertical frameworks will differ depending on the size of the organization and hospital structure. For example, in larger organizations there may be intermediary management positions between the Departmental Leads and Divisional Medical Director such as Clinical Services Leads who are operationally accountable for groups of services (Figure 3).

In addition to the vertical relationships, the ICU Clinical Director has horizontal relationships with the ICU Nurse Lead, other Clinical Directors and Service Managers within the hospital (Figure 4). Externally the ICU Clinical Director will have links with ICU Clinical Directors from other hospitals. The relationship with the ICU Nurse Lead and Service Manager is an important one as together they form the ICU management team and have overall responsibility and accountability for the service. Each will have a different expertise and be able to contribute to how the ICU service can be run most effectively and cost efficiently. For example, when reviewing cost effectiveness of a therapy on the unit, the ICU Clinical Director's main focus might be on improving patient outcomes, that of the ICU

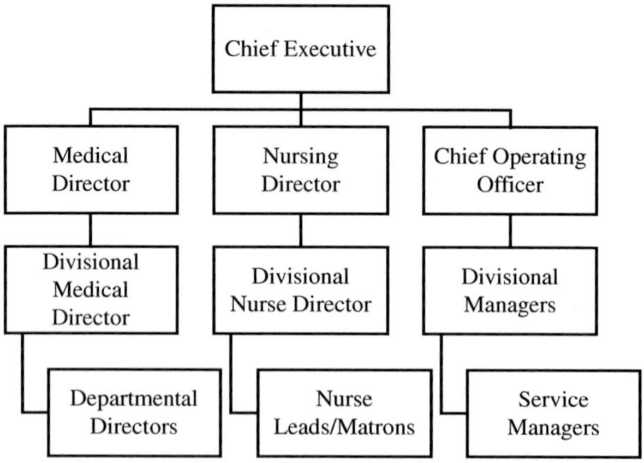

Figure 3. An example of a hospital leadership hierarchy.

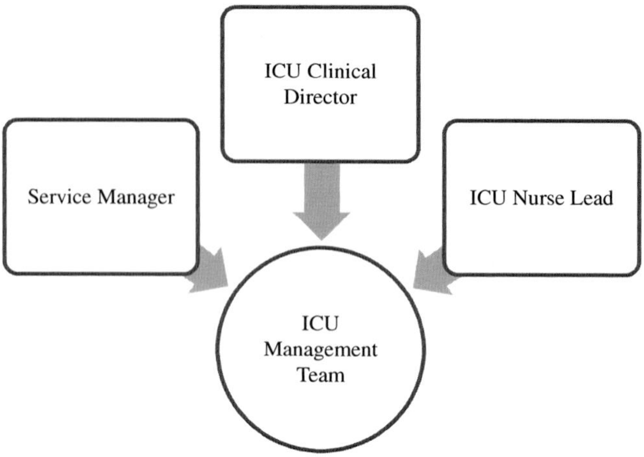

Figure 4. The ICU management team.

Nurse Lead overall unit safety, and that of the Service Manager the likely impact on the ICU budget.

Historically, ICU Clinical Directors have tended to have greater political influence in organizational management compared to other Departmental Directors due to the large number of staff employed and relatively large budget apportioned to ICUs.

The roles and responsibilities of the ICU Clinical Director can be simplistically divided into four key areas: financial management, clinical governance, human resource management, and strategic planning. In reality, the role is often much larger, encompassing other elements such as operational planning, rota management, case scheduling, complaints investigation, and cross departmental multi-disciplinary, liaison lead depending on the size of the ICU and number of clinicians.

Financial management

The ICU Clinical Director works closely with the Service Manager to manage the ICU budget. In most developed countries, the ICU budget accounts for a relatively large proportion of the hospital budget (up to 20%). The ICU budget needs to be closely monitored for variances. If substantial variances do occur, a more detailed analysis is required. By far the largest costs for ICUs are staffing costs. An increase in staff turnover, vacancy or sickness resulting in a greater reliance on temporary staff use, often at higher costs, frequently results in a deficit in the ICU budget. For this reason it is important for the ICU Clinical Director and Service Manager to have a good understanding of the factors that impact on staff recruitment, the sickness rate, and retention. Procurement is another important area of financial management. Here, the ICU Clinical Director needs to work closely with the ICU Nurse Lead and Service Manager to ensure that evidence-based practices are being followed, and best prices are being negotiated in drugs and consumables. This also includes purchasing decisions about new equipment as well as capital replacement for old equipment.

Clinical governance

This encompasses activities such as risk management, guideline and policy development, audit and quality review, and service improvement.

Human resources

The ICU Clinical Director and ICU Nurse Lead are responsible for staff recruitment, staff support and mentorship, teamwork and conflict management, external networking, task allocation, appraisals and job plan reviews, managing performance, and addressing complaints.

Strategic planning

This involves data gathering and planning of how to develop and shape the service. It is important for the ICU Clinical Director to collaborate with ICU colleagues, the hospital management team, and Directors of other departments to set priorities for the service. To be successful, the unit's strategic plan needs to align with the strategic goals of the organization and to have a term, medium, and long-term (five year) outlook.

ICU Clinical Director Job Description

ICU Clinical Directors should be given a job description to outline their roles and responsibilities clearly. A job description helps the ICU Clinical Director to understand the scope of their role and to ensure they meet the expectations of senior management. It also allows for the setting of objectives against which a regular performance review can occur. The role of the ICU Clinical Lead should have adequate dedicated time and be appropriately financially remunerated.

Role of the ICU Educational Lead

The role of the ICU Educational Lead commonly involves activities such as junior doctor appraisals, managing rotas, educational program development, mentorship, career guidance, performance management, and recruitment. This may extend into roles outside the unit such as national recruitment, curriculum development, examination, and courses. Within the unit the ICU Educational Lead takes overall responsibility for education in the unit. For many countries this involves ensuring that the program offered in the unit complies with national training standards. The role of ICU Education Lead may expand beyond post-graduate training to undergraduate training, fellowships and work experience/observerships. The ICU Lead for Education will commonly work collaboratively with the Nurse Educators to develop a comprehensive multi-disciplinary training program of education for the ICU.

Role of ICU Research Lead

The role of the ICU Research Lead varies according to the particular parental organization (research active or not) but generally involves facilitating and coordinating the research activities in the unit. This includes participation in multi-centre studies, creation of research portfolios, and development of a local research program that reflects the unit's patient population and ethos. Typically the role will involve grant applications and other methods to secure research funding, research governance, ethics, overseeing study conduct, supervising projects run by research nurses, research fellows, and post-doctorate students.

Role of ICU Clinical Governance Lead

The role of the ICU Clinical Governance Lead includes an overview of factors affecting patient safety, including risk management, investigation of serious untoward events/critical incidents, review of audits, and service evaluation projects. It should also include ensuring that the team is aware of patient safety alerts and that they are acted upon.

Does Good Leadership Impact on Unit Performance?

Leadership impacts on patient safety and outcome in critical care.[18,19] For example, Reader *et al.* were able to identify team leadership behaviours used by senior clinicians that correlated with improved patient safety.[18] Similarly, trauma and resuscitation team leaders who set clear expectations for their team member behaviours, demonstrate a positive attitude, are flexible to change, delegate leadership authority as task load lessens, but provide increased guidance for complex/novel tasks and set high standards for good teamwork through their own cooperative behaviours that would have better outcomes.[18]

In nursing, greater positive feelings towards the unit's leadership team and the work environment impacts closely on nurse job satisfaction, retention, staff sickness, vacancy levels, and burnout. Nurse leaders that seek and value contributions from staff, promote a climate where information is disseminated effectively, promote shared decision-making, and influence coordination of work which provides a stable nursing workforce. Good communication and shared vision and close collaboration a between nursing staff and clinicians enhance patient outcomes, multi-professional relationships, opportunities for learning, and greater staff satisfaction.

Behaviours of leaders have been shown to impact on organizational culture and staff morale. Good leadership can improve efficiency, operational delivery and financial performance.[19] In units where leaders promote and support a culture of safety, encourage a shared vision for the unit and drive for excellence in patient outcomes, staff satisfaction and engagement has been shown to be high and collaborate teamwork better.[19] Similarly, strong leadership is essential to driving change and for quality improvement activities to be successful.

A commonly asked question is "How does one identify if a service is well lead?" Although there are currently no specific indicators for measuring leadership, surrogate markers can be used to assess the quality of medical and nursing leadership in a unit. Indicators that measure patient safety, operational delivery and financial performance can be used. These indicators could also be used to compare and benchmark the quality of leadership in different units. Some examples of indicators are shown in Table 4.

The Art of Delegation

While there are those who are able to keep tight control of almost every aspect of the function of an ICU, this is simply not realistic for the vast majority of leaders in what is an ever burgeoning environment. In addition, refusal to share responsibility soon leads to disillusionment and disengagement amongst those members of the team who would otherwise be keen to participate in decision-making. Thus, effective delegation is a key skill for a good leader. The art of delegation lies in knowing which tasks should be delegated and to who. Effective delegation maximizes efficiency and organizational productivity and allows staff to grow, develop new skills and feel valued as members of the team.[20]

Delegation is a fine balancing act and staff require support, information and the authority to proceed.[20] Delegation is a five step process: the first step involves the identification of the task to delegate. A good starting

Table 4. Examples of quality indicators for leadership.

Structure	Staff	Staff vacancy Staff turnover Staff sickness Staff appraisal rates Staff satisfaction Staff mandatory training completed
	Environment	Environmental cleanliness Equipment serviced Stock levels for consumables Unit compliance with building regulations Environmental safety
Processes	Infection	Catheter-related blood stream infection Ventilator-associated pneumonia (VAP) Other unit acquired infections (e.g. MRSA, *C. difficile*)
	Adherence to policies/ guidelines	Availability of protocols/guidelines Hand hygiene compliance Antibiotic stewardship Ventilator bundle compliance Central line bundle compliance Thromboembolism bundle compliance Weaning protocol compliance Low tidal volume ventilator compliance Record of regular protocol/guidelines update
	Clinical governance	Critical incidents Complaints/complements Quality improvement/audit projects Quarterly clinical governance meetings
Outcomes	Unit outcomes	Standardized mortality ratio
	Operational delivery	Cancelled operations Late night discharges Readmissions with 48 hours Accidental extubations Non-clinical transfers out due to unit capacity issues Patient satisfaction
	Financial management	Variance from budget

point is to consider those tasks that the leader was involved in earlier in their career. Other tasks that should be delegated include those in which specific staff have more experience than the leader. This does not mean that the leader relinquishes accountability, but that the default decision should rest with the individual selected to do the task. Routine tasks should be distributed evenly throughout the team, preferably interspersed with those that are more interesting and thought provoking. However, it is equally important that certain tasks, such as staff motivation, team-building, praising, performance reviews, and promotion, are never delegated as to do so as it undermines their perceived importance. Second, the leader needs to select the appropriate person carefully. Third, good communication is crucial. The individual should be given clear instructions about what is expected of them and clear completion timelines. The individual should have the necessary information, resources and be empowered to carry out the task autonomously. Fourth, while the leader should be there to offer support and feedback as needed, it is important that the delegation comes with ownership and accountability — being routinely second guessed by the boss is demoralizing and demotivating. Finally, the leader should evaluate the delegation process after the task has been completed and give feedback.

Learning to delegate effectively takes time and practice. One of the main concerns amongst leaders about delegation is that by giving others the authority, the leader loses control. This is not necessarily the case. By training staff to apply the same criteria as the leader would do themselves (with clear information and explanation) staff can exercise control of the task on the leader's behalf.

Institutional Leadership/Management Support

It is an absolute requirement that the institution offers sufficient support to the Clinical Lead for them to succeed in their role. Inadequate allocation of time, reimbursement and administrative resource risks a poor outcome for all concerned. Individuals forced to operate under conditions of high pressure with minimal support rapidly become disillusioned and potentially burnt out. It is vital that there is an explicit statement of the level of available support in advance of the role being filled.

Leadership training

There are now a number of courses that seek to address the deficit in training that has previously existed. While there are few specifically targeting critical care medicine trainees and junior consultants, there are many more targeted at the healthcare sector in general. These range from one day courses to a Master's degree in Business Administration. Given that many of the skills involved in both leadership and management are not innate to the majority of clinicians, support at an institutional level and the opportunity to attend these courses is crucial for those aspiring to be involved in the running of ICUs.

Choice of leader

The choice of unit leader has traditionally followed two paths. The first is essentially a rotational allocation, through which all those appointed to a senior (specialist) level will have an expectation that they will spend some specified period as unit Clinical Lead, following which it will be someone else's "turn". While democratic in its application, this method carries a high risk of the appointment of unsuitable individuals. It does, however, carry the benefit of restricting appointments to a fixed term, limiting the damage caused by such appointees. The second is by competitive appointment. This is advantageous in that it results in the appointment of an interested individual, and providing there is sufficient competition and that the appointment process is not flawed, that individual should be best suited to the post. The process also creates a sense of legitimacy that rotational leadership does not.

Succession planning

Failing to succession plan and allowing individuals to continue in role beyond the point at which they are useful to the development of the unit risks a state in which the unit director becomes overly used to the privileges and status that comes with being group leader, and may lose sight of the fact that the no one individual is bigger than the institution that they serve. Overly long appointments also risk the growth of 'group thinking' and burn out. While one cannot be prescriptive about how long a given individual should remain in role, it is important that succession planning is seen to take place early on (particularly if the replacement is likely to come from within the organization). This involves identification of those with an interest and aptitude, and offering them training opportunities and progressive exposure to increased levels of responsibility. This creates an expectation that there will be change in leadership at a given point (which will need to be fulfilled), maintaining motivation in others in the team and helps minimize the risk of excessive time in the role.

The career beyond unit leadership

As part of succession planning, one needs to consider what will become of the "ex-leader". Graduated and visible handovers should hopefully lead to an understanding from all concerned that there is a new lead in place. This must include senior leaders within the institution, who must be seen to be supportive of the change. If not, there is always a risk that the previous incumbent will continue to act as a surrogate "parallel" lead, undermining his or her replacement. Consideration of this possibility in advance and clarity around the new role and expectations/objectives for the previous lead will also help to obviate the risk. Obviously, the specifics of a new role will be personality and institutional requirement dependent, but need to be defined.

To conclude, leadership requires the leader to be flexible in their approach depending on the circumstance. Having a good understanding of the various leadership styles and theories allows individuals and organizations to adapt and exhibit flexibility depending on the situation. For organizations, this may involve selecting leaders with certain characteristics according to context or encouraging leaders to show versatility depending on the circumstance. Leaders should be given a job plan, sufficient time and resources to undertake the role and the opportunity to undertake training in preparation for the role.

References

1. Giordano R (2010). Leadership needs of medical directors and clinical directors. Kings Fund, London. Available at: http://www.kingsfund.org.uk/publications/leadership-needs-medical-directors-and-clinical-directors (Accessed 29 January 2015).

2. Ackerly DC, Sangvai DG and Udayakumar K (2011). Training the next generation of physician-executives: an innovative residency pathway in management and leadership. *Acad. Med.*, 86(5), 575–579.
3. Stogdill R (1974). *Handbook of Leadership: A Survey of Theory and Research.* Free Press, New York.
4. Bennis W (1989). *On Becoming a Leader.* Addison-Wesley, Reading, MA.
5. Bennis W and Nanus B (1985). *Leaders: The Strategies for Taking Charge.* Harper & Row Publishers, New York, NY.
6. Fitzpatrick M (1996). Leadership... wherever patients and families are. Presented at the National Teaching Institute, May 20, Anaheim, CA.
7. Health care leadership model: The nine dimensions of leadership behavior. NHS leadership Academy (2013). Available at: http://www.leadershipacademy.nhs.uk/resources/healthcare-leadership-model/ (Accessed 29 January 2015).
8. Taylor CA, Taylor JC and Stoller JK (2008). Exploring leadership competencies in established and aspiring physician leaders: an interview-based study. *J. Gen. Intern. Med.*, 23(6), 748–754.
9. Lewin K, Lippit R and White RK (1939). Patterns of aggressive behavior in experimentally created social climates. *J. Soc. Psychol.*, 10, 271–301.
10. Blake RR and Mouton JS (1964). *The Managerial Grid.* Gulf Publishing Company, Houston, TX.
11. Hersey P and Blanchard KH (1969). *Management of Organizational Behavior — Utilizing Human Resources.* Prentice Hall, New Jersey.
12. Goleman D, Boyatzis RE and McKee A (2002). *Primal Leadership: Realizing the Power of Emotional Intelligence.* Harvard Business Press, Boston, MA.
13. Burns JM (1985). *Leadership.* Harper Collins, New York.
14. O'Toole J, Galbraith J and Lawler EE (2002). When two (or more) heads are better than one: the promise and pitfalls of shared leadership. *Calif. Manage. Rev.*, 44(4), 65–83.
15. Day DV, Gronn P and Salas E (2004). Leadership capacity in teams. *The Leadership Quart.*, 15(6), 857–880.
16. Kotter JP (1990). What leaders really do. *Harv. Bus. Rev.*, 68(3), 103–111.
17. Yukl G (2006). *Leadership in Organizations*, 6th Edition. Pearson Prentice Hall, Upper Saddle River, NJ.
18. Reader TW, Flin R and Cuthbertson BH (2011). Team leadership in the intensive care unit: the perspective of specialists. *Crit. Care. Med.*, 39(7), 1683–1691.
19. Baggs JG, Schmitt MH and Mushlin AI (1999). Association between nurse–physician collaboration and patient outcomes in three intensive care units. *Crit. Care. Med.*, 27(9), 1991–1998.
20. Covey SR (1990). *The 7 habits of Highly Effective People, Powerful Lessons in Personal Change.* Simon & Schuster, New York.

Governance

Stephen M. Pastores
*Professor of Medicine in Clinical Anesthesiology,
Weill Cornell Medical College and Program Director,
Critical Care Medicine Fellowship,
Department of Anesthesiology and Critical Care Medicine,
Memorial Sloan-Kettering Cancer Centre,
1275 York Avenue, C-1179, NY, USA*

Key Points

1. The rising patient demand for critical care medicine (CCM) services at a time of intensivist workforce shortage and mandates from external organizations to improve on the efficiency and quality of care are posing significant challenges for critical care (CC) leaders across the United States (US).
2. The organization and management of CCM services are keys to intensive care unit (ICU) performance and may impact patient outcomes and healthcare costs.
3. The traditional model of CCM as a division or service of a department is not typical for many European countries where freestanding CCM departments are commonplace.
4. Many aspects of ICUs need governance including patient management, protocol institution, technology acquisition, education, training, and interactions with other hospital areas.

5. Recent guidelines highlight the importance of process of care and ICU structure to improve outcomes particularly in the understanding and use of process improvement methodology to assess the impact of changes in ICU structure.

Introduction

Governance refers to "the processes of interaction and decision-making among the actors involved in a collective problem that lead to the creation, reinforcement, or reproduction of social norms and institutions.[1]

More than 5 million patients are admitted to ICU annually in the US. Between 2000 and 2010, CCM beds increased 17.8% (88,235–103,900) in nearly 3,000 acute care hospitals with ICU beds.[2] CC is expensive. In 2010, CCM in the US accounted for 13.2% of hospital costs, 4.1% of national health expenditures, and 0.74% ($108 billion) of the gross domestic product.[2]

In recent years, CCM leaders across the US have been increasingly faced with the rising patient demand for CCM services at a time of intensivist workforce shortage and mandates from external organizations to improve on the efficiency and quality of care.[3–7] CCM leadership must also respond to the need to educate new generations of CCM physicians and non-physician care providers (nurse practitioners and physician assistants) in the ICU, standardize care and technologies in hospitals with many ICUs, optimize ICU integration within the hospital, and participate in cost control, research, and fundraising initiatives.[7]

The organization and management of critical care (CC) services are key components that contribute to ICU performance and may impact patient outcomes and healthcare costs.

Evolution of CC as a Stand-Alone Department

In the US, ICUs are traditionally under the direction of academic or hospital departments. For example, medical and coronary care ICUs are associated with the department of medicine. Surgical ICUs are linked to the department of surgery, neurocritical care units reside under the department of neurology or neurosurgery and cardiothoracic ICUs belong to departments or divisions of cardiothoracic surgery. This model has persisted today in many large academic medical centres with several ICUs. Intensivists in these ICUs often have multiple departmental appointments and may be full-time or part-time ICU clinicians and hospital-based or voluntary staff members. Whereas large academic institutions have closed model ICUs (i.e. intensivists have exclusive or primary authority for patient triage, ICU admission and discharge decisions, and patient care), in non-academic hospitals, the majority of ICUs are open units with many requiring CC consultation and intensivists comanaging patients with the primary attending physicians.

In contrast, the traditional model of CCM as a division or service of a department is not typical for many European countries where freestanding CCM departments are commonplace.[8] In United Kingdom, most ICUs are integrated medical-surgical ICUs and the vast majority of intensivists have an anaesthesiology background. In Canada, most ICUs are also combined medical-surgical units; however, the intensivist staff in many academic centres come from varying training backgrounds (e.g. anaesthesiology, surgery, internal medicine, emergency medicine) similar to the US.

Until very recently, many US hospitals have not fully understood CC as a stand-alone discipline.[9] Hospitals view the ICUs as part of established and distinct services, divisions or sections within well-established and easily identifiable departments. Additionally, CCM physician billing often flows through departmental or non-hospital billing systems, thus hospitals are unaware of the intricacies of CCM billing or the potential receipts. In university hospitals, the intricacies of CCM recruitment, job activities, and billing may be even more complex.

Hospitals in the US are now beginning to look at CCM differently than in the past. This has occurred with the evolution of CCM as a distinct specialty, Institute of Medicine (IOM) reports of avoidable hospital deaths, and the marketing of CCM to hospitals through the Leapfrog Group and Institute for Healthcare Improvement (IHI) initiatives and telemedicine vendors.[6,10,11] There has been a strong push to control ICU costs, standardize technologies, provide 24/7 in-house attending physician coverage and rapid response team services, improve throughput from the emergency department and post-anaesthesia care unit, and comply with quality assurance (QA) mandates at local, state or national levels. Hospitals are required to report on their initiatives to track and decrease their rates of ventilator-associated events, central line associated bloodstream infections and severe sepsis, among others.

Additionally, US hospitals are now exposed to hospitalists and are recognizing the benefits of having hospital-based clinicians who provide full-time service to the hospital, enhance throughput, control costs and enable the application of evidence-based protocols. With this evolution of the inpatient care model, hospitals can now understand the concept of intensivists providing full-time service to the hospital especially in conjunction with evidence supporting intensivist-led, high-performing multi-disciplinary teams dedicated to the ICU in improving patient care and ICU management.[12,13] Finally, hospitals are becoming more aware of the CCM specialty and the need to craft distinct CCM privileges.

What Needs to be Governed?

Many aspects of ICUs need governance including patient management, protocol institution, technology acquisition, education, training, and interactions with other hospital areas. The question is whether governance should or can be provided at the local ICU level, the departmental level or at the hospital level.

New CC medicine models

Hospitals are now more willing to examine their ICU infrastructure and clinical staff and perhaps take on "battles" to pull the ICUs away from departments and place them into a hospital-based environment and political and administrative infrastructure. Within this new paradigm, hospitals must figure out what is done in their various ICUs especially if the hospitals are frustrated when trying to gain data from their ICUs, determine the actual ICU functions and relations with other hospital areas, and compliance with mandatory QA initiatives and reporting. Hospitals are recognizing that the previously perceived specialty ICUs may have more in common with other ICUs than previously thought and actually if the ICUs were grouped together, rather than functioning as separate entities, the hospital could benefit in many ways.

From the hospital's perspective, a critical care organization (CCO) offers an excellent opportunity to bring together all ICUs under one leadership with defined accountability. Added advantages include improved opportunities to contain costs, implement local and national patient safety and quality initiatives through protocols, standardize technologies across ICUs with resultant savings from volume based equipment and supply purchases, warranties, and staff training, enhanced CCM research, and improved recruitment or retention of faculty through a more stable environment.[7]

Over the past decade, larger academic medical centres (AMCs) in the US with many specialty ICUs have begun to create freestanding CCM departments or other hospital-based CCO (e.g. centres, institutes, and service lines) similar to those that have been developed for other specialties or care categories (e.g. cardiovascular disease, transplant, or cancer). With the exception of a few single centre descriptive reports,[14,15] data on CCOs are relatively sparse.

Using a survey questionnaire of physician directors of CCOs, a descriptive multi-centre study on the structure, governance, and experience to date of CCOs in hospitals in North American AMCs was recently reported.[7] The CCOs were identified through a web search over a one-year period (April 2013–April 2014) using several search terms (i.e. CC or IC Department, Centre, System, Institute, Operations Committee, Service or Product Line or CC Hospital). The search was supplemented with personal e-mail correspondence, face-to-face discussions, telephone communication, and referral from responding CCO directors. For study purposes, the CCO had to have an advanced governance structure that is headed by a physician with primary governance over the majority if not all of the ICUs and CC operations in the AMC.

We identified very few CCOs (n = 27) in North America. 27 CCO physician directors from 23 individual AMCs (19 sites in the US and four in Canada), out of 24 (89%) completed the survey. Nearly 80% of the CCOs were created in the last 15 years. The majority of the CCOs (67%) were located in larger urban AMCs (>500 beds) and 79% were primary university medical centres. Majority of the CCOs were called departments, centres, or systems. The transition to a CCO was initiated by the hospital administration in 46% and/or existing CCM service or division in 42%

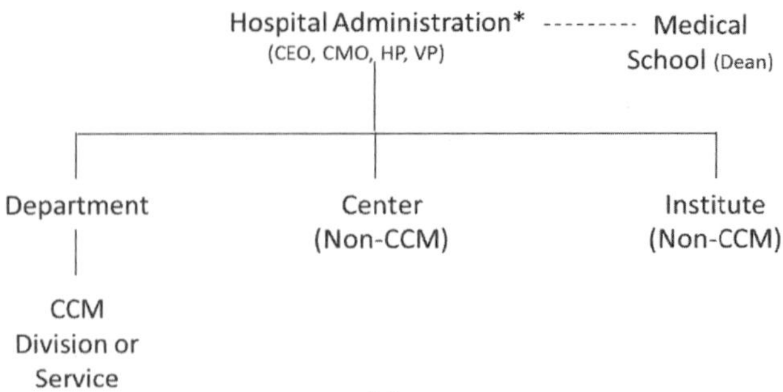

(a)

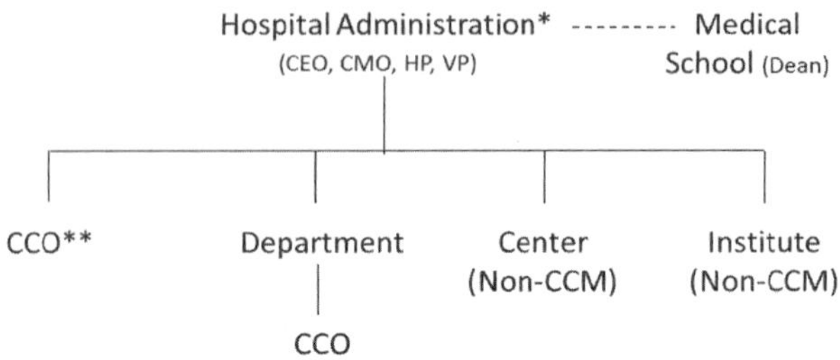

(b)

Figure 1. (a) The traditional model that exists in most hospitals today. This includes hospital departments, centres, or institutes. CCM is usually a division or service of an existing department, and the CCM division or service chief reports to the departmental chair. (b) The evolving model of CCM governance where the (CCO can be developed as a stand-alone organization at an equivalent level to existing hospital departments, centres, or institutes. Alternatively, the CCO may be a component of an existing department. Of note, in both A and B, the departmental chairmen, centre, institute, or CCO directors may report to various members of the hospital administration and to the medical school dean if a medical school is associated with the hospital.
Reprinted with permission.[7]
*CEO: Chief Executive Officer, CMO: Chief Medical Officer, HP: Hospital President, VP: Vice-President.
**CCO: Department, Centre, Institute, System, Service Line, Critical Care Hospital, or Operations Committee.

and by consensus of department chairmen in 13%. There were various models of CCM governance, reporting structures, hospital support, and general satisfaction. Almost 90% indicated that their CCO governance structure was either moderately or highly effective, and are still evolving. On average, there was six ICUs per hospital with an average of four ICUs under CCO governance. In-house intensivists were present 24/7 in 49%;

non-physician advanced practice providers (nurse practitioners, physician assistants) in 63%; hospitalists in 21%; and telemedicine coverage in 14%. Nearly 60% indicated that they had a separate hospital budget to support data management and reporting, oversight of all ICUs, and rapid response teams.

The relatively small number of CCOs that currently exist in the US were attributed to several factors including, perhaps, the reluctance of department chairmen to give their ICUs up to a CCO as they perceive potential loss of billing, triage, patient, and staffing control. Furthermore, CCM has been very intertwined with other disciplines in terms of fellowship training and attending staffs (i.e. medicine, pulmonary, anaesthesiology, surgery, neurosciences, and paediatrics) due to the absence of a unified CCM fellowship track and certification examination. Thus existing departments have come to believe that their ICUs and intensivists especially in specialty ICUs have little in common with each other. Finally, very few CCM graduates have the necessary skill set to champion the creation and lead CCOs despite CCM fellowship program training in management and team leadership.[7,16,17] Additional studies are needed to better understand the factors that can foster the growth of CCOs.

CC policies and rules

The 2001 and 2015 updated guidelines for CC delivery, clinical roles, and best practice model in the ICU from the Society of CCM are excellent resources for how ICUs should be administered.[13,18] The 2001 guidelines[18] proposed the following recommendations:

(1) Medical interventions should be provided by intensivists leading multi-disciplinary groups.
(2) Patient care should be directed by ICU teams using a "closed" format in which dedicated CC teams take ownership of all aspects of care in the ICU.
(3) ICU physicians should be available for medical and administrative tasks without competing clinical responsibilities.
(4) ICU physicians and nurses should have CC credentials.

Table 1. Recommendations from the Society of CCM task force on models of CC.

• An intensivist-led, high-performing, multi-disciplinary team dedicated to the ICU is an integral part of effective care delivery.
• Process improvement is the backbone of achieving high-quality ICU outcomes.
• Standardized protocols including care bundles and order sets to facilitate measurable processes and outcomes should be used and further developed in the ICU setting.
• Institutional support for comprehensive quality improvement programs as well as tele-ICU programs should be provided.

(5) Care teams should include CC pharmacists and full-time respiratory care practitioners as well as ICU physicians and nursing staff.
(6) ICU governance should be conducted by multi-disciplinary groups.

The 2015 guidelines[13] highlighted the importance of process of care and ICU structure to improve outcomes and offer four important recommendations (Table 1). An essential component to improve ICU outcomes is an understanding and use of process improvement methodology to assess the impact of changes in ICU structure.

Among the most important universal policies and rules for ICU governance are the admission, discharge, and triage process including having policies for management and leadership, multi-disciplinary team members, patient types, processes, and procedures and policies to guide patients' flow throughout their hospital stay, and telemedicine coverage, if applicable. There should be clear directives to prevent conflicts and patient care delays; a process to deal with conflict, and provisions for escalation to higher levels; policies for rounds and team hand-off reports, nurse driven protocols, and order writing.[17]

CC audit and reporting

All ICUs need to develop key performance indicators, monitor, audit and improve those parameters in a dynamic process. This requires standardization, improvement, and innovation.[19] Performance parameters are greatly influenced by patient demographics, comorbidities, type and severity of acute illness, cumulatively referred to as case mix. Variation in care in the ICU and among different ICUs with similar case mix can only be done if indicators are compared on regular basis. Process driven and protocol based management should eliminate ambiguity and ensure better outcome. Such approach is not possible unless care provided is quantified and gap between current level and desired level is assessed followed by improvement initiatives taken to bridge the gap. Selection of indicators and monitoring the same should therefore, be considered the most vital and challenging task to bring continuous improvement in the performance level of the ICU.[19]

In 2002, the Joint Commission released the six core performance measures (ventilator-associated pneumonia prevention, stress ulcer prophylaxis, deep vein thrombosis prophylaxis, central line-associated bloodstream infection; ICU length of stay (LOS), and hospital mortality) for the ICU.[20] The Acute Physiology and Chronic Health Evaluation, version IV (APACHE IV) score was selected for risk adjustment of two outcome measures (ICU LOS and inpatient mortality). However, the implementation of these performance measures was put on hold in 2005 to allow alignment with the requirements established. In 2010, the Joint Commission divided its performance measures into accountability and non-accountability measures. This approach places more emphasis on an organization's performance on accountability measures — quality measures that meet four criteria designed to identify measures that produce the greatest positive impact on patient outcomes when hospitals demonstrate improvement: research, proximity, accuracy, and adverse events. Only one (ICU venous thromboembolism (VTE) prophylaxis) of the nearly 50 accountability measures was specific to ICU care. In 2012, Joint Commission accredited hospitals were required to meet a new performance improvement requirement that established compliance with an 85% composite target rate for performance on accountability measures. However, effective 2015, this standard was temporarily suspended and hospitals now have more flexibility in selecting accountability measure sets and the method for submitting measurement data to the Joint Commission (i.e. chart-based measure data, electronic clinical quality measures, or a combination of both).

Other organizations such as the Agency for Healthcare Research and Quality, National Quality Forum, the Institute for Healthcare Improvement, the Leapfrog Group, Keystone Centre for Patient Safety and Quality, and

Table 2. Quality indicators that need monitoring by ICU leadership.

- Rate of delayed admissions.
- Rate of delayed discharges.
- Premature discharge.
- ICU readmission rates at 48 hours.
- Cancelled surgical cases.
- Emergency department by-pass hours.
- Standardized handover system for discharge.
- Daily rounds by multi-disciplinary teams.
- Resource allocation and reporting.
- 24 hour availability of a consultant level intensivist.
- Adverse event reporting system.
- Reporting and analysis of standardized mortality ratios.
- Rate of central venous catheter-related infections.
- Rate of unplanned extubations.

group purchasing organizations (e.g. Veterans Health Administration and Premier, Inc.) have also promoted similar national initiatives in the CCM quality improvement movement with an eye to linking quality of care to pay for performance.

A listing of the quality indicator measures that need to be monitored by ICU leadership is shown in Table 2.

Conclusions

The rising patient demand for CC services coupled with an intensivist workforce shortage has put a tremendous strain on CC and the healthcare delivery system in the US. With the evolution of CCM as a distinct specialty and its prominence in national safety and quality reports and marketing initiatives, hospitals are beginning to view CCM in a different light. This is evidenced by the recent strong push to control ICU costs, standardize technologies, provide 24/7 in-house intensivist coverage and rapid response team services, improve throughput from the emergency department and post-anaesthesia care units, and comply with QA mandates at local, state or national levels. In the midst of all of these, hospitals are now examining their ICU infrastructure and clinical staff and starting to separate their

ICUs away from their traditional departments and placing them into a hospital-based institute or centre with political and administrative infrastructure and envisioning additional profits with these initiatives.

The slow but steady increase in the number of CCO (departments, centres, institutes, service lines) is paving the way for new CCM leaders to be inserted into the hospital organizational hierarchy at par with department chairs and introducing innovative and proactive marketing strategies for the medical and lay communities. At this time, there are many differences between the few operating CCM systems as the models vary and their maturity level continues to evolve. Others struggle in deciding how CCM fits into existing service lines as a care component instead of a unique program and how to address the academic issues and governance model for hospitals that are affiliated with medical schools.

Top hospital leadership support and CCM leadership in quality care and patient safety, a willingness to allocate resources, the development of support mechanisms, the active support and involvement of physicians, management commitment and accountability during implementation will be required for CCM service lines to succeed.

References

1. Hufty M (2011). Investigating policy processes: the governance analytical framework (GAF). In *Research for Sustainable Development: Foundations, Experiences, and Perspectives,* Wiesmann U and Hurni H (eds.). Geographica Bernensia, Bern, pp. 403–424.
2. Halpern NA and Pastores SM (2015). Critical care medicine beds, use, occupancy, and costs in the United States: a methodological review. *Crit. Care Med.*, 43(11), 2452–2459.
3. Angus DC, Shorr AF and White A (2006). Committee on Manpower for Pulmonary and Critical Care Societies (COMPACCS): critical care delivery in the United States: distribution of services and compliance with Leapfrog Recommendations. *Crit. Care Med.*, 34, 1016–1024.
4. US Department of Health and Human Services Health Services and Research Administration: The critical care workforce (2006). A study of the supply and demand for critical care physicians. Health Services and Research Administration, Washington, DC. Available at: ftp://ftp.hrsa.gov/bhpr/nationalcenter/criticalcare.pdf.

5. Halpern NA, Pastores SM, Oropello JM and Kvetan V (2013). Critical care medicine in the United States: addressing the intensivist shortage and image of the specialty. *Crit. Care Med.*, 41, 2754–2761.
6. Pastores SM, O'Connor MF and Kleinpell RM (2011). The accreditation council for graduate medical education resident duty hour new standards: history, changes, and impact on staffing of intensive care units. *Crit. Care Med.*, 39, 2540–2549.
7. Pastores SM, Halpern NA and Oropello JM (2015). Critical care organizations in academic medical centers in North America: a descriptive report. *Crit. Care Med.*, 43, 2239–2244.
8. Offenstadt G, Moreno R, Palomar M and Gullo A (2006). Intensive care medicine in Europe. *Crit. Care Clin.*, 22(3), 425–432.
9. Grenvik A and Pinsky MR (2009). Evolution of the intensive care unit as a clinical center and critical care medicine as a discipline. *Crit. Care Clin.*, 25, 239–250.
10. Kohn LT, Corrigan JM and Donaldson MS (2000). Committee on Quality of Health Care in America, Institute of Medicine. *To Err Is Human: Building a Safer Health System.* National Academy Press, Washington, DC.
11. Committee on Quality of Health Care in America, Institute of Medicine (2001). *Crossing the Quality Chasm: A New Health System for the 21st Century.* National Academy Press, Washington, DC.
12. Wilcox ME, Chong CA and Niven DJ (2013). Do intensivist staffing patterns influence hospital mortality following ICU admission? A systematic review and meta-analyses. *Crit. Care Med.*, 41, 2253–2274.
13. Weled BJ, Adzhigirey LA and Hodgman TM (2015). Critical care delivery: the importance of process of care and ICU structure to improve outcomes: an update from the American College of Critical Care Medicine task force on models of critical care. *Crit. Care Med.*, 43(7), 1520–1525.
14. Bekes CE, Dellinger RP and Brooks D, (2004). Critical care medicine as a distinct product line with substantial financial profitability: the role of business planning. *Crit. Care Med.*, 32(5), 1207–1214.
15. Irwin RS, Flaherty HM and French CT (2012). Interdisciplinary collaboration. The slogan that must be achieved for models of delivering critical care to be successful. *Chest*, 142(6), 1611–1619.
16. Gasperino J, Brilli R and Kvetan V (2008). Teaching intensive care unit administration during critical care medicine training programs. *J. Crit. Care*, 23(2), 251–252.
17. St. Andre A (2015). The formation, elements of success, and challenges in managing a critical care program: part 1. *Crit. Care Med.*, 43(4), 874–879.

18. Brilli RJ, Spevetz A and Branson RD (2001). American College of Critical Care Medicine task force on models of critical care delivery; the American College of Critical Care Medicine guidelines for the definition of an intensivist and the practice of critical care medicine. Critical care delivery in the intensive care unit: defining clinical roles and the best practice model. *Crit. Care Med.*, 29, 2007–2019.
19. Ray B, Samaddar DP and Todi SK (2009). Quality indicators for ICU: ISCCM guidelines for ICUs in India. *Indian J. Crit. Care Med.*, 13(4), 173–206.
20. Specifications Manual for National Hospital Quality Measures — ICU (2005). Available at: http://www.jcaho.org/pms/core+measures/icu+manual.htm.

Design and Role of the Intensive Care Unit

Neil A. Halpern
Chief, Critical Care Medicine
Professor of Medicine in Clinical Anesthesiology
Department of Anesthesiology and Critical Care Medicine
Memorial Sloan-Kettering Cancer Centre, NY, USA
Professor of Clinical Medicine, Weill Cornell Medical College, NY, USA

Diana C. Anderson
Architect, Royal Architectural Institute of Canada

Key Points

1. Intensive Care Unit (ICU) specific design is a complex process and requires a multi-disciplinary team that includes both clinical and expert design-based professionals.
2. The layout of an ICU is arguably the most important design feature affecting all aspects of critical care (CC) services.
3. The core of the ICU experience is the patient room, conceptually subdivided into patient, caregiver, and family/visitor zones.
4. Central clinical support zones within the ICU act to bind the patient rooms and other supportive areas together, with the overall goal of supporting bedside care.

5. Deploying advanced informatics into the modern ICU electronically integrates the patient with all aspects of care.

It is highly probable that hospital-based intensivist leaders will be asked at some point in their careers to participate in efforts to design new ICUs or renovate old ones. After all, in 2010, there were approximately 6,100 ICUs with over 104,000 beds in the 3,100 acute care hospitals in the United States (US).[1] There are a wide array of design issues ranging from the politics of ICU design, to configuring the ICU space and finally implementing smart informatics.

Concept to Occupancy

ICU as a hospital resource

The ICU provides care for the hospital's most critically ill patients and is therefore a necessary resource for an acute care hospital. In large hospitals, there are usually a high percentage of hospital beds dedicated to CC and multiple specialty ICUs (e.g. medical ICU, surgical ICU, coronary care unit, cardiothoracic ICU, neurosurgical ICU, burn ICU, paediatric ICU, and neonatal unit).[2] In contrast, in many of the smaller community hospitals, fewer beds are allocated to CC and there are fewer ICUs. Often there is one large multi-purpose adult ICU that handles all types of critically ill patients. However, there are many variations on how many and what types of ICUs exist in medical centres. Similarly, the individual ICUs within a centre may have standardized design, technologies, locations, staffing models, etc., versus no standardization among the ICUs at all. These variable circumstances are based upon the facility's age, space availability, CC evolution, and overall approaches to ICU design and management.

From the perspective of a hospital's table of organization, an ICU may be viewed as a departmental resource rendering care to a specific group of patients versus a hospital-based resource applying care to all critically ill patients.[3] For example, the cardiothoracic surgical department "owns and operates" a cardiothoracic ICU. The location of this ICU, and its design and function may be targeted to the specifics of this selective group of patients and the necessary departmental throughput. The cardiothoracic ICU would then be located near the operating rooms, post-anaesthesia care unit and step-down units, and not near other ICUs. Alternatively, the ICU may organizationally "belong" to hospital administration or function under a critical care organization (CCO) (e.g. critical care medicine (CCM) Department, Institute or Centre). In these latter models, all ICUs may be co-located, and their designs, technologies and functions standardized. Locating all ICUs near each other, which commonly occurs in newer ICU towers, permits the efficacy of shared services (e.g. waiting rooms, staff lounges, pharmacy, laboratory, and logistics).

Principles of ICU design

Four core principles should guide ICU specific design. First, designing an ICU is a complex and time-consuming process. Secondly, an ICU is a semi-autonomous mini hospital. Thirdly, the design requires balance between innovation and functionality, space and physical limitations, desire, and cost. Lastly, the design should combine technology, security, and healing.

These principles should support the growing notion of evidence-based design (EBD), which borrows from work done in evidence-based medicine to observe, quantify and analyze the way people use buildings carefully. EBD is the process of basing decisions about the built environment on credible research to achieve the best possible outcomes. EBD innovations optimize patient safety, quality, and satisfaction, as well as improve workforce safety, satisfaction, and productivity, with the additional benefit of operating cost savings and energy efficiency.[4,5]

Building the ICU design team

ICU design can succeed only if there are common goals between the CCM team and the hospital administration to design, provide adequate space, and fund a "spectacular" ICU.[6] ICU design projects are ideally guided by a design team with a core membership that reflects the responsibilities of the group. Hospital projects of this scope commonly have a project manager; however, successful ICU design requires that the committee be co-chaired by the CCM clinical chief and the facilities project manager. Ideally, only architects with a prior track record of excellent ICU design experience should be engaged.

The committee should start the design process by utilizing existing guidelines, recommendations and expert opinions to gather core knowledge of ICU design.[7–13] A primary source is the Guidelines for Design and Construction of Hospitals and Outpatient Facilities published by the Facility Guidelines Institute's (FGI).[14] These guidelines recommend minimum program, space, risk assessment, infection prevention, architectural detail, surface and furnishing needs for clinical and support areas, as well as minimum engineering design criteria for plumbing, electrical, heating, ventilation, and air-conditioning (HVAC) systems. The FGI document is designed to meet minimum standards for design and construction and has been adopted by most states in the US, in addition to being used in other countries. The second is the Society of Critical Care Medicine (SCCM)'s guidelines for ICU design that describe universal functions that need to be accommodated in the modern ICU.[7] SCCM also maintains a digest of the ICU design award winners and includes architectural design drawings, pictures and videos of outstanding ICUs from throughout the world.[15,16] Finally, the ICU team may choose to "benchmark" or visit selective ICUs, meet with the staff and inquire for themselves what worked best.

Design timeline

Both the hospital and the ICU design committee must recognize that from design origination to occupancy may take several years.[6] Design committee meetings should occur regularly. Provision of continuously updated schematics and computerized renderings of the various design concepts by the architects speed the design process along. Full scale mock-ups of the patient rooms (with devices and finishing's) are even more helpful as they allow for an experiential rather than an observational experience. The design process is iterative; therefore, the committee must balance the time necessary to figure out the best possible layout and design versus forward momentum to avoid delays, project fatigue, and cost overruns.

The Vision

Useful design specific deliberations can only begin after basic ICU issues are addressed and a vision for the new ICU has been articulated.[6,9] Issues include the location and purpose of the unit, the planned number of beds, the apportionment of space between patient and support areas, the logistics of unit function (centralized or decentralized) and whether a step-down unit will be associated with the ICU. The vision of the new ICU should reflect the big-picture focusing on the desired atmosphere and feel, approach to patient and family care, workflow, technology, environment, the ICU's physical and logistical relationships with the remainder of the hospital.

Renovation or New Construction

Renovations are different than new construction. Renovations of existing ICUs are usually limited in scope and may range from a cosmetic upgrade to a total overhaul. Renovations are often more complicated than new build because of the restrictions of building in an older space (i.e. existing floor to ceiling heights, structural depths, and locations of elevators and staircases). Renovations also require the updating of existing space to current building codes. In new space, however, the design begins with a clean slate and of course, new construction is built to current code. The design committee may also be looking at more than one ICU at a time. If multiple ICUs are being built within a new facility, the hospital should carefully assess the ICU placements in order to maximize workflow and efficiencies.

It is important to recognize that once the ICU is completed, major design changes will probably not be implemented for a long time, if ever. Therefore, the design must account for long-term functionality. As future ICU upgrades will primarily occur in the informatics or technology worlds, the ICU should be equipped with extra networking and electrical capabilities.

ICU Technologies

Medical devices today are actually informatics platforms.[12] For example, the purchase of infusion pumps or mechanical ventilators should include the costs of software licenses and updates. Additionally, connectivity and interactions with existing hospital systems should be considered. New technologies should be tested in a simulation environment prior to purchase and deployment. Testing should encompass device networking, connectivity and interoperability, and middleware functionalities. A well-disciplined testing approach will reveal technological gaps between current and new systems, thus guiding purchases and preventing avoidable errors.

Optimally, the technologies in a new ICU should be standardized with those across the entire enterprise of CC beds. Standardization permits efficiencies in education and assignment, device maintenance, and purchasing.

ICU technologies are usually purchased and installed months before an ICU is opened. Early purchase, while seemingly well-organized, may lead to the acquisition and installation of devices that are at the end of their timeline. Thus, non-obsolescence agreements (replacement of older platforms with current ones) should be included with these purchases to prevent an ICU from opening with obsolete technology.

Ramifications and Expectations of the New ICU

The ramifications of a new ICU design on workflow, staffing, logistics, and informatics etc. must be assessed. More staffing may be needed for more beds and additional training to utilize new technologies. Hospital administrations may be of the belief that new ICUs provide a large return on investment (ROI) and will result in improved outcomes, cost savings, infection prevention, and enhanced staff and family dynamics. These expectations may be unrealistic as such outcomes are dependent on many variables beyond the ICU design and technologies themselves.

Construction

Tours of ICU construction sites are quite beneficial for both ICU design groups and the future end users. These visits may identify unanticipated problems and allow for early remediation. The ICU should also be photographed throughout its construction. A pictorial record will provide a knowledgeable background for repair and retrofitting as well as for presentations to the staff in order to maintain an upbeat attitude.

Occupancy, Post Occupancy Evaluation, and Issue Correction

Moving day anxiety is diminished with pre-occupancy preparations including move simulation. Non-ICU staff and the family members of current ICU patients should be made aware of the moving date in order to minimize their anxiety as well. The post-occupancy evaluation (POE) process should be developed to identify major issues and plan for short and long-term fixes as unanticipated problems are recognized. When implemented in healthcare design, the research findings of POEs can positively impact patient and visitor experiences and satisfaction, create supportive work environments for staff and caregivers, and help achieve organizational objectives.[17]

ICU Design

The layout of an ICU is arguably the most important design feature affecting all aspects of critical care services including patient privacy, comfort and safety, staff working conditions, throughput, logistical support, and family integration. Layout determines the location and configuration of different spaces and/or functions within an ICU, the relationship of internal and external spaces and how their functions relate. Within the physical limitations of the space, designers have applied various types of layouts (square, circular, triangular, and rectangular schemes, or any combination) (Figure 1) to solve throughput challenges of patients, staff and visitors, circulation between clean and used supplies, equipment and the end users.[11,13,16] The choices are usually dictated by the physical layout of the

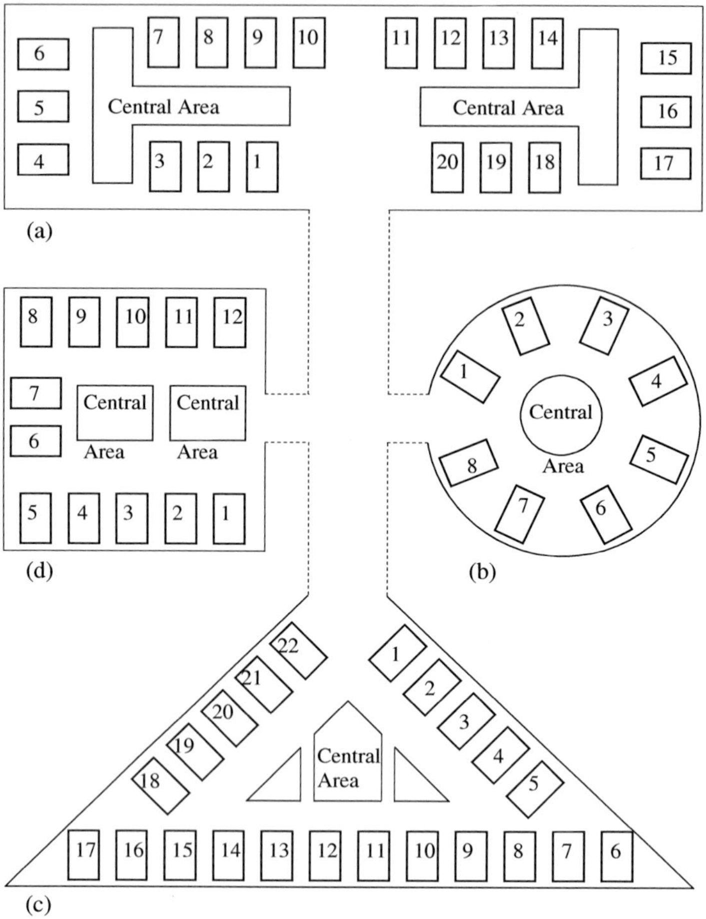

Figure 1. ICUs can be planned in many configurations: (a) rectangular, (b) circular, (c) triangular, and (d) square. Reprinted with permission from CHEST.[11]

facility and the location of fixed hospital components such as windows, staircases, elevators, and plumbing. Nevertheless, the ICU design group may have a certain degree of latitude in the specific elements of the floor design. These decisions may also be guided by considerations that address safety versus efficiency, supportive versus functional environments, revenue generating ICU patient rooms versus central supply and logistical spaces.[19]

The ICU patient room

The core of the ICU experience is the patient room.[8,9,11,13,18] As per the various guidelines, the patient rooms should accommodate one patient only. Each room should offer privacy, infection prevention and control, a healing environment and have access to outdoor views through windows. Each room should be similarly designed and equipped to function as an autonomous area. Concomitantly, the rooms should be fully interwoven into the ICU and hospital fabric.

Infrastructure

Most of the patient room's infrastructure involves components not usually familiar to clinicians. This includes HVAC systems, electrical, plumbing, lighting, flooring, connectivity and communications, bathrooms and sinks, etc. The team's clinical members should be knowledgeable enough to ascertain whether the core infrastructure will meet the needs of the end users.

The primary decision that guides the room's utilization involves the selection of the medical utility distribution systems. The choices are divided between fixed headwalls or floor mounted columns versus mobile articulating columns (booms) mounted to the ceilings or walls (Figure 2). The medical utility distribution system brings the hospital's supportive infrastructure (medical gases, vacuum, plumbing, electrical, and data jacks) to the patient. Additionally, the medical utility distribution system provides the venue for installing medical devices (physiological monitors, mechanical ventilators, infusion pumps), communications and entertainment systems. The stationary systems are less expensive than the mobile systems; however, the mobile booms offer greater flexibility, patient access, and bed movement. Regardless of the system selected, much thought has to go into positioning of all the outlets and medical devices.

Bedside medical technologies

Core ICU room medical devices optimally include the ICU bed, physiological monitor, mechanical ventilator, infusion and feeding pumps, pneumatic compression devices, patient lift, computers, chairs for patient and

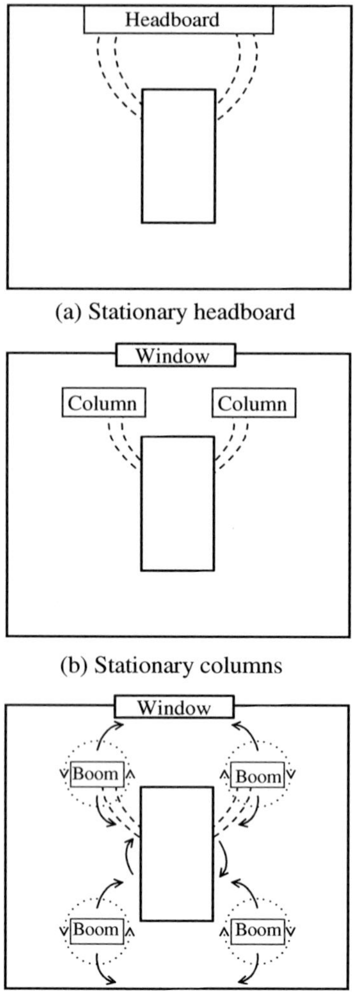

(c) Mobile articulating arms (booms)

Figure 2. ICU utilities and equipment are mounted on (a) a stationary headboard (b) stationary (left side) or rotating (right side) columns, or (c) mobile articulating columns (booms). The booms can be attached to the walls or ceiling, at any corner of the bed and swivel and move horizontally or vertically. Reprinted with permission from CHEST.[11]

visitors, overbed tables, laboratory specimen label printer, nurse call intercom station, webcam, entertainment system, storage areas, and waste disposal bins. The design team should also address point of care testing (POCT) and ultrasonography and whether these devices should be placed in each room or stored centrally.

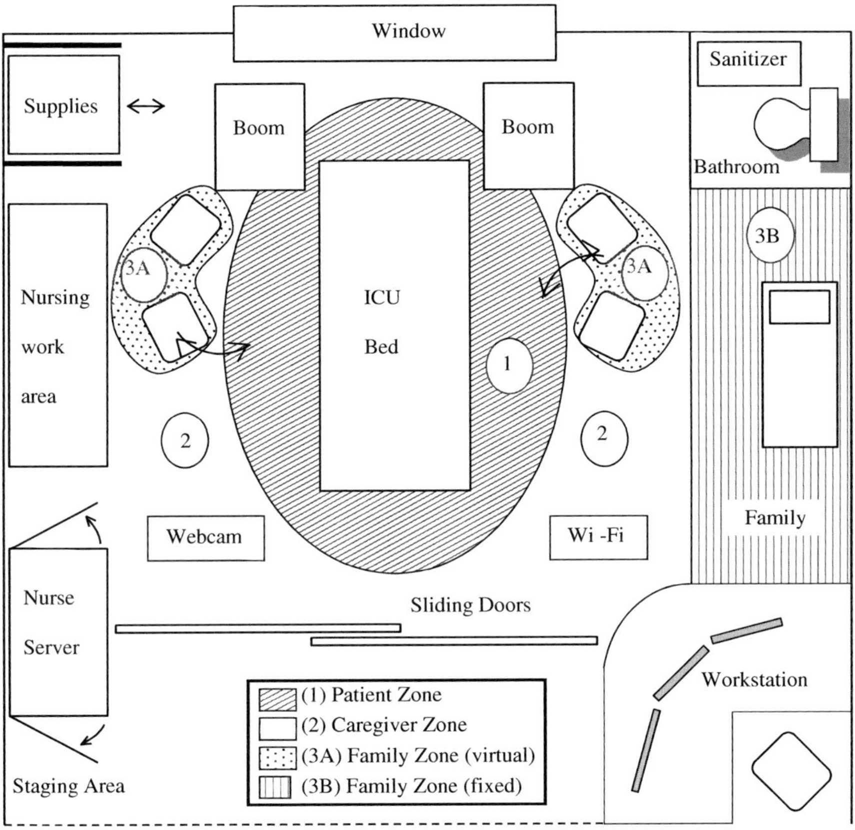

Figure 3. The ICU patient room is commonly divided into three zones: patient (1), caregiver (2), and virtual (3A) or fixed (3B) family zones. This figure also demonstrates a nurse sever with bidirectional access, work area, logistical support space, booms, bathroom, webcam, Wi-Fi antenna, and a workstation and staging area directly in front of the patient's room. Reprinted with permission from CHEST.[11]

Zones

Conceptually, each ICU room can be subdivided physically or virtually into three overall zones: patient, caregiver, and family (visitor) (Figure 3). The room's focal point is the patient bed. Installing all medical equipment on the medical utility distribution system clears the floor and facilitates ready access to the patient by family and staff. Elements of the caregiver zone include work areas for medication preparation, surface space, computers and displays, and storage areas. The family zone should incorporate electrical outlets, access to the hospital wireless communications systems as well as comfortable chairs, and if possible long-term visiting furniture (chair-sofa-bed, table, light, sink, locker, and refrigerator).

Room logistics and waste management systems

The patient room must have adequate storage spaces for supplies, medications, linens, and waste management systems. Storage is achieved through a mix of permanently based secured and non-secured drawers, cabinets, and/or mobile carts. Permanent "nurse servers" (cabinets with bidirectional and secure access from both outside and inside the room) should also be considered. The ability to access the nurse servers from outside the room improves privacy and infection control.

Whereas in the past a toilet may have been located inside cabinetry within the patient room, ICU patient rooms must now have direct access to separate enclosed bathrooms.[14] These bathrooms should have either sanitizers to clean reusable bedpans or macerators to destroy single-use bed pans. Even with bathrooms, portable commodes are still necessary. Rolling carts or stationary containers should be available in each patient room for trash (standard, infectious, sharps) and soiled linens.

Room environment

Evidence has demonstrated that the physical environment affects the physiology, psychology, and social behaviours of all those who experience it.[20] Thus, the patient room environment must promote healing and serenity and address sound, light, temperature, visuals, and entertainment.

Sound is controlled through a mixture of minimizers of both physical sound and sound transit (sound-absorbent finishings and ceiling tiles, acoustic baffling in the walls, sound-proofed windows, and sound attenuators in the HVAC system). Noise is also mitigated through sound cancelling headphones or sound masking in the patient's room. Sound from entertainment systems can be projected through entertainment displays, nurse call handsets, directional speakers, or wireless headsets. Additionally, control of alarms emanating from devices and sounds from communications systems should be sought. Pilot projects are now underway to transform stark device alarms to more calming sounds.

Natural light is essential to the well-being of patients and staff. Thus, ICU patient rooms are now all required to have windows.[7,14] Windows should be anti-glare and have sunlight reducing shades, preferably with electronic controllers. The room itself should have multiple lighting arrangements to accommodate patient and staff needs.

ICU artwork can be mounted on the ICU walls, embedded in privacy curtains and ceiling tiles, electronically projected on video displays, or integrated into televisions or television/computers. Entertainment may also be provided through visor based video displays. The patient room should also have a venue for the display of get well cards and family pictures.

Electronic and computer based integration of the environmental systems (e.g. light, shades, temperature, artwork) and entertainment systems facilitates efficient patient and staff centred control of the room. Environmental profiles can then be tailored to day and night, procedures or no procedures, and individual patient needs. Multi-parameter sensors that monitor temperature, humidity, light, sound and provide alerts for uncomfortable environmental circumstances also help track and maintain the healing environment.

Front of ICU room

The front of the ICU patient room is the interface of the room with the ICU hallway. Beyond providing entry to the room, this space controls privacy, transmission of sound, infection, smoke, and allows for patient observation and monitoring. The front of room options include curtains, framed glass doors with integrated privacy solutions (integral blinds, electronic glass (e-glass) or curtains behind the glass doors). The curtains are more economical to install than the glass systems; however, the efficacy of curtains in controlling sound, infection or smoking is limited. The electronic glass systems are easy to clean but should be purchased with long-term warranties; options for the glass control, color, and opacity adjustment should be considered. Signage in the front of the room can include erasable whiteboards or programmable electronic displays.

The rooms may open directly onto the hallway, be set back or have a hybrid design. Opening directly to the hall provides the largest possible room; however, setting the room back may provide a staging area that incorporates handwashing systems, storage space, coat hangers, and identification systems. A hybrid design may provide the best of both worlds.

Patient observation and monitoring is facilitated by the incorporation of a clinical workstation (decentralized) in the front of the room. These spaces are generally designed as one per room or one per two rooms, and provide direct patient visibility and local patient monitoring. Such workstations should have access to bedside physiologic data (mirrored on displays or web-based) and the electronic medical record.

Central areas

The central areas of the ICU bind all the patient rooms as well as other supportive areas together and help develop overall unit cohesiveness. The goals of the central areas are to support bedside care, provide access to central nurse stations, logistical support areas, and offer a welcoming and warm atmosphere. Core design is commonly governed by the hospital's and ICU's approaches to centralized or decentralized care and logistics.

Central (nursing) stations

Administrative, clinical, and social interactions commonly occur at the central stations. In a small ICU, one centrally located station may suffice; in contrast, multiple central stations may be needed in a large ICU with several bed pods. The layout of these areas is affected by the physical arrangement, space availability and overall bed configurations (Figure 1).

Optimally, unobstructed views of the ICU beds should be available from the central stations. In reality, however, such views are commonly precluded by the ICU layout. Regardless of the layout, bedside webcams, centrally based physiologic monitoring stations or other data displays are strongly suggested. The composition of the central stations includes greeting desks, quiet work and conferencing areas, offices, and restrooms. Other technologies include nurse call communication stations, telephones, grease boards, computers, high-definition image review stations, multi-modality printers (if paper is used), laboratory specimen label printers, pneumatic tube stations, nourishment stations, emergency alerts, and cut-off switches for ICU utilities.

Corridors

ICU corridors provide pathways for transit around the ICU and promote physical and social unity. However, physical barriers (staircases, elevators, supportive conduits, and closets) can limit optimal corridor design. If possible, designated hallways for patient and supply transport augment patient privacy and visitor distraction.

The corridor finishings, artwork, sound control, and lighting set the emotional tone for the ICU. These considerations are very important as hallways are used to conduct rounds, impromptu clinical consultations and family meetings, and provide a track for patient mobilization. Some ICUs have also included large alcoves for devices and carts and respite areas for ICU visitors within the hallways.

ICU Logistics Spaces, Supplies, and Medical Devices

Providing appropriate storage space for supplies, medical devices, and procedure carts usually proves to be challenging for ICU design teams. Rightsizing the storage areas (central and bedside) requires clarity in the approaches to centralized (hospital and ICU) and decentralized (bedside) storage and correct assumptions of ICU supply utilization of consumables. Storage spaces may include stationary or track based shelving, closed supply cabinets, or rolling exchange carts. Storage units and expensive supplies should be outfitted with electronic inventory management systems as part of real-time locating systems/solutions (RTLS). Additionally, central storage spaces must be able to handle supplementary medical devices (e.g. infusion pumps, ventilators, specialty monitoring or imaging devices). Similarly, properly positioning these spaces in the ICU may prove to be challenging. Storage spaces should be accessible to transport or cargo elevators and be fairly close to the patient care areas. When space allocation and storage location are not handled well, ICU hallways are always cluttered.

The ICU design may also grapple with the designation of ICU space for permanent imaging and procedural suites versus using the space for additional beds. This discussion is evolving as imaging technologies (e.g. mobile CT scanners) have become more economical and mobile today than in prior years.

Pharmacy

Hospitals may have centralized or decentralized pharmacy and medication distribution systems and staffing models. Thus, like ICU logistics, the ICU pharmacy systems must be coordinated with the hospital's pharmacy and ICU bedsides. Options include a fully equipped satellite ICU pharmacy versus a pharmacy area with minimal resources. Both alternatives commonly utilize decentralized self-contained and secure automated medication disposing units. Medications may also be stored in secured cabinets at the ICU bedside.

ICU Laboratory Testing and POCT

A combination of POCT and centralized laboratory testing is usually required for the ICU. POCT focuses primarily on whole blood analyses. POCT platforms are either small, using a single cartridge per test or larger, using multi-use cartridges. The smaller devices are amenable for positioning at each ICU bedside. The larger devices are commonly placed in defined ICU locations (ICU stat laboratory or central station) or on carts. A combination of POCT modalities and locations may be used depending on the ICU workflow, necessary testing, available space, and resources. POCT is never a complete replacement for the central laboratory; therefore, pneumatic tube stations are still required to transport specimens to laboratories outside the ICU area.

Staff Lounge and On-Call Suites

Beyond patient-centred care, the ICU design must address the impact of space on staff efficiency, job satisfaction and multi-disciplinary teamwork, as ICU clinicians regularly face extreme stress. Thus, well-designed staff lounges and on-call suites located within the ICU provide a place close to patient care, for staff to relax and recharge during their breaks from ICU care. The lounges should be able to accommodate the average number of staff on breaks and be tastefully decorated to provide a warm and useful environment. Lighting should be from outside windows; comfortable seating and tables with entertainment as well as access to the electronic medical record and ICU communications should be incorporated. Bathrooms, changing areas, lockers and scrub dispensers, napping alcoves, and nourishing stations complete the lounge furnishings.

In ICUs that maintain 24/7 clinician availability, sleeping accommodations in on-call suites should also be provided. These quarters should be outfitted with computers, nurse call stations, and entertainment systems, as well as bathrooms and showers.

Family Lounge (Visitor Waiting Room)

ICU visitors, like staff, need a healing environment close to the ICU to relax in between visits with their loved ones. Soft lighting, warm colors, nature themed artwork (either real or virtual), and quiet background entertainment set a serene tone. Large windows, with outdoor patio access as available, are also beneficial. A modicum of privacy should be provided using small groups of comfortable chairs that are separated by dividers. Informatics support may include wireless Internet access, computers, and charging stations. Nourishment areas as well as bathrooms, lockers, and coat hangers should be the norm. The inclusion of consultation rooms and social work offices helps promote family meetings and social support. Long-term sleeping accommodations, if possible, provide a space for visitors who prefer to remain nearby.

Conference Rooms

Staff meetings, educational programs and family meetings are sustained through the construction of multi-purpose conference rooms within the ICU environment. The seating capacities of these rooms should be based upon predicted usage. Furnishings should include comfortable seating, conference tables with built-in informatics access, audio–visual–video systems, wireless access, smart boards, electronic attendance, scheduling systems, food preparation, and storage areas.

Universal Support Services

Universal ICU support services should be integrated into all aspects of the ICU and hospital systems. This coordination maintains continuity across the enterprise and avoids duplication of efforts that may or may not be complimentary.

Infection Prevention and Control

Strategies for infection prevention and control rely upon infrastructure systems that provide clean air (air-cleansing systems, room-based air exchanges, and airborne infection isolation), clean water (plumbing for sinks inside and outside each patient room), waste sequestration and elimination in patient rooms, housekeeping, and environmental closets. Additionally, non-porous, well sealed and easy-to-clean surfaces and finishings, hand sanitizers and fluid dispensers should be used throughout the ICU. Advanced modalities include electronic surveillance of handwashing, copper or silver "self-cleaning surfaces" in conjunction with surface surveillance monitors, and the use of environmental decontamination systems (e.g. ultraviolet light, hydrogen peroxide dispersion, and continuous air disinfection).

Nevertheless, serious infections remain an ICU problem even in the setting of optimal infection control design measures. Effective infection control also requires an ICU culture and workflow that believes and promotes infection deterrence. Ultimately, the ICU may even include superisolation zones that group highly infectious patients together with designated ICU traffic patterns. Additionally, the ICU may have to put protocols in place that address colonization and decontamination of smart phones.

Staff Communications

Communicating technologies (telephones, smart phones, nurse call intercom systems, pagers, and bidirectional transmitters) are integral to the

ICU informatics environment. These devices may all be integrated into one communication platform (e.g. within a nurse call system, a primary communication platform, or an alarm system) and provide point-to-point and global messaging, telephone and alarm communications and real time locating of staff. Even in these advanced settings, landline telephones and overhead speakers continue to be of value in providing reliable ICU communications.

Signage and Wayfinding

Good signage is necessary for efficient wayfinding. Directional signs should be easily visible and clear in their message; destination signs should be clear in room identification and purpose. Efficient signage is vital for visitors and non-ICU staff, especially in large ICUs with multiple pods. Computerized renderings of the ICU corridors provide the core framework for developing efficient directional signs. Signs also provide information and can include the ICU designation (e.g. surgical ICU), management names (e.g. ICU director and nurse leader), and visiting hours. Advanced electronic signage systems with kiosks may be integrated into the hospital and produce directional wayfinding from hospital entrances to the ICUs.

Security, Fire, and Safety

The ICU design must address security and fire safety. Electronic identification card coded access should be used for staff at all secure doorways. Time-limited electronic access may also be distributed to ICU visitors. The ICU "front door" optimally should be staffed by dedicated clerks. However, staffing limitations commonly preclude full-time greeters; therefore, other systems for visitor identification (e.g. closed-circuit televisions with electronic buzzers) should be installed at ICU entrances. Overall, the ICU is optimally monitored by a mix of hospital-based video cameras and locally based webcams. The ICU should also have a plan and the necessary equipment for evacuation of patients in the setting of a major disaster.

Beyond the basic fire safety devices (smoke detectors, automated sprinklers, fire extinguishers) and fire and smoke alerting systems (fire alarm pull-stations, sound or light alerts, and overhead speakers), four design elements help ensure the safety of the ICU in the settings of fire and smoke. The first involves selection of products and furnishings with a low fire load and minimal release of heat and toxic smoke. The second addresses the construction of compartments that are fire and smoke-rated. The third is the use of protective technologies within the HVAC systems to prevent the spread of smoke and other products of combustion from one area to another. The last is the integration of experienced fire safety officers into the ICU design process.

Advanced Informatics

Deploying advanced informatics into the modern ICU requires great attention to detail and goals.[12] The primary objective should be to electronically integrate the patient with all aspects of care. The second goal is to transform all patient related data into actionable information using smart technologies. The biggest challenges in this endeavor are coordinating the products of multiple vendors into one platform that will meet the ICU needs and be fully synchronized with hospital informatics systems.

Creating the Smart ICU

The smart ICU infrastructure necessitates the development of a connectivity envelope around the patient which encompasses the patient, medical devices, healthcare staff, as well as pharmacologic and other care elements.[12] This requires the installation of a robust wire and wireless infrastructure at each bedside, connectivity hardware within the patient room to connect and communicate with data sources, the placement of automatic identification tags on data sources for tracking purposes, the attachment of transmission units on medical devices to transmit their data and provide interoperability between the medical devices, and finally the placement of middleware (the software that connects medical devices with the hospital's operating systems and provides specialized applications) on hospital and ICU networks between the medical devices and the hospital servers.

ICU middleware is categorized by the Food and Drug Administration (FDA) as either Class 1 medical device data systems (MDDS) or Class 2 devices. MDDS devices maintain data storage, manage, transfer, display and also convert proprietary device languages into interoperability standardized formats. Class 2 applications additionally offer active patient monitoring and alarms, and thus are more intensely scrutinized by the FDA.

Applications inherent in ICU middleware include (Figure 4) transforming hospital- and ICU-based data and alarms to actionable information, managing devices, applying RTLS, creating smart displays, providing decision support, and facilitating telemedicine programs. All ICU middleware should be interfaced with the hospital's bed management system to automatically populate middleware applications, should meet hospital privacy protocols and have off-site backup systems.

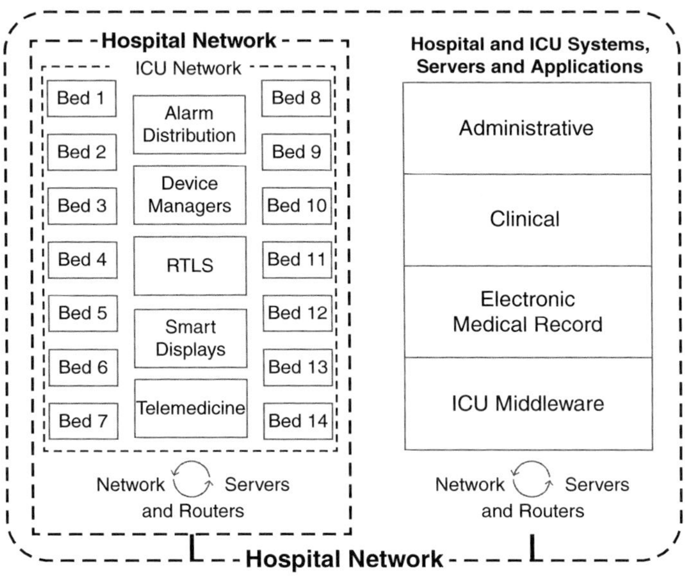

Figure 4. Two networks (ICU and hospital) are interlinked. Bedside devices are connected directly to either network and linkage is accomplished through servers, gateways, and routers. Middleware at both the ICU and hospital levels provides advanced applications for the ICU. RTLS: Real-time locating solutions. Reprinted with permission from CHEST.[12]

Advanced ICU Informatics Concepts

Three concepts are integral to advanced informatics. The first is the linkage or association of the patient with the medical devices and the data generated by those devices. Association protocols usually focus on either a "patient-centric" approach using the patient's unique medical record number or a "location-centric" approach using the patient's location. The location-centric solution appears more popular because it is simpler to implement than the patient-centric method; however, the latter solution always attaches the data to the patient regardless of patient movement within the hospital. The second concept is the application of interoperability between systems. Interoperability implies that the data generated by one device can be clearly understood by the receiving device. This requires data alignment between the proprietary data output languages of the medical devices and the recipient middleware. Without interoperability, the data produced by the medical device may not be integrated into the electronic medical record even though the devices are connected to the hospital network. The third concept addresses time synchronization between all medical devices, middleware and the hospital network. Time synchronization allows for a medical record that has correct time stamps for all data.

Medical Devices are Informatics Platforms

Medical devices are informatics platforms. Thus, software and hardware upgrades to ICU systems should be carefully assessed in simulation laboratories that duplicate the ICU informatics infrastructure. A gap analysis between current and proposed capabilities should always be performed. Budgeting for the systems must also include annual software upgrades and licensing agreements.

ICU Applications

Alarm systems

Alarm middleware captures device alarms, filters them as per hospital protocols and transmits them to handheld devices or other displays. Through these processes, device-generated alarms can be transformed into important and actionable information delivered to the providers in real-time, who can then act upon the data. The most sophisticated of these systems process streaming raw device data and create personalized patient alarms.

Virtual device communities

Stand-alone medical devices can be linked together through device middleware to generate a virtual device community. The virtual device community provides a venue for global and simultaneous monitoring of all devices and additionally for data storage, alarm transmission, and report generation. This middleware also allows for remote viewing capabilities (local telemedicine) by clinicians, and a portal for software upgrades and device monitoring by the vendor.

Real-Time Locating Systems

RTLS middleware offers a large variety of solutions for workflow efficiencies of all assets (staff, patients, equipment, consumables, and patient rooms). RTLS are most commonly used to locate tagged devices (mobile outset tracking) and to provide notification if devices leave designated areas. RTLS can also track the usage of consumable-tagged supplies to inventory and direct patient utilization. Within the ICU, RTLS can be integrated into nurse call systems and used to monitor patient and staff movements, compliance with hand washing protocols, and overall monitoring of the environment and housekeeping needs.

Data integration, smart displays, and decision support

Using middleware applications, data can be integrated from a host of data sources including the electronic medical record (EMR), bedside devices, bed management systems, RTLS, imaging servers, webcams, and decision support systems to support smart displays, real-time intelligent algorithms and monitors, and data sniffers (automated systems that search for preselected data elements). The smart displays supplement standard vender supplied stations (e.g. physiological monitoring central stations) and enable clinicians to rapidly monitor and identify changes in patient conditions through the use of customized graphical and tabular views, and intelligent algorithms. These displays efficiently present preselected historical and current data and minimize the need for clinicians to retrieve data from disparate systems and sort things out for themselves. Real-time intelligent algorithms and data sniffers profile patients and automatically identify patients at risk for clinical deterioration, alert staff and provide clinical support. Decision support systems are available for the management of sedation, infection and antibiotic control, nutrition, insulin infusions, and outcome predictions.

Telemedicine

Informatics systems provide the framework for telemedicine through the use of interfaces and bidirectional communications to transmit data, clinician orders, video and voice between the various ICU areas (e.g. patient room and waiting room) and the telemedicine vendor's bunker (e.g. proprietary EMR, decision support system, and alarm notification solution). These solutions are applicable whether the hospital outsources telemedicine to a third party at either an on- or off-site location, or internally to the hospital's own telemedicine team. Alternatively, the hospital can install web-based middleware that interfaces with hospital systems and allows the CC team to review all hospital and ICU systems and various handheld platforms.

References

1. Halpern NA and Pastores SM (2015). Critical care medicine beds, use, occupancy and costs in the United States: a methodological review. *Crit. Care Med.*, 43(11), 2452–2459 [Epub ahead of print].
2. Halpern NA and Pastores SM (2006). Changes in critical care beds and occupancy in the United States 1985–2000: differences attributable to hospital size. *Crit. Care Med.*, 34, 2015–2112.
3. Pastores SM, Halpern NA, Oropello JM, Kostelecky N and Kvetan V (2015). Critical care organizations in academic medical centers in North America: a descriptive report. *Crit. Care Med.*, 43(10), 2239–2244 [Epub ahead of print].

4. Ulrich RS, Zimring C and Barch XZ (2008). A review of the research literature on evidence-based healthcare design. *HERD*, 1, 61–125.
5. Sadler BL, DuBose J and Zimring C (2008). The business case for building better hospitals through evidence-based design. *HERD*, 1, 22–39.
6. Halpern NA (2014). Innovative designs for the smart ICU: part 1: from initial thoughts to occupancy. *Chest*, 145, 399–403.
7. Thompson DR, Hamilton DK and Cadenhead CD (2012). Guidelines for intensive care unit design. *Crit. Care Med.*, 40, 1586–1600.
8. Hamilton DK and Shepley MM (2010). *Design for Critical Care: An Evidence-Based Approach.* Elsevier Ltd., Burlington, MA.
9. Kesecioglu J, Schneider MM, van der Kooi AW and Bion J (2012). Structure and function: planning a new ICU to optimize patient care. *Curr. Opin. Crit. Care*, 18, 688–692.
10. Valentin A and Ferdinande P (2011). ESICM working group on quality improvement. Recommendations on basic requirements for intensive care units: structural and organizational aspects. *Intens. Care Med.*, 37, 1575–1587.
11. Halpern NA (2014). Innovative designs for the smart ICU: part 2: the ICU. *Chest*, 145, 646–658.
12. Halpern NA (2014). Innovative designs for the smart ICU: part 3: advanced ICU informatics. *Chest*, 145, 903–912.
13. Rashid M (2014). Two decades (1993–2012) of adult intensive care unit design: a comparative study of the physical design features of the best-practice examples. *Crit. Care Nurs. Q.*, 37, 2–31.
14. Guidelines for Design and Construction of Hospitals and Outpatient Facilities (2014). The Facilities Guidelines Institute, 2014 Edition. ASHE (American Society for Healthcare Engineering) of the American Hospital Association, Chicago, IL.
15. Award Winning ICU Designs (2016). How to build a better facility for patients and caregivers. Society of Critical Care Medicine. Available at: www.sccm.org (Accessed 1 September 2015).
16. Cadenhead CD and Anderson DC (2015). Critical care design: trends in award winning designs. World Health Design. Availabe at: http://www.worldhealthdesign.com/critical-care-design-trends-in-award-winning-designs.aspx (Accessed 16 September 2015).
17. Pati D and Pati S (2013). Methodological issues in conducting post-occupancy evaluations to support design decisions. *HERD*, 6(3), 157–63.
18. Evans J and Reyers E (2014). Patient room consideration in the intensive care unit: caregiver, patient family. *Crit. Care Nurs. Q.*, 37, 83–92.

19. Stroupe JM (2014). Design for safety in the critical care environment: an evidence-based approach. *Crit. Care Nurs. Q.*, 37, 103–114.
20. Drews FA (2013). Human factors in critical care medical environments. In *Reviews of Human Factors and Ergonomics*, Vol. 8, Morrow DR (ed.). SAGE Publications Thousand Oaks, CA, pp. 103–148.

Part II

Staffing and Staff Development

Staffing Models

Timothy G. Buchman

Director, Emory Critical Care Centre
Professor of Surgery and of Anesthesiology,
Emory University School of Medicine
Editor-in-Chief, Critical Care Medicine (2015–2020)

Key Points

1. The fundamental expertise is critical care (CC) nursing, which requires on average no fewer than one nurse for every two critically ill patients around the clock.
2. CC physicians (intensivists) are dispersed unevenly with respect to geography and time. Intensivists are in short supply in the USA but somewhat more plentiful elsewhere.
3. It appears more important that critically ill patients have the benefit of a CC consultant, less important that the intensivist consultant be physically present around the clock.
4. Advanced practice (non-physician) providers, including both nurse practitioners and physician assistants (PAs) in CC, are at least as safe and effective as physician trainees in augmenting and extending the coverage of intensivists.
5. Telemedicine (tele-ICU) can also extend the coverage of intensivists. Although telemedicine appears safe and clinically effective, the costs and benefits have yet to be fully determined.

Introduction

Safe and effective care of the critically ill patient is a complex task that engages diverse clinical, technical, and administrative professionals. In order to achieve the triple aim of better outcomes, better experience of care and lower costs, these professionals must be organized and managed.

The evolution of professional staff models and their potential futures has varied internationally. While the principles of staffing are global, solutions to the challenge of CC staffing are inevitably local and necessarily leverage whatever resources are most plentiful. One size fits one.

History

CC is widely considered to have originated in post-operative units early in the 20th century. Dr. Walter Dandy (a neurosurgeon practicing at Johns Hopkins in Baltimore) in 1923 decided to cohort his post-operative patients in a common location to leverage the experience and clinical skills of a small group of nurses. The unit had three beds but no specialized technology: stethoscopes and sphygmomanometers were the contemporary tools.

Five years later, heavy expensive technology appeared: the negative pressure ventilator (the "iron lung"). This was the first effective treatment to combat the respiratory failure of paralytic poliomyelitis. The polio epidemics took root in the western world as rapid transoceanic travel by sea and air became commonplace. Polio ("infantile paralysis") afflicted primarily children and in great numbers. Reports that the negative pressure ventilators could save at least a few lives led to the inception of several large wards where multiple patients could be attended by clinical personnel focused on caring for similar (and otherwise healthy) patients with a single system failure. However, these were by definition chronic care facilities: patients would spend months and years (and occasionally decades) supported by the devices.

Team-based care was born of a tragedy, the Cocoanut Grove nightclub fire in Boston, Massachusetts on 28 November 1942. Approximately 1,000 celebrants were toasting the victory of the Holy Cross football team over rival Boston College when fire broke out. The exits were locked and more than 400 died immediately of burns and asphyxiation. Survivors were taken to two local hospitals, the Massachusetts General Hospital and Boston City Hospital. Wartime hospital disaster committees had preassigned space and personnel in their emergency plans, which were quickly activated. Similar to polio victims, the surviving victims were generally young and previously healthy. Similar to the polio victims, they shared a common pathology. Different from the polio situation, the injuries were acute and the patients therefore required rapid and aggressive, yet consistent care. It quickly became apparent that debriding and dressing the complex burn wounds required a physician–nurse team approach, and further that the skills of the team rapidly improved with experience. As a matter of practical necessity, doctors and nurses were organized into task-focused groups. With team-based care, no patient who survived ten minutes at the Massachusetts General Hospital died within 12 hours, and 32 of 39 survived the first week. The success of this team-based care gained the attention of military physicians who were dealing with the many casualties of World War II.

As that war ended and civilian travel resumed, poliomyelitis returned with a vengeance. In the summer of 1952, the centre of the epidemic had seemingly shifted to Scandinavia. The Blegdam hospital in Copenhagen saw more than 3,000 cases, including many hundreds of children with respiratory paralysis. Unfortunately, iron lungs were scarce locally and the likelihood of a child with respiratory symptoms dying approached 85%. The chief anaesthesiologist proposed an alternative, namely tracheotomy and ventilation with a canister of soda lime interposed to absorb carbon dioxide. Several hundred nurses and medical students were pressed into service as human ventilators to support the hundreds of children who would receive this lifesaving therapy. Physician–nurse team care again proved extraordinarily effective. Perhaps more importantly, the experience led directly to the invention of the mechanical ventilator.

Early mechanical ventilators were bulky and heavy so could not be moved easily. Patients were brought to the machines, not vice versa. Importantly, as the polio epidemic waned (especially with the introduction of the Salk vaccine in 1953), the mechanical ventilator technology was used in respiratory failure more generally. The late 1950s and early 1960s witnessed rapid proliferation of respiratory care units where patients could be ventilated. New skills around use of the machines and the delivery of inhaled medications led to the creation of a new role, the "inhalation therapist", later becoming an integral member of the CC team as respiratory therapists.

Equipment-driven consolidation of space and personnel led to the creation of other types of care units, including coronary care units (pacemakers and defibrillators) and renal units (dialysis machines). These were staffed with specially trained nurses yet lacked a full-time physician staff.

In 1956, Dr. Peter Safar, an Anaesthesiologist working at the Baltimore City Hospital, determined that his patients would benefit from continuous presence of a physician with expertise in cardiac and pulmonary care, with special lifesaving skills such as endotracheal intubation and cardiopulmonary resuscitation (CPR). He organized his intensive care unit (ICU) such that qualified physicians and specialized nurses were present at all times and moreover followed standard protocols and procedures addressing the most common problems he encountered.[1] Bear in mind that the monitoring tools of CC had changed little since Walter Dandy's unit four decades earlier: those early physicians had little more than physical examination and the tools in their doctor bags to make diagnoses.

The next 15 years witnessed massive technological advances. Shock units were conceived, abetted by the invention and proliferation of bedside monitors led largely by Dr. Max Harry Weil. Indwelling arterial and central venous access routes were described and became commonplace, paving the way for the use of vasoactive infusions. The balloon-tipped pulmonary artery catheter was introduced by William Swan and Jeremy Ganz in 1970, and with it the ability to estimate cardiac output by thermodilution. Management of the technology at the bedside and interpretation of the data became essential competencies for CC nurses. Insertion of the invasive devices and medical decision-making including titration of therapies required near-continuous presence of physicians. By the early 1970s, the competencies required in the ICU — the knowledge, skills, and attitudes required for safe care of critically ill patients — were beyond those of the average clinician. The specialty of CC medicine was born.

Along with it, a specialty society was born. The Society of Critical Care Medicine (SCCM) was launched by 29 physicians in 1970. Dr. Weil became the first president, Dr. Safar the second. Pertinent to staffing models, the SCCM was deliberately (and at the time uniquely) organized to welcome not just physicians but every member of the multi-professional team contributing to care of the critically ill.

The nursing profession organized itself relatively quickly. In the USA, the American Association of Critical Care Nurses (AACN) evolved from the cardiovascular nurse society in 1971 and five years later offered the first certification examination leading to the Credential of Critical Care Nurse (CCRN). The credential is promoted in several ways, and many nurse unit directors (and their hospitals) advocate for their clinical staff to study and sit for the examination. Awards of CC excellence often include the percentage of staff with this credential as a metric.

While pharmacy and nutrition support services have lagged a little behind nursing in CC specialization and recognition, there exist tracks and certifications. Pharmacy has CC residencies that lead to specialty certification in CC yielding fewer than 100 graduates annually in the USA. Nutrition support staff, typically registered dieticians, can avail themselves of internships focusing on CC.

The USA physician community planned a joint accrediting body, the American Board of Critical Care Medicine (ABCCM). Training would follow primary training in one of several specialties but there would be a common pathway leading to certification in CCM. Unfortunately, one of the component boards backed out of the agreement and the plan for a common pathway dissolved. As a consequence, CC medicine in USA is less a specialty than a collection of sub-specialties, for example anaesthesiology CC, surgical CC, and so on.

Challenges of Staffing Critical Care

Against this backdrop of desired attributes, core strategy and secular trends, CC leaders face challenging strategic decisions around professional staffing (licensed staff: physicians, nurses, therapists, pharmacists, and others who are appointed to hospitals). Certificated staff such as secretaries, medical assistants, practical nurses, and others are surely important to the operation of CC units. However, they are typically in greater supply as technical and trade schools matriculate and graduate new classes in response to changing demand.

The decisions around professional staffing are challenging because their training aligns poorly with either present or projected demand for their services. In a famous example, the COMPACCS workgroup reported 15 years ago that secular trends (including the aging of the post-war "baby boom" population and the inevitable retirement of the first generation of CC physicians) would lead to CC physician shortfall in the USA.[2] The projected gap was confirmed in a subsequent study sponsored and reported by the federal government.[3] However, training programs did not group in number or size to meet the projected demand. As a consequence, even large medical centres in desirable urban areas are progressively short of qualified CC physicians.

CCN in the USA faces three intersecting pressures. First, the average age of a bedside nurse in the USA rose steadily as fewer young people were entering and staying in the nursing profession. Second, training to competency at the bedside is prolonged compared to other areas of clinical nursing, with most trainers suggesting that it takes at least two years for a newly graduated nurse to be safe "solo" at the bedside of a critically ill patient. Third, critical care nursing experience is effectively a pre-requisite to alternative (and more lucrative) nursing careers as, for example, a certified registered nurse anaesthetist (cRNA) or acute care nurse practitioner (ACNP). These three pressures have tended to siphon CCNs away from the bedside.

CC pharmacy provides yet another example of misaligned demand and supply. There are ample studies showing the value of a CC pharmacist to patient safety and ICU operations. Still in the USA, compensation for retail pharmacists exceeds that of hospital-based pharmacists. The predictable consequence is that there is a shortfall in CC pharmacist manpower.

These and similar shortfalls create specific and predictable pressures around staffing, all related in some way to limited budgets framed against the need to provide continuous, safe and competent care to aging and progressively complex patients. Profession by profession, various resolutions have emerged. Yet there are certain themes that are common to all of the resolutions, themes that bear awareness and reflection.

The first theme is that CC is a continuous, around-the-clock activity yet the professional staff's lives are typically organized around the more ordinary schedules of weekdays, weekends, holidays, sleeping at night (not by day) and so on. All CC professions have to solve the puzzles of allocating not only numbers but also experience and expertise of the staff to the continuous and sometimes suddenly increased demands of critically ill patients.

The second theme is that training is nearly as continuous as care itself. In nearly every ICU, there is always the "new person" — whether a newly graduated nurse, a physician-in-training, or someone who has just recently joined the professional staff and requires acclimatization. In every ICU (without exception) there is continuous learning and verification of that learning. Nurses have skills days and there are various 'merit badges' to be acquired (such as the Advanced Cardiac Life Support credential that requires recertification every two years) by nurses and physicians alike. Each new (or replacement) technology requires substantial commitment to a training strategy around use, interpretation and troubleshooting of that technology. Training therefore must be planned as part of staffing and hardwired into schedules and budgets.

The third theme is practice to the "top of one's licence". Chronic shortages in the various professions and the costs of hiring those who are available converge into an expectation that those who have direct clinical care responsibilities will do every clinical activity permitted by law, job description, and local credentialing. Indeed, the pressure is so great that 'creep' is common: nurses especially find themselves pressured into taking decisions and actions that are properly the domain of their physician colleagues.

The fourth — and potentially the most important — theme has to do with the balance between management and leadership. CC units require both, often in different measure and at different times from the different professions. It follows that the appointment of leaders — medical director, nursing director, etc. — should be made with utmost care to ensure ICU leadership is sustained.

Nurses

An ICU can operate without therapists, pharmacists and even physicians. No ICU can operate without the continuous presence and actions of qualified nurses.

Measurement of nurse activity was and remains common in CC. Perhaps the best known system of measurement is the Therapeutic Intervention Scoring System. This score, originally developed around 1974, was intended to report and provide a basis for balancing nursing workload among the diverse patients who might be in an ICU.[4] The original TISS described 57 activities with points assigned for each activity. There have been modifications to include fewer or greater activities. Regardless of version, TISS has been widely studied and validated. The studies reach convergent and consistent conclusions. First, there is a practical limit to the number of tasks that a nurse can perform during a tour of duty (shift). Second, there is a sufficiently tight relationship between the number of tasks required by a given patient and their clinical outcome that TISS emerged as among first risk-stratification systems, seven years before the first version of the familiar acute physiology and chronic health evolution (APACHE) system appeared.

Put simply, the number of interventions reflects the severity of illness and therefore is a reflection of both intensity of care required and the likely outcome. The subtlety is that while TISS is an intervention scoring system, only some (but not all) of the interventions must be performed by a nurse. Task reassignment is common. For example, TISS includes chest physiotherapy, intratracheal suctioning, and aspects of ventilator management. Most or all of these tasks can be (and commonly are) reassigned to a respiratory therapist so that nurse time can be invested elsewhere. That therapist can then provide specific care to a relatively larger number of patients. Similar task gerrymandering occurs across other professions and professionals: pharmacists, physical therapists, dieticians who are granted specific authorities, responsibilities, and resources.

The most important tasks of the CCN — learning the patient's physiology, monitoring the patient for anomalies, engaging the family, and generally being guardian of the patient's safety and well-being in an increasing technical environment — cannot be delegated or reassigned. This leads to practical limits on CC staffing. Absent the various professionals listed in the prior paragraph (respiratory therapists, physical therapists, and so on), critically ill patients who require continuous surveillance and pharmacological and/or mechanical support of failed organs require 1:1 nursing. With those professionals to assist, critically ill patients generally require at least 1 nurse for every 2 patients. There are notable exceptions. For example, care of patients with unique requirements (e.g. a patient with Ebola virus disease who must be attended by nurses wearing special protective suits)may increase the required nursing complement to up to 6 nurses per patient.[5] Reciprocally, patients who require frequent (versus continuous) monitoring to sense deterioration might be safely cared for in a ratio of 1 nurse to as many as 3–4 patients.

There are population level data worldwide to suggest that nursing ratios leaner than 1 nurse for every two patients are associated with (preventable) harm.[6] There are also population level data to suggest that certain patient flow events — for example, a discharge made during unsocial hours in order to accommodate a new admission — are also associated with preventable harm. Such patient flow events clearly impose additional work on nursing staff (the discharge process, a room clean, an admission process). When this additional work occurs at times of thinnest staffing (nights), there is a statistically significant increase in adverse outcomes.[7]

Collectively, these data point to minimal flexibility around ICU nurse staffing ratios. Given the relative shortage of CCNs, the major staffing issue confronting ICU nurse managers is locating sufficient nurses to meet those ratios. Even when the nursing positions in a unit roster are filled (and that is rare in the USA), gaps inevitably appear and every unit relies on reserves. In order of preference, nurse managers seem to request (a) their own ICU nursing staff to take "overtime" shifts; (b) nurses from other ICUs within the hospital to fill in; (c) float pool nurses; and (d) locum tenens ("traveling") nurses. This order reflects decreasing familiarity with ICU-specific and hospital-specific processes. While internal overtime is preferred by most ICU nurse leaders, there are limits and consequences to its use. Overtime, while typically paid at "time-and-a-half", is limited by convention (and in some locales by regulation) to half of the regular work schedule.

Physicians

In contrast to nursing, patterns of physician staffing vary around the world. Some nations specify physician staffing patterns with the same precision that nursing staffing patterns are described. These specifications typically identify different tiers of ICU capability and assign both nursing and physician minimum training and staffing level appropriate to the complexity of patients cared for in each tier. Other nations are silent on the number and training of physicians required to care for patients in CC units.

From the perspective of USA history, a third of a century elapsed between the inception of CC (Johns Hopkins Hospital, 1923 under the direction of Dr. Walter Dandy) and the first dedicated physicians assigned to ICU duty (Baltimore City Hospital, 1956, under the direction of Dr. Peter Safar). Three more decades would pass until sufficient data were gathered to support a standard of continuous availability of at least a minimally qualified physician.[8] Curiously, the standard was not issued by accrediting agencies, professional groups or regulatory bodies. Rather, it emerged from a business roundtable. Given that a substantial portion of the cost of medical care for Americans was borne by (and paid by) corporate America at the time that the standard was initially issued, hospitals took notice.

It quickly became apparent that the high-intensity staffing standard could not be met with the then-existing cadre of CC physicians and that it would never be met even in the most optimistic estimates of the number of physicians who would enter the CC training pipeline.[9] With that realization, American physicians and their hospitals have taken three approaches:

- Assert and demonstrate that the stringent standard of intensivist availability can be relaxed without harm to patients.
- Train and deploy advanced practice providers to fill the gaps that have appeared in providing care to critically ill patients.
- Develop and deploy technologies enabling telepresence so as to distribute scarce physician cognitive resources over a larger geographic "footprint".

Standards of intensivist availability

It is a truism that acute, emergent, and critical illness does not respect "ordinary working hours". Some disciplines and professional societies that overlap with and rely on CC services have established and adhere to rigorous staffing standards and response times (trauma teams, interventional cardiology teams, stroke teams are three common examples). However, standards around physician staffing of ICUs are local, voluntary, and largely pragmatic in the sense that there "must be enough business to justify continuous specialist physician presence". The desirability of continuous intensivist presence to complement such teams when the patient arrives in the ICU is evident.[10] Justification is another matter and typically easier in large urban hospitals with multiple ICUs.

Specialty hospitals (for example, orthopaedic hospitals, long term acute care hospitals) and smaller general hospitals that serve rural populations may have fewer and less sick patients who can ordinarily be cared for in one of two models. One model has on-site generalist physicians, typically hospital-employed physicians (hospitalists) who have familiarity with and competence in basic CC. Another model relies on telephonic consultation with off-site physicians backstopped by on-site emergency medicine physicians who can provide emergent care (such as endotracheal intubation or tube thoracostomy).

Teaching hospitals that keep one or more physician trainees on site while attending intensivist physicians are available telephonically represent a variant in the continuum between continuous presence of a qualified intensivist and limited availability of a non-intensivist physician. Studies addressing the outcomes of these models have been performed and widely discussed.

The most consistent finding is that continuous presence of a qualified intensivist is not required to achieve optimal outcomes provided there is on-site presence of senior physician trainees who are empowered to act according to plan and have qualified intensivists immediately available by telephone for advice. For example, the Wallace study discerned no difference when night-time attending intensivists were at home provided an advanced (fellowship-level) trainee was available on site supported by additional trainees (residents) so long as the attending intensivist had been available to make a plan in the daytime.[11] The Wilcox meta-analysis showed that some engagement of a qualified intensivist to see the patient and make a plan — either as the attending physician or as consultant — significantly reduced mortality and length of stay.[12]

The problem arises that there are insufficient numbers of intensivists in the USA. Both the COMPACCS study and the HRSA study projected a gap between supply and demand.[2,3] Despite modest increases in the production rates of physicians qualified to provide critical care in the USA, demand continues to outpace this supply. There are two reasons. First, the demographics are overwhelming: for the past five years and for the next 15 years, around 10,000 Americans reach retirement (Medicare) age each day. Second, the attrition of physicians from the ranks of practicing intensivists is substantial. Part of the attrition reflects the retirement of the generation of new physicians who were attracted to CC in the early years (awake ventilation, pulmonary artery catheter-guided hemodynamic management, bedside dialysis via Scribner shunts) when multiple organ support became a reality. Simple mathematics shows that those physicians are now in the seventh and eighth decades of their lives. The other part of the attrition reflects the fact that critical care medicine is a part-time profession for many if not most intensivists in the USA: pulmonology, operative anesthesiology and emergency surgery are common complementary activities, and those often have better hours, better compensation and lower risk of 'burnout'.

While the numerical shortage is less severe in some nations (e.g. England) and there is a surplus of qualified intensivist physicians in others (e.g. Australia), care delivery is commonly challenged by a maldistribution of personnel and their availability. In other words, intensivist physicians tend to be concentrated in urban centres and their availability is highest during weekday hours. Still, critical illness does not respect geography, the calendar or ordinary day-night cycles and therefore "coverage" challenges every community of physicians charged with maintaining quality, value and access to CC.

In the past, the complementary problems of insufficient intensivist numbers and their maldistribution in time and location had been solved by promoting trainees to roles of greater authority and responsibility. That solution remains viable in some nations where training in CCM is prolonged over many years. In some cases, these physicians may even graduate from their training programs yet remain employed as house physicians while awaiting appearance of a vacancy in a consultant/professor post. In other parts of the world, particularly the USA, reliance on trainees to fill gaps has diminished. There are fewer trainees. The trainees assigned to the ICU are progressively junior. Their work hours are restricted. Expectations of instructor-at-the-elbow supervision have increased. It is apparent that both saturation of the intensivist job market where staff are plentiful as well as reassignment of trainees that limit number, seniority or hours away from ICUs where intensivist staff are thin lead to a similar result: fewer trainees available to fill coverage gaps.

Advanced Practice Providers

Over the past decade, the gaps have been increasingly filled with advanced practice (non-physician) providers who have been trained and credentialed to provide CC. A few PAs have worked in specialty ICUs (such as cardiothoracic surgical ICUs) since the 1980s. However, use of advanced practice providers in CC settings remained rare until about a decade ago. Perhaps the strongest catalyst for the advanced practice provider role was the development of the ACNP credential by the AACN in the mid-1990s. On the heels of the credential came the development of accredited training programs that commonly recruit trauma, emergency and CCNs to develop and verify competencies and return them to the bedside as practitioners.

As graduates of these ACNP programs returned to the bedside, it became apparent that additional training was required to achieve both comfort and competencies as CC providers. It was also apparent that additional training was required of graduates of PA programs. This supplemental training has taken one of three forms: simple apprenticeships; structured "on-the-job (OJT)" training; and formal residencies in CCM.[13]

There is substantial evidence that these advanced practice providers provide care that is equal to or superior to the care provided by physician trainees.[14] Multiple studies in diverse settings have uniformly demonstrated the clinical quality and effectiveness of their care.[15]Moreover, they are cost-effective substitutes for physicians. Such alternative staffing models are attractive and, at this point, firmly embedded in CC practice in the USA. They have already started to spread to Europe.

Tele-ICU

Video telephony, the audiovisual link between two participants over a closed circuit, was conceived in the 1920s and publicly demonstrated at the 1964 World's Fair in New York City as the "Picture phone". Rapid technical advances enabled higher resolution cameras and larger displays, and a decade later initial experiments were implemented using early audio-visual systems for CC consultation. The need to establish both clinical and economic effectiveness was apparent, and that step required more than a quarter-century.

Telemedicine for CC enjoyed early adoption in the USA, then levelled off at about 8% of the total ICU beds.[16] USA Veterans Administration has invested heavily in telemedicine, including tele-ICU care. In contrast, the very first tele-ICU centre opened in 2015 in London. Early scepticism about the clinical usefulness of tele-ICU has faded: remote support of a bedside team has consistently been shown to reduce adverse events, shorten lengths of stays and generally improve the quality of care.[17]

Rather, the debate centres around costs. Estimates of the costs of CC telemedicine vary widely owing to inconsistent cost accounting strategies, but there is no question that the costs have been substantial in all instances and prohibitive in some. Fortunately, an objective accounting strategy is emerging that will bring some rationale to balancing cost with benefit.[18] The new strategy looks at the actual costs of providing tele-ICU care and examines the aggregate impacts in a clinical effectiveness model using tunable parameters that can identify a break-even point. While tele-ICU incurs hardware, software, facility and licensing costs, those costs are dwarfed by the cost of the labor to staff the tele-ICU. Most tele-ICUs allocate one nurse for every 30–50 beds covered, and one physician for every 100–150 patients covered. For a 24 × 7 coverage model that allows for illness, time off and so on, 150 beds would require the services of 15–25 full time equivalent nurses and 5 full time equivalent intensivist physicians. Even so, a recent review suggests that while tele-ICU implementation incurs substantial costs, it may be cost-effective when the intensity of application is high and in sicker patients.[19]

Of note, studies of the cost and effectiveness of tele-CC have focused on the location of the intensivist — either at the bedside or in the remote facility. Reports are emerging that show length-of-stay (but not mortality) benefit of nurse-only surveillance at a remote site.[20] There has been no study reported to date looking at the effect of a remote intensivist supporting an advanced practice provider at the bedside, although such a model is in place and has been accumulating data since May 2014 at Emory University.

Leadership staffing

CC delivery systems depend on the training, recruitment and deployment of costly and scarce personnel. Every profession that serves critically ill patients is challenged to ensure a steady supply to meet the needs of aging and progressively complex patients. Direct, hands-on care by CCNs is the foundation of all CC and their ranks must be expanded to keep pace with patient needs. Wherever possible, their effectiveness can be extended by shedding tasks to other professionals (respiratory therapists, pharmacists, nutrition support staff, physiotherapists) provided those tasks lie appropriately within scope of practice. Shortages and maldistribution of CC physicians, previously mitigated through extensive use of physician trainees, is increasingly offset through substitution by advanced practice non-physician providers who come from PA and nurse practitioner backgrounds. The introduction of this new class of providers has sustained the quality of care. Telepresence, while costly, has the potential to expand the supervisory reach of intensivist physicians.

Choosing among the various staffing options will require extraordinary management skills supported by deep understanding of hospital administration, healthcare economics, and the labor force. Those staffing choices, once made, will require extraordinary leadership if they are to be safely and securely implemented. The leadership challenge is much more than a matter of reallocating tasks and roles. The leadership role requires rethinking the value and execution of every aspect of CC, reshaping the workforce to serve the needs of patients not the traditions of professions, and guiding each team member towards a novel allocation of responsibilities and actions while sustaining communication, cohesion and a common vision.

References

1. Safar P and Grenvik A (1971). Critical care medicine. Organizing and staffing intensive care units. *Chest*, 59(5), 535–547.
2. Angus DC, Kelley MA and Schmitz RJ (2000). Current and projected workforce requirements for care of the critically ill and patients with pulmonary disease: can we meet the requirements of an aging population. *JAMA*, 284(21), 2762–2770.
3. Duke EM (2006). US Department of Health and Human Services, Health Resources & Services Administration (HRSA) report to Congress: The Critical Care Workforce. A study of the supply and demand for critical care physicians. Available at: http://bhpr.hrsa.gov/healthworkforce/supplydemand/medicine/criticalcaresupply.pdf.
4. Cullen DJ, Civetta JM, Briggs BA and Ferrara LC (1974). Therapeutic intervention scoring system: a method for quantitative comparison of patient care. *Crit. Care Med.*, 2(2), 57–60.
5. Johnson SS, Barranta N and Chertow D (2015). Ebola at the National Institutes of Health: perspectives From Critical care nurses. *AACN Adv. Crit. Care*, 26(3), 262–267.
6. Sakr Y, Moreira CL and Rhodes A (2015). For the extended prevalence of infection in intensive care study investigators. The impact of hospital and ICU organizational factors on outcome in critically ill patients: results from the extended prevalence of infection in intensive care study. *Crit. Care Med.*, 43(3), 519–526.
7. Neuraz A, Guérin C and Payet C (2015). Patient mortality is associated with staff resources and workload in the ICU: a multicenter observational study. *Crit. Care Med.*, 43(8), 1587–1594.
8. Pronovost PJ, Angus DC and Dorman T (2002). Physician staffing patterns and clinical outcomes in critically ill patients: a systematic review. *JAMA*, 288 (17), 2151–2162.
9. Kahn JM, Matthews FA and Angus DC (2007). Barriers to implementing the Leapfrog Group recommendations for intensivist physician staffing: a survey of intensive care unit directors. *J. Crit. Care*, 22(2), 97–103.
10. Burchardi H and Moerer O (2001). 24 hour presence of physicians in the ICU. *Crit. Care*, 5(3), 131–137.
11. Wallace DJ, Angus DC and Barnato AE (2012). Night-time intensivist staffing and mortality among critically ill patients. *N. Engl. J. Med.*, 366(22), 2093–2101. Erratum in *N. Engl. J. Med.*, 367(9), 881.
12. Wilcox ME, Chong CA and Niven DJ (2013). Do intensivist staffing patterns influence hospital mortality following ICU admission? A systematic review and meta-analyses. *Crit. Care Med.*, 41(10), 2253–2274.

13. Luckianow GM, Piper GL and Kaplan LJ (2015). Bridging the gap between training and advanced practice provider critical care competency. *JAAPA*, 28(5), 1–5.
14. Kleinpell RM, Ely EW and Grabenkort R (2008). Nurse practitioners and physician assistants in the intensive care unit: an evidence-based review. *Crit. Care Med.*, 36(10), 2888–2897.
15. Edkins RE, Cairns BA and Hultman CS (2014). A systematic review of advance practice providers in acute care: options for a new model in a burn intensive care unit. *Ann. Plast. Surg.*, 72(3), 285–288.
16. Kahn JM, Cicero BD, Wallace DJ and Iwashyna TJ (2014). Adoption of ICU telemedicine in the United States. *Crit. Care Med.* 42(2), 362–368.
17. Lilly CM, Cody S and Zhao H (2011). Hospital mortality, length of stay, and preventable complications among critically ill patients before and after tele-ICU reengineering of critical care processes. *JAMA*, 1, 305(21), 2175–2183.
18. Yoo BK, Kim M, Sasaki T, Melnikow J and Marcin J (2016). Economic evaluation of telemedicine for patients in intensive care units. *Crit. Care Med.*, 44(2), 265–274.
19. Venkataraman R and Ramakrishnan N (2015). Outcomes related to telemedicine in the intensive care unit: what we know and would like to know. *Crit. Care Clin.*, 31(2), 225–237.
20. Kahn JM, Gunn SR and Lorenz HL (2014). Impact of nurse-led remote screening and prompting for evidence-based practices in the ICU. *Crit. Care Med.*, 42(4), 896–904.

Staff Training and Development

Graham R. Nimmo
Consultant Physician in Intensive Care Medicine and Clinical Education, Western General Hospital, NHS Lothian, Edinburgh, UK

Mike C. Clapham
Honorary Consultant Intensive Care Medicine and Education, Queen Elizabeth Medical Centre, B15 2TH, Birmingham, UK

Key Points

1. Training and education underpin all of our activities in critical care (CC).
2. Learning needs should be based on evaluable clinical practice i.e. what is required to do the job.
3. Theory, practical skills, and clinical behaviours are all important elements in a blended learning approach to CC.
4. So-called soft skills including communication, team work, and decision-making can be the hardest to do, learn, teach, and evaluate. Clinical simulation has a major role as an educational modality for this.
5. Continuing professional development for all staff groups improves patient care, staff job satisfaction and long-term staff retention but requires support both in terms of time and funding.

Introduction

The Bombay Hospital motto adapted from a quotation from Mahatma Gandhi reminds us that "A patient is the most important person in our hospital. He is not an interruption to our work: he is the purpose of it. He is not an outsider in our hospital: he is part of it. We are not doing a favor by caring for him: he is doing us a favor by giving us the opportunity to do so".[1]

All that we learn, teach and do should be for the benefit of our patients and their families. In adopting this philosophy in training and education, and by putting it into practice, staff and students can maximize benefit. There is a wide variation in the provision, delivery and quality of CC in who delivers this care but staff training, learning and education are pivotal to the provision and enactment of day-to-day, and night-to-night, CC everywhere. The 24/7 and often, unpredictable nature of CC needs to be surfaced and addressed in the writing of curricula and in the development of educational materials and teaching programs.

Medical staffs make up a small proportion of the team delivering hands on critical care (CC) to individual patients, the vast majority of clinical staff being nurses. Training, education, and development of all staff groups and grades as a team, is pivotal to the delivery of sustained safe, effective, and high quality care. The issues can be tackled from the perspective of general educational theory with practical solutions, easily applicable on a relatively small scale. The design and delivery of the curriculum of the standalone Faculty of Intensive Care Medicine (FICM) Physician IC Training program[2] in the UK provides illustrations of possible approaches. The ideas are not original to the FICM; they are based on the best ideas from around the world adapted to local requirements. One key issue was that the curriculum had to be credentialed nationally by the regulatory body, the General Medical Council. A non-medical syllabus and curriculum for Advanced Critical Care Practitioners (ACCPs) including nurses and physiotherapists, was also developed,[3] from which there were some key lessons.

The term IC is used to cover all CC areas. Core educational principles, explicit strategies, processes for teaching, learning and very importantly, how the learning is assessed, involve the unpacking of knowledge, skills and behaviours, which encourages a blended learning approach combining all of these. Real life, pragmatic, practice-based training and assessment is applicable to all staff groups and, hopefully, will be useful and useable no matter which CC context or country the reader is in. The complementary and parallel contributions of clinical skills training and immersive, whole patient simulation as tools for training in the clinical setting should be blended together to avoid the pitfalls identified by Florence Nightingale over a 100 years ago when she wrote: "theory without practice is ruinous to nurses".[4] This also applies to doctors and other healthcare professionals.

A Pedagogy of CC Training

The starting point for any training or educational intervention is to define the learners in their clinical, CC context to inform the development and definition of learning objectives. Ask: "who are the learners?" Look at the clinical environment in which they work and the activities that they are involved with. Remember that learners are from different backgrounds and have varying levels of experience and therefore different learning needs. Since the staffing of CC is multi-professional, with different models of practice and professional responsibilities across the team, it will be natural to define both generic and specific intended learning outcomes. For medical staff there may be a national curriculum, or syllabus such as that of FICM in the UK, or an internationally developed guide such as Competency Based Training in Intensive Care in Europe (CoBaTRICE).[5] In nursing training there are multiple curricula across countries often based in individual higher educational institutions. Undergraduates and postgraduates also learn in CC but this text relates to staff who are in clinical practice with established professional registration.

The curriculum house model

Knowing what you want to teach is pivotal. This should be allied to what the learners need to know. There needs to be clearly defined educational objectives and intended learning outcomes. These objectives and outcomes must be evaluable as well as being utterly transparent to both learner and trainer. This applies just as much to locally developed, in practice, training as it does to a national curriculum or syllabus. The mechanism of the achievement of the learning, and the methods and practicalities of assessment, should also be explicit.

Consider the curriculum house as a method of identifying learning needs based on evaluable clinical practice, i.e. what is required to do the job. It can be used in developing a national training program or for the creation of a local teaching package for a clinical skill. The house is a metaphor that can be used by trainers and teachers as a platform from which one has to identify the core elements required for any educational intervention. It allows visualization of the relationships between these different elements and provides a checklist for the content, delivery, and assessment strategy for the educational intervention. It can be used to define intended learning outcomes. This model is based on the one used when all of the postgraduate medical programs in Netherlands were reformed.[6] This involved a three step design process: structuring the content; choosing activities which are information rich in order to define exemplary evaluable professional activities (EPAs); and having created this assessment toolbox, matching it to a professional framework, in this case the CanMEDS roles.[7] This approach can be utilized in the development of curricula in any professional context. Taking the UK FICM curriculum for ACCPs[3] (Figure 1) as an exemplar of the application of this approach, it can be seen at the top of the house the overall goal of producing competent, capable practitioners is emphasized. In order to realize this goal a process of educational diagnostics is necessary, whereby the operational competencies required to fulfill the clinical role for which the learners are training are identified. The knowledge, skills, attitudes, and behaviours involved in the job are defined from the exemplary professional activities. The training materials, methods and learning activities are developed from, and based on the requirements of learning these.

The FICM (UK) ACCP handbook[3] states:"This curriculum identifies the aims and objectives, content, experiences, outcomes, and processes of postgraduate specialist training leading to a Postgraduate Diploma/Masters qualification in Advanced CC practice or equivalent. It defines the structure and expected methods of learning, teaching, feedback, and supervision. It sets out what knowledge, skills, attitudes and behaviours the ACCP trainee will achieve. A system of assessments is used to monitor

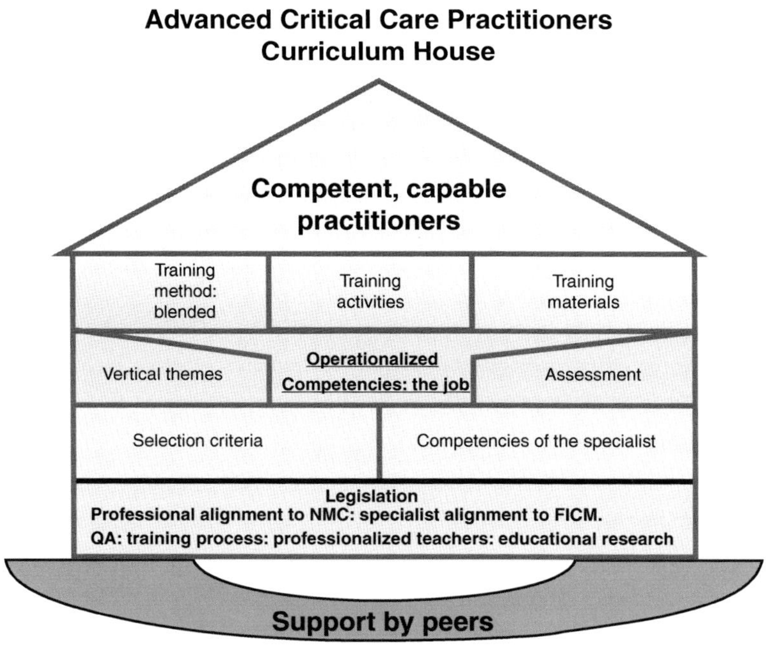

Figure 1. Curriculum house in developing a national or regional program for ACCP.

the ACCP trainee's progress through the stages of training. The objective of the program is to produce high quality patient-centred practitioners with appropriate knowledge, skills and attitudes to enable them to practice in Intensive Care Medicine (ICM)".

The ACCP syllabus was developed using this Curriculum House approach. The training program utilizes a spiral learning approach. Basic principles are learnt and understood early on and are then revisited and expounded later, and then further developed as time in training is accrued. This approach is also applied to the acquisition of skills, attitudes, and behaviours. The outcome is to attain clinical mastery at the level required to commence autonomous practice in a specific job by the end of training. Knowledge, skills, attitudes, and behaviours metaphorically spiral upwards. Following qualification, the continuing professional development of the ACCP follows the same model, although different practitioners will progress at different rates. The Royal College of Physician and

Surgeons of Canada has defined the different roles of the doctor in the CanMEDS domains[7] (Table 1). These could also form a foundation for the development of similar systems for other healthcare professionals.

Ways of Learning

There is a plethora of learning methods and locations and some of these are listed in Table 2. A number of the crucial elements are.

Table 1. The CanMEDS domains.[7]

Medical Expert
Communicator
Collaborator
Leader (formerly Manager)
Health Advocate
Scholar
Professional

Table 2. Locations and methods for learning.

Learning locations
Bedside
Operating theatre/room (OR)
Clinic
Classroom
Lecture theatre
Skills/simulation lab
Learning methods
Tutorial
Workshop
Seminar
Journal club
Morbidity and mortality meeting
Problem based learning /Enquiry based learning
E-learning: lectures, on-line tutorials, modules (interactive web based materials)
Gaming
Clinical skills practical training
Simulation

Learning from experience and practice

Clinical learners spend a large proportion of time in the workplace engaged in experiential learning during supervised clinical practice. Learning involves closely supervised clinical practice until competence is achieved.

Learning from feedback

Learning from experience can be optimized when feedback is available from staff, patients and families, and carers. More formalized and structured feedback from consultant trainers and other experienced teachers can be utilized to facilitate the formative experience. This feedback should be quick, reliable, relevant, accurate, and unambiguous. It should recognize both good practices and areas for development and improvement, and identify methods to achieve these; ways of providing feedback are described later.

Training with peers

Training can be enhanced when groups of learners study or work together, partly through the immediate discussions which occur, and also by stimulating reflection on practice by the individuals involved. Some of the educational techniques which can be utilized in this way are detailed later.

Learning in formal situation

Tutorials, lectures, regional, national courses and conferences remain an important resource both for those in training and for continuing professional development (CPD).

Personal study

Ideally time should be made available for personal study and for self-directed learning. However, in many countries, study leave time and budgets are limited or non-existent, and healthcare professionals will study in their own non-clinical time. It could be argued that this independent study is a natural component of professional life, and certainly for those clinicians sitting high stakes examinations or writing dissertations and theses, it is an absolute pre-requisite for success. Independent learning can be enriched and supported by educational interventions delivered by newer learning technologies such as web-based resources and podcasts and interactions through social media where discussion for a are utilized.

Teachers and Trainers

CC training should be delivered by clinical subject matter experts who also have educational expertise in clinical training, teaching, and education. Ideally they should have undergone formal training in teaching and education.

Educational contracts

The development of a learning agreement that incorporates the expectations of both the learner and the trainer helps to focus activities and provides goals for achievement and for training.

Learning using clinical skills training

A list of standard clinical skills can be found in Table 3. Figure 2 demonstrates how the curriculum house approach can be used to develop individual clinical skills training: the Skills House approach.[8] The mastery method of complex skills simulation training has been effectively described by McGachie and colleagues (Figure 3) and is recommended for clinical skills training in CC.[9] This approach significantly improves performance, and when the simulated training takes place within the clinical environment, authenticity, context, and meaning are added to the learning experience.

Learning using simulation training

Simulation lends itself very well to training and education for acute clinical situations. It is an excellent learning environment to explore interactions

Table 3. Directly observed procedural and practical skills.

Evaluable practical clinical skills
General
Hand washing
Vital signs measurement: respiratory rate, pulse, cuff blood pressure, conscious level, temperature
Basic airway management, basic life support
Bedside glucose measurement
Urinary bladder catheterization
Gastric tube insertion
Venepuncture, blood cultures, cannulation, intravenous fluid, and drug administration
Arterial blood gas sampling
Pleural aspiration, chest drain insertion, lumbar puncture
Advanced
Airway management: intubation, ventilation
Advanced life support: defibrillation, cardiac pacing
Invasive monitoring: arterial cannulation, central venous cannulation
Intra-osseous access
After Nimmo and Shippey[10]

and behaviours such as team work, decision-making, handover and other elements of communication which are so important in the acute clinical setting (Figure 4).

Simulation training in CC may shift emphasis from the readily accessible (although undeniably important) learning of practical skills to those non-technical skills that are described as soft skills involving communication, team work, decision-making, and situation awareness. In reality they are harder to do, to learn, to teach and to evaluate than practical skills.[10,11]

These non-technical skills have been well defined in anaesthesia, CC and other disciplines[12,13] and these taxonomies include:

- Team working and behaviours.
- Situation awareness.
- Clinical decision-making.
- Preparation and planning.
- Communication.

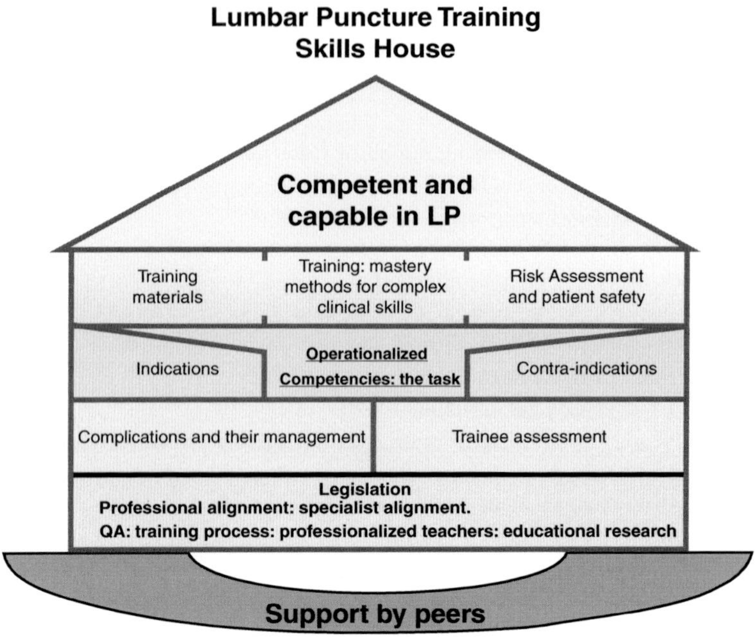

Figure 2. Developing a local clinical skills teaching package.

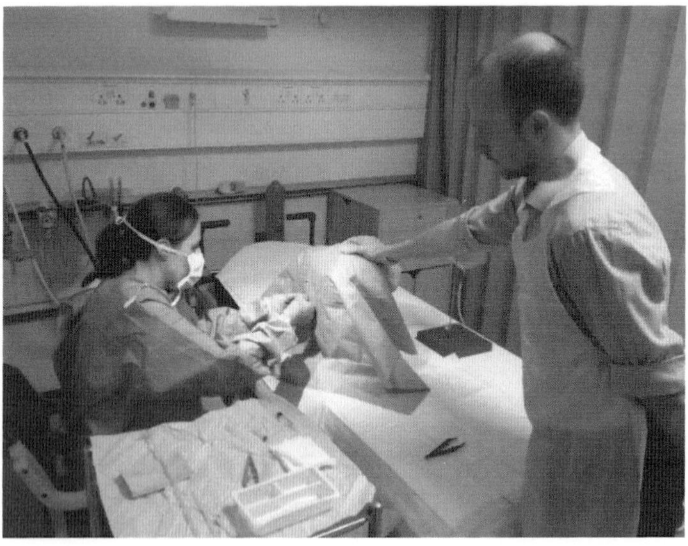

Figure 3. Lumbar puncture training in the clinical skills mastery program, South East Deanery, Scotland.

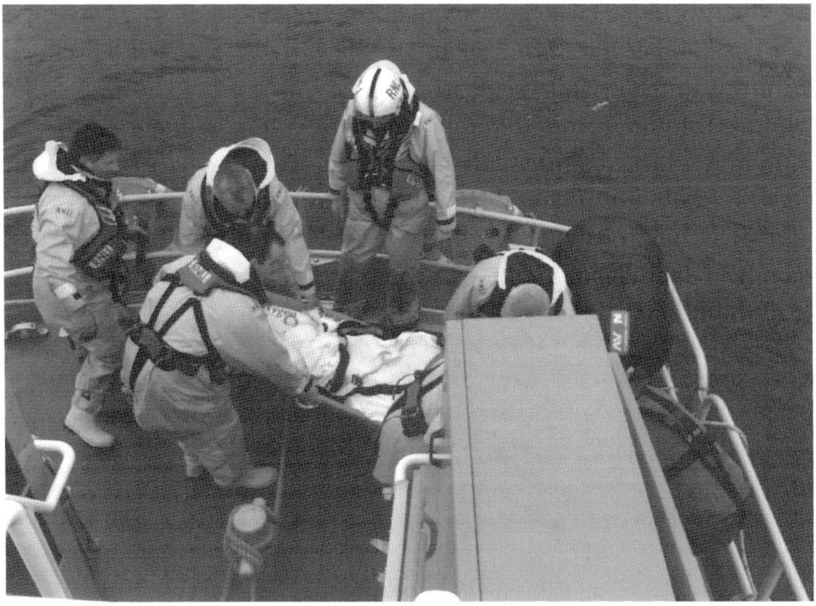

Figure 4. An example of *in situ* simulation (on a lifeboat).

It is increasingly recognized that high quality, safe, and effective CC is not only dependent on adequate knowledge and skill but on other factors such as communication, leadership, and followership, which can influence clinical outcome. These so-called non-technical skills are recognized as fundamental in the fields of patient safety, clinical error, and critical incident prevention. These skills (or the absence of them) can be observed very well in the simulated clinical environment, and with skilled debriefing the learner can appreciate and adopt changes in behaviour that have the potential to improve clinical outcomes. Simulation lends itself to the development of teaching and learning of these skills. Technical improvements in simulator technology have allowed more complex simulated conditions to be constructed and have facilitated the introduction of high fidelity simulation into ICM training. This has led to the development of *in situ* simulation within the clinical intensive environment. This ranges from fundamentals such as emergency airway management in the critically ill adult to the management of neonates, infants, and children who require extracorporeal membrane oxygenation.[14]

Some important ground rules for simulation

Define ***why*** you are going to teach using simulation (Table 4). It is a very powerful tool for learning (Table 5). Most of the time participants hope to learn from simulation, not to be assessed. A safe and constructive educational environment should be created.

Consider ***where*** you are going to use your simulator. This will allow you to decide what you will need in the way of space, and supporting equipment such as audio-visual recorders, projectors and computers. Does this equipment need to be portable?

Decide ***when*** you are going to do it: a simulated patient scenario may last an hour, but will take 10 times that to prepare. In order to sustain ongoing training this will need dedicated recurring time, preferably built into trainers' job plans. Finding the physical space to do this on a busy intensive care unit (ICU) may also be a great challenge.

Table 4. Why simulation?

- Repetition of practice.
- Allow 'safe' errors with support.
- Can stop and start.
- Unusual situations.
- Time for debriefing.
- Timing of acute presentations: planned events.
- Need to gain experience.
- Gap between knowledge and experience.

Table 5. Fundamentals of simulation.

Trainers and teachers.

- Designing scenarios and courses.
- Developing and delivering both.
- Facilitated debriefing.
- Following it up.
- Preparation.
- Action.
- Debriefing.
- Reflection and reflexion.

Get involved with your local, regional or national simulation centre. This should allow you to gain experience and expertise in all aspects of simulation. It will also allow you to develop simulation teaching networks to share ideas and materials, and will support you and your colleagues in educational professional development. Start small and build up.

More work is needed to clarify the impact of *in situ* clinical skills and simulation training on patient outcomes, and from a learner perspective, skill retention/decay, and the requirement for updates and refreshers.

Continuing professional development

The following is an extract from the General Medical Council (GMC) guidance on CPD[15] and relates to the areas which should be included:

"20. You must remain competent and up to date in all areas of your professional practice.

21. The content of your CPD is for you to determine in discussion with your appraiser. The resulting PDP will influence many of your learning objectives.

22. Our Good Medical Practice Framework for appraisal and revalidation provides a useful structure for discussing your CPD during appraisal. Your CPD activities should take account of the domains and attributes in the Framework. But you don't have to match your CPD against every element of the Framework. The domains are:

    a. Knowledge, skills, and performance,
    b. Safety and quality,
    c. Communication, partnership, and teamwork,
    d. Maintaining trust.

23. You should look for developmental opportunities across all four domains and not confine your learning to the areas of your practice in which you feel most comfortable.

24. Unless you have given us specific undertakings or had conditions attached to your registration as a result of involvement in our fitness to practise procedures we will not prescribe the CPD activities you should take part in.

25. However, from time to time, we will identify and publicize issues that we believe may be relevant to the CPD of all doctors or to particular groups of doctors. These issues might relate, for example, to particular developments in medical practice, to aspects of professionalism arising from our research and regulatory activities, or to relevant changes in the law. It will be up to you, in discussion with your appraiser, to decide whether those issues are relevant to your own practice and whether they should be addressed through your CPD".

These activities inform appraisal discussions. This is readily applicable to the professional development of nursing and other allied health professionals. In addition there are models for career progression and CPD in advanced practice which may be useful in identifying aspects of a healthcare professional's personal development plan.[16] This could include a number of activities which are engaged in parallel with clinical work such as:

- Research and audit.
- Quality improvement and patient safety.
- Teaching and education.
- Management and leadership.

Assessment

Examinations are set by Higher Education Institutions and by national bodies such as specialist societies, faculties, and colleges. In UK most professional medical examinations have been developed and run by the Medical Royal Colleges.

Workplace based assessments

A system that is applicable across the range of CC training and practice, and applicable to a wide range of professions, is that of workplace-based assessments (WPBAs). These can be incorporated into the everyday clinical routine, and have the validity of being grounded in real clinical practice (Table 6). Assessment by the direct observation of work is based

Table 6. Available assessment methods as set out in UK FICM curriculum.[1]

Assessment	Minimum No.
DOPS	8
ACAT	4
CBD	2
I-CEX	2
(MSF (including self-assessment exercise within specified domains)	1
Expanded Case Summary — 2,000 words max. (to standard of case presentation in departmental meeting)	1
Logbook Summary — demonstrating activities, patient involvement, practical procedures and critical incidents. *Note*: No patient identifiable material should be stored or presented.	1
Records of reflective practice — 500 words max.	2
Summary of all formal teaching sessions and courses attended	1

on the belief that an expert is able to make a judgment about the quality of an expert process by watching its progress. This is the methodology of the motor vehicle driving test and there is a long history of the use of observational assessment in the accreditation of practice.

A pragmatic approach to the choice of assessment methods can be adopted but direct observation of clinical practice, and focused discussion on real cases in real time are validated and are readily available tools.

ICM WPBAs are Mini Clinical Evaluation Exercise (CEX) (I-CEX), Directly Observed Procedural Skills (DOPS), Case-based Discussion (CBD) and Acute Care Clinical Assessment Tool (ACAT). These methodologies have a practical utility attested to by experience in their use and at least some objective evidence that if correctly applied they have validity and reliability. Multi-Source Feedback (MSF) is another well validated assessment tool for global performance, particularly in more complex areas such as team work. It is important that focused, formative verbal and written feedback is provided for each WPBA. WPBAs provide an opportunity for instantaneous, structured formative feedback to the trainee or learner.

MSF is an objective, systematic collection of feedback of performance data, using a structured questionnaire, on an individual ACCP trainee.

This is derived from a number of stakeholders in their performance and will typically include a mixture of healthcare professionals and possibly others.

Directly Observed Procedural Skills

Practical skills and capability are assessed in real-time with the assessor directly observing the clinician undertaking a practical procedure. Table 3 contains a list of these which is not exhaustive. Performance is assessed and feedback is provided.

Acute Care Assessment Tool

The ACAT is designed to assess the learners' capability in managing a body of work over an extended period of time such as a clinical shift. The assessment may focus on a number of non-technical skills such as prioritization and planning, task management, decision-making, and team work. In the CC environment this will usually be over a shift period and the assessment may focus on a variety of areas including record keeping, time management, team work, handover quality, and team leadership.

The Clinical Evaluation Exercise

This is used to assess a trainee's skill in real clinical encounters with patients. It involves the assessor directly observing a trainee in a real clinical situation such as the initial assessment and treatment of a patient with sepsis in the admissions unit. It is designed to assess a variety of skills such as history taking, examination, communication skills, and clinical judgement.

Case-based Discussion

CBD can be used for a variety of training and assessment purposes as indicated in the curriculum section of this document. It will often focus on patient management. CBD is also used for assessing both generic and clinical, knowledge and skills needed for effective practice, e.g.

evidence-based practice, maintaining safety, teamwork, clinical research methodologies.

Choosing Appropriate Assessment Instruments

In examining operational competencies, using the curriculum house approach, particular knowledge, skills, and behaviours are defined. From these the appropriate allocation of cognitive, psychomotor and behavioural learning outcomes to the specific WPBA instruments can be achieved. During a training program the learner will progressively build a portfolio of evidence to demonstrate that he or she has mastered the required competencies.

How many WPBAs and how do they fit into a training program?

The purpose of WPBAs is not to tick off each individual competence but through a process of supervised apprenticeship to provide a series of snapshots of work from the general features of which it can be inferred whether the trainee is making the necessary progress, not only in the specific work observed, but in related areas of the application of knowledge and skill. Given the inherent time restriction within a training program, a minimum number of WPBAs should be specified, but these numbers should be viewed as an absolute minimum. The actual number of observations of work required will depend on the individual trainee's progress and guidance from their supervisors; trainees should be encouraged to undertake as many WPBAs as they feel is needed to support their acquisition of competence.

It must be stressed that there is no single, valid, reliable test of competence and review of all the evidence, and triangulation of performance measured by different instruments, is required before drawing conclusions about a trainee's progress.

A note on observational assessments

Assessment by the direct observation of work is based on the belief that an expert is able to make a judgement about the quality of an expert process by watching its progress. This is the methodology of the motor vehicle driving test and there is a long history of the use of observational assessment in the accreditation of practice. WPBAs provide instantaneous feedback to the trainee.

Summary

Training and education are pivotal to the delivery of high quality CC.[17] An approach to the development of local or system wide education has been described and a number of educational tools and assessment strategies have been detailed. These approaches can also be applied to CPD and maybe important in underpinning revalidation and relicensing in professional practice.

References

1. Available at: www.bombayhospital.com/.
2. Available at: http://www.ficm.ac.uk/curriculum-and-assessment.
3. Available at: http://www.ficm.ac.uk/advanced-critical-care-practitioners-0.
4. Vicinus M and Nergaard B (1990). *Ever Yours, Florence Nightingale: Selected Letters.* Harvard University Press, Cambridge MA, 385–387.
5. Available at: www.cobatrice.org/.
6. Scheele F, Teunissen P and Van Luijk S (2008). Introducing competency-based postgraduate medical education in the Netherlands. *Med.Teacher*, 30, 248–253.
7. Available at: www.royalcollege.ca/canmeds/canmeds2015.
8. Available at: www.csmen.scot.nhs.uk/resources.aspx.
9. McGachie W, Issenberg S, Barsuk J and Wayne D (2014). A critical review of simulation based mastery learning with translational outcomes. *Med. Educ.*, 48, 375–385.
10. Nimmo G and Shippey B (2016). *Clinical Skills in Intensive Care.* Webb A, Angus D, Finfer S, Gattinoni L and Singer M. *Oxford Textbook of Critical Care*, 2nd Edition. Oxford University Press, Oxford.
11. Shippey B and Nimmo G (2016). *Simulation in Intensive Care.* Webb A, Angus D, Finfer S, Gattinoni L and Singer M. *Oxford Textbook of Critical Care*, 2nd Edition. Oxford University Press, Oxford.
12. Available at: www.abdn.ac.uk/iprc/ants/.
13. Reader T, Flin R, Lauche K and Cuthbertson B (2006). Non-technical skills in the intensive care unit. *Brit. J. Anaesth.*, 96, 551–559.

14. Nimmo GR, Wyllie G and Scarth J (2008). Critical events training for neonatal and paediatric extracorporeal membrane oxygenation. *J. Intens. Care Soc.*, 9(1), 20–22.
15. Available at: http://www.gmc-uk.org/education/continuing_professional_development/26745.asp.
16. Available at: www.advancedpractice.scot.nhs.uk.
17. Nimmo GR and Fox-Robichaud A (2007). Education and simulation techniques for improving reliability (QI) of care. *Curr. Opin. Crit. Care*, 13, 737–741.

Leadership and Organizational Development

Carlos Daniel Scheinkestel
Director Intensive Care & Hyperbaric Medicine, The Alfred Hospital Adjunct Clinical Professor, School of Public Health and Preventive Medicine, Monash University
Debby King-Rowley
Director Burlington Group, Melbourne, Australia

Key Points

1. The team must have direction and vision: it is hard to know how to get there if you do not know where you are going.
2. Build a superior team, in which the members trust one another, complement each other's strengths and compensate for each other's limitations, have common goals larger than the individual goals, and produce extraordinary results.
3. Break down the silos: the intensive care unit (ICU) must be well integrated and responsive to the needs of the hospital and aligned with organizational purpose, strategy, and business goals.
4. Attract, inspire, nurture diverse, and committed staff who are open-minded to new ideas and approaches and wish to continually improve, while ensuring that the expectations are clear and that each member of the team has responsibilities and is held accountable for them.

5. Create a culture of equity and transparency in workload, work conditions and finances, dealing with all issues, thoroughly, openly and promptly, without fear of tackling difficult issues and create an environment in which the challenges, rewards and the culture mean that people are motivated, enjoy coming to work and are enthused to target higher and higher levels of departmental achievement.

Introduction

In 2005, the Intensivists at the Alfred Hospital, Melbourne, some highly regarded and experienced, functioned as individuals in a silo within the broader organization.

While the ICU had pockets of prominence, as a department it lacked stature both within the organization and externally, and possessed no vision for the future. The pockets of achievement related to a few individuals rather than the department, which had few processes in place, and in which practice was inconsistent, budget overruns the norm, training and education average, and patient outcomes suboptimal. The Intensivists had little to do with each other, those achieving did not actively encourage the growth of the others and the ICU had little engagement with the rest of the organization and its input was rarely sought. The ICU doctors and nurses saw themselves as distinct entities, disconnected from the rest of the hospital, and this attitude was inculcated in the doctors and nurses in training.

Based on the team performance curve discussed by Katzenbach and Smith in The Wisdom of Teams,[1] the Intensivists were a classic example of a 'pseudo-team', i.e. a group for which there could be a significant, incremental performance need or opportunity, but they had not focused on collective performance and were not really trying to achieve it; they had no interest in shaping a common purpose or set of performance goals, even though they called themselves a team. Consequently, the ICU failed to achieve its tremendous potential and related poorly with the rest of the hospital.

The situation then, however, was not dissimilar to that still existing in many, if not most, ICUs today. Disappointingly, one of the main outcomes of a workforce summit held by the Australian New Zealand Intensive Care Society (ANZICS) and the College of Intensive Care Medicine (CICM) at the end of 2014 published in the Intensivist, the newsletter of ANZICS,[2] was an acceptance that "there should not be significant changes to the current role of an Intensivist". Strong views expressed at the summit, stated Intensivists should remain within the ICU, just care for critically ill patients, not high dependency unit (HDU) type patients, and resist roles outside of the ICU.

In our ICU, the situation was critical, as so much of the hospital's highly specialized patient case mix requires a high performing ICU. Approximately 30% of the Hospital's funding is associated with an ICU stay. In our hospital, a poorly performing ICU not only becomes the bottleneck for patient flow through the organization, but a financial liability.

In 2007, working as a group, the Intensivists set out to correct this pattern of behaviour and changed the situation through the implementation of numerous self-initiated targeted interventions. Most of these went against the trend of accepted practice in our region and we remain to be one of the very few ICUs in our region to have made such changes.

As a result of concerted and orchestrated effort, the ICU now functions as a cohesive team, delivering world's best practice and innovative and seamless patient care. It is well integrated with the hospital, and is now considered to be a pre-eminent department both within the hospital and in the wider medical community. It is an exemplar site of organizational development and management.

The transformation from where we were to where we are now is described as a practical approach to organizational change based on the interventions we used.

There is more than one way to achieve cultural change and organizational transformation. We are not suggesting that ours is the only way, nor that ours is the right way, but the way we have done things has worked well for us. Not everything may be applicable to other units, but we are sure some aspects of what we have done may be adopted or adapted and used elsewhere to benefit organizational development.

The Challenge

The challenge for us was to develop a highly motivated, skilled and engaged workforce of responsible and accountable professionals who would "*work together in an extraordinary way, as a "superior team", who would trust one another, complement each other's strengths and compensate for each other's limitations, who would have common goals that were larger than the individual goals, and who would produce extraordinary results*".[3]

To move from being a pseudo-team to becoming a superior team, a number of goals would have to be achieved, including:

- Developing effective communication skills, both within the team and with external parties, to improve professional relationships and breaking down the silos.
- Building bridges with the rest of the organization and alignment with organizational purpose, strategic, and business goals.
- Implementing processes to achieve the best possible patient outcomes.
- Establishing processes for managing and reporting on staff and financial performance.
- Enhancing our training and education in order for the ICU to become the premier place in Australia for Critical Care (CC).
- Elevating the ICU's research program so as to be recognized as an international centre of excellence in research, supporting a broad range of research activities.
- Growing a culture of quality improvement, continually improving performance by regular review of all aspects of service, changing strategies as required.

We wanted to be able to attract, inspire, and nurture diverse and committed staff who would be open-minded to new ideas and approaches and who wished to continually improve their skills and knowledge in an environment where the delivery of best practice, cost-effective, responsible CC, with wise management of human and material resources was the norm.

While leadership, direction, motivation and sometimes push were provided by the director, the Intensivists collaborated to meet the need for change and to develop strategies to achieve the goals. Collectively, the strategies are displayed graphically depicting groupings of specific interventions that the ICU implemented (Figure 1).

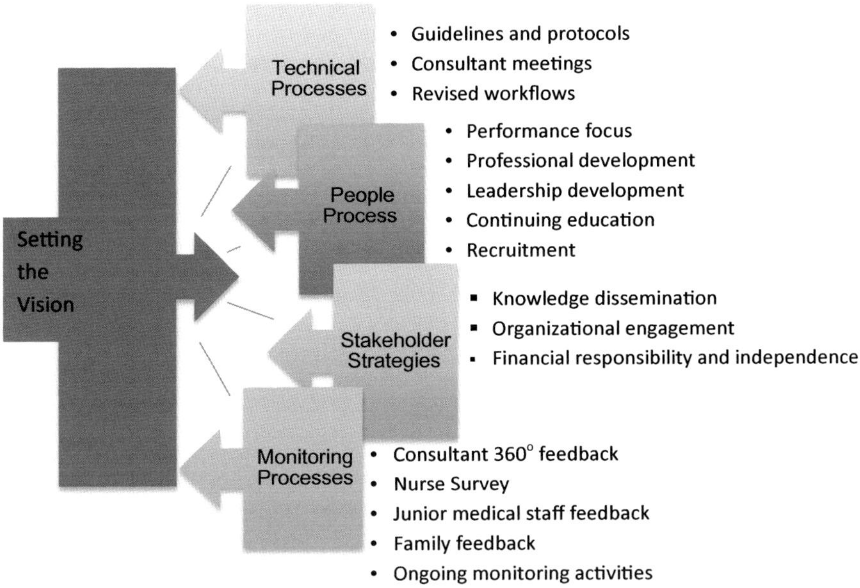
Technical Processes
• Guidelines and protocols
• Consultant meetings
• Revised workflows
People Process
• Performance focus
• Professional development
• Leadership development
• Continuing education
• Recruitment
Setting the Vision
Stakeholder Strategies
▪ Knowledge dissemination
▪ Organizational engagement
▪ Financial responsibility and independence
Monitoring Processes
• Consultant 360° feedback
• Nurse Survey
• Junior medical staff feedback
• Family feedback
• Ongoing monitoring activities

Figure 1. The Vision sets the stage and is the driving force for the interventions. The interventions' primary role is to contribute to the achievement of the vision. Information gathered through the formation and implementation of the interventions also serves to help update/morph the vision as needed.

The Vision

The first step in the transformation process was to set a vision for the Intensivists — one that would articulate an exciting, ennobling future image of the ICU and that would enlist others by appealing to shared aspirations.[4] While all staff needed to be part of the process, the Intensivists were targeted initially as they would have the biggest impact on cultural change in the department. Collectively, the Intensivists developed a mission statement to clearly articulate the ICU goals and aspirations (Figure 2).

After agreeing the vision, the Intensivists then systematically addressed the gaps, capitalizing on their individual strengths. Each Intensivist took on a portfolio, becoming responsible and accountable for progress in that area.

Demonstrating strong support for the vision, and wanting to ensure that the ICU remained at the leading edge with best but proven technology,

Figure 2. Alfred ICU mission statement.

Department of CC

Mission statement

As CC specialists, *our primary responsibility* is to provide safe, appropriate, high quality care and comfort to all Alfred patients with any form of critical illness and to support those that care for them.

- *Clinical care*: Our aim is to provide best possible patient outcomes through the practice of excellent, evidence-based, compassionate and consistent team-oriented intensive care medicine (ICM). In every situation, the wishes of the patient and the hopes of those around them will be balanced with the likelihood of success and suffering. Our practice will include dignified end-of-life care if treatment becomes futile.
- *Communication*: To keep our patients and their relatives well-informed. To communicate effectively with our colleagues and other hospital staff.
- *Support*: To build positive relationships within and outside our department. To support our colleagues in our clinical and academic pursuits so that we can attract, inspire, and nurture diverse and committed staff who wish to continually improve their skills and knowledge.
- *Teaching*: To facilitate critical care (CC) teaching of all CC and hospital staff. We wish the Alfred to be the premier place for CC training in Australia.
- *Research*: To maintain the Alfred CC as an international centre of excellence in research. To encourage and support a broad range of research activities. To present regularly at CC conferences nationally and internationally.
- *Management*: To deliver best-practice, cost-effective, responsible CC with the wise management of human and material resources.
- *Quality Assurance*: To continually improve our performance by regular review of all aspects of service so that we change our strategies if required. To set both long and short-term goals on an annual basis, which we strive to accomplish by working together.
- *Values*: To apply the following values to all aspects of our work: compassion, honesty, commitment, respect of personal beliefs and differences. To remain open-minded to new ideas and approaches.

the Intensivists committed to financially support the ICU, donating a percentage of private practice income back to the department, with specific criteria for expenditure. Having these funds available has enabled us to initiate and implement a wide range of interventions, moving us closer to achieving our vision and stretching us to think even further to the future.

Implementation of the Vision: The Interventions

The four categories of interventions that have helped us align with our vision span the technical side of our work as Intensivists, people processes that guide the selection and development of staff, stakeholder engagement strategies and ongoing monitoring to ensure a culture of continuous improvement.

Technical processes

Guidelines and protocols

Prioritizing delivery of best practice, quality clinical care with reduced mortality and morbidity, the team developed, audited and ensured compliance with evidence-based guidelines for the most common conditions and developed a number of critical checklists. Building on the resulting success of the initial sets of guidelines and protocols, the team has recently set elimination of unnecessary variation in clinical practice as a departmental objective.

Our clinical outcomes, not only standardized morbidity ratio (SMR) and adverse events but all our key performance indicators (KPIs) (hand hygiene, central-line associated bloodstream infection (CLABSI), Falls, pressure injuries, medication errors) are the subject of continuous scrutiny and our processes are regularly changing in order to achieve best outcomes.

Consultant meeting

Processes and systems of care were established to deal with all issues, thoroughly, openly and promptly, without fear of tackling difficult issues, to ensure problems did not recur, and that our practice was as good as possible. This required expansion of the weekly team meeting, not only to perform a detailed mortality and morbidity review, but to discuss any other issues. When required, Intensivists would voluntarily take accountability for an issue, draft solutions and present to the group for input and subsequent implementation. Initially these sessions were chaired by the director, but routinely, the senior members of the department now chair the meeting.

This meeting is prioritized above all others, with all Intensivists and the Nurse Manager participating, and senior trainees encouraged to attend. As a result the department is very dynamic, and continuous improvement characterizes the culture, resulting in the ICU nursing leadership referring to ICU as the Intensive Change Unit.

The dynamic nature of the Department unintentionally has become a disincentive for medical sabbaticals, since then on return to the Unit; the fact that so much has changed can be quite unsettling. We have dealt with this spin-off consequence by specifying that during sabbaticals, the Intensivists need to remain in regular contact with the department, receiving and reading minutes of the consultant meeting, and scheduling teleconferences to discuss major issues and inform the department of the progress of the sabbatical and the realization of the stated objectives.

Revised workflows

Careful analysis of workload was undertaken and roster changes introduced, matching workforce to workload to improve patient care. Previously, weekdays were covered on a day by day basis with the Intensivist on for the day also being on call for the night. As our funded beds and complexity of patients increased, this became a sub-optimal solution. With continuity of care a priority, days are now rostered in blocks of 7 and nights in blocks of 2 and 3. Weekdays can be split into blocks of 3 and 4 if required, but not less than that. Weekends were initially covered by 2 consultants, but we now have 5 consultants rostered on and a 6th for the night. The voluntary implementation of night shifts and increased consultant numbers on weekends provided extended hours of in-house consultant cover, while simultaneously improving work–life balance. We admit more patients between 6pm and 6am than we do between 6am and 6pm. Thus before the new workflows were introduced, being on call usually meant working all day, getting calls and frequently recalled during the night and having to work again the next day. With the new night shift, it means that the nights are distributed amongst the group and when you do nights, you do not do days, making both the days and nights much more tolerable.

On weekends we had reduced numbers of consultants but the workload was overwhelming and you needed several days to recover. With increased consultants on weekends, the workload is much more manageable and fatigue much less of a problem, thus also decreasing the risk for error.

In addition, we formally roster an additional Intensivist as back-up. As our workload with Extra Corporeal Membrane Oxygenation (ECMO) increased (Intensivists do the cannulation percutaneously) and we commenced ECMO retrievals, it became clear that the additional workload could not be absorbed by the existing rostered staff, so an additional member of the team is rostered to be available for these emergencies. This Intensivist is also available to step in to cover unscheduled leave or assist if workload becomes excessive. This addition to the roster was done without additional funding, at the expense of non-clinical time. The team considered it important to provide this resource in order to improve patient care but it has also improved conditions for the consultants.

This year as admissions increase further, the workload is again becoming a risk, and we have voluntarily split the department into four pods instead of three to manage the work better. This has in fact created an additional year of ward service, which has been absorbed by the group with only a small increase in consultant numbers.

These changes are seen by the group as improvements not only for patient care but for the Intensivists as individuals and were implemented voluntarily with no additional claims on the organization.

Similar roster changes were instituted for junior medical staff, while complying with "safe working hours".

Through these waves of change, the team fostered a culture of equity and transparency in workload, work conditions and finances with all private practice income being billed by a company and evenly distributed amongst the group.

People Processes

Performance focus

The team grew and benefited from dialogue on the concepts of responsibility and accountability, and through each team member taking responsibility and being accountable for specific portfolios. ICU restructured to focus on its key performance areas and main stakeholders by appointing five deputies heading up: trauma, general, cardiothoracic (our main patient groups), plus quality improvement and research and education.

Further restructuring occurred to ensure that all consultants worked a set minimum number of clinical days per annum. Those with minimal appointments were offered the choice of significantly increasing their commitment to the department or leaving, and those with larger fractional appointments but less than 0.66 EFT, were incrementally replaced by full timers.

The team established processes to continually evaluate and improve performance through regular review and feedback of all aspects of service. Utilizing strengths within the team, the consultants developed new models of care and new services, like ECMO retrievals from local and remote sites.

Sabbaticals were revamped to incorporate departmental input to ensure they fit in with departmental goals and needs.

With active participation of the team, a comprehensive annual 360° performance review for the Intensivists was devised (Table 1) and implemented. All junior medical staff, nursing leadership, peers, and more than 100 external consultants who have regular interaction with the ICU are asked to participate and provide feedback on all the ICU consultants. Usually, this means that between 80 and 100 people provide feedback on each consultant yearly. Clear expectations were set for levels of performance (initially top 33%, subsequently top 25%) with any deficiencies being actively managed and coached, both internally, and when required, by external non-medical consultants. As a last resort, if performance failed to improve to set standards, contracts were not renewed.

In this way, the Intensivists are able to continually improve performance, the external parties appreciate having their input sought (particularly because issues raised are always dealt with) and the interactions between ICU and the broader organization are further enhanced. Yearly team summaries are shown in Figure 3.

Professional development

The greatest factor in achieving organizational change is the ability to enthuse the group to target higher and higher levels of departmental

Table 1. Questionnaire for annual Intensivist 360° performance review.

If I needed ICU I would like to be managed by this consultant
Has a good knowledge base
Has a thorough and organized approach to patient management
Deals effectively with patient's relatives
Readily initiates direct communication and deals effectively with other consultants (inc. external units, departments) for complex patient management issues
Provides effective supervision of junior staff
Deals well with nursing staff
Builds effective working relationships and cooperation between work areas
Is readily approachable and available for advice or personal presence when required
Tackles the necessary issues even if difficult
Is effective at helping others to develop and achieve their potential
Has initiative is self-driven is proactive and solution focused
Is an effective teacher
Is productive and timely with non-clinical work
Is an asset to the unit
Is able to achieve objectives set for the department
Shows dedication and commitment to the unit
Embraces continuous improvement and cultural change
Demonstrates vision for the department
Is able to motivate others to achieve the objectives set for the department
Creates an environment that enables high performance from all, within the department
Has taken an active role within the hospital for the benefit of the ICU & or Hospital
Brings new ideas to the unit and is instrumental in implementing change
Seeks out opportunities for improvement and change

- Last six questions only apply to directors.
- Not every group gets the same questions — i.e. peers, external consultants, nursing leadership and junior medical staff, each get different combinations of the questions below

achievement. This is never easy, as it requires hard work, not only in the technical areas with which we are all familiar, but also in non-technical skills. Second to the desire to do this, is the ability and skill to achieve it, and key to this was to provide the tools and skill sets required, many of

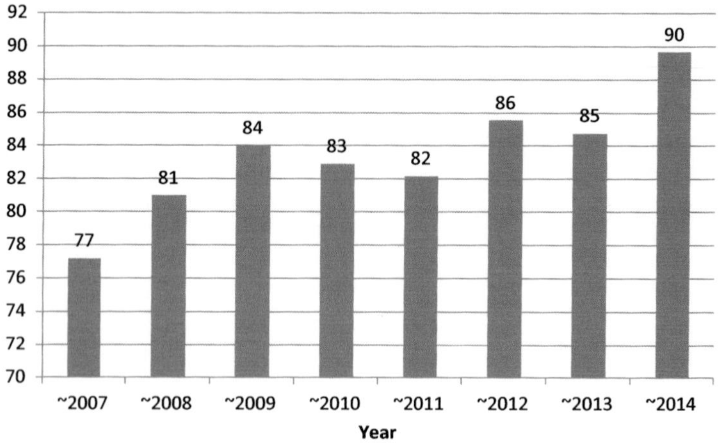

Figure 3. Team performance review results showing improvement over the years.

which were totally new to the group and not usually covered in either medical or specialist training.

As much if not more emphasis is placed on the department's continuing professional development as on the Individual's. An expert group of organizational change consultants were engaged and together we planned the team's annual development strategies which were delivered through a yearly series of workshops.

The foundations for the development work were laid through use of several assessment tools including the Myers–Briggs Personality Type Indicator (MBTI), the Thomas–Kilmann Conflict Mode Instrument (TKI) and the Belbin Team Roles. Based on the team's profiles, in the initial stages we focused on improved communication skills, managing egos, leveraging the diversity in the team and achieving sustainable excellence. We also acquired techniques to enhance leadership, manage change, deliver and receive feedback, and become proficient in systems thinking. As the team matured in our interactions, we delved into the deeper areas of immunity to change at a personal level, the make-up of individual value systems and their subconscious influence on behaviour patterns, and the role of the inner-critic in limiting our further development. This year, we spent time on the concept of "the Intensivist plus", complex-adaptive systems and business concepts such as why some organizations flourish while others succumb.

With a successful development program underway for the Intensivists, a program was developed to benefit the senior doctors in training, targeting clinical leadership, mentoring, coaching, teamwork, and negotiation skills. This was combined with the expansion of their role to include a rotation through the "hospital clinical lead" an innovative new role in the restructure of the hospital at night, independent of the ICU.

A similar program was then set up for the nursing leadership group, centred on communication skills, giving and receiving feedback, leadership, conflict management and responsibility and accountability.

Embedding of skills learnt in the various workshop series was supported through the development of formalized Mentoring and Coaching relationships for:

- deputy directors with newly appointed consultants.
- all consultants and senior trainees.
- senior trainees and junior trainees.
- senior associate nurse managers and new associate nurse managers.
- senior nurses and newly employed nurses.

These relationships provide guidance to the medical and nursing staff as they move into new roles, ensuring clarity of expectations and support in meeting those expectations.

The team work between Nurses and doctors was further aided by simulation sessions, both planned and impromptu to improve technical competence but more importantly to enhance non-technical skills, including teamwork, decision making, and operational performance.

Leadership development

More recently, all of the directors undertook further development based on insights from assessments using the Leadership Circle, a 360° assessment that differs from others as it measures not only leadership competencies but also the inner assumptions that drive behaviour. The assessment was used to inform them on what they are doing, why they are doing it, and key opportunities for development. Through a series of 6 sessions of 1-to-1 intensive coaching, the directors were able to identify simple things of which they were not previously aware, and now with focus, they are making visible differences that are enhancing effectiveness in their leadership capabilities and impact.

Two of the deputies have also undertaken further university studies achieving "Professional Certificates in Health Systems Management", through a formal degree program offered by the University of Melbourne in partnership with the Victorian Department of Health Redesigning Hospital Care Program.

Continuing education

All Intensivists have formal ICU qualifications, and some have secondary specialties including physician, anaesthetist and emergency medicine. Formal subspecialty qualifications include renal, respiratory, clinical pharmacology, toxicology, cardiology, and infectious diseases. They all have academic appointments with Monash University.

While maintaining high levels of multi-skilling, which are required on night shifts when the consultants must be able to competently handle all types of patients, as part of the motivation for working in the ICU, all consultants are encouraged to develop further skills in areas of interest to them.

The diversity enhances the overall performance of the team, and is evident in areas of their pursuit over the past few years. Nine consultants have formal qualifications in echocardiography, two have university qualifications in education, one in clinical ultrasound, one has a masters of biostatistics, five have qualifications in clinical simulation, one a Master's degree in public health and nine are Advanced Life Support (ALS) instructors.

New skills currently being acquired by the team include Information Technology, Social Media, Lean Thinking, and Six Sigma.

Recruitment

According to change guru, John Kotter,[5] one of the keys for consolidating improvements in organizational change is to recruit people who can implement the vision. In keeping with this principle and building on the commitment to work as a team to achieve the vision, recruitment of new Intensivists was retargeted. Candidates were screened looking for the specific skillsets required to achieve the vision concentrating on identified gaps in the existing team, and building on those already present that were critical for our development. In addition, an articulated hiring criterion was generated around enthusiasm to work in a high performing team and to assist goal achievement.

Therefore, some of the usual interview questions were discarded in favor of those probing cultural fit and ability to function well in a team environment. This took a little adjusting for those non-Intensivists on the interview panels.

Stakeholder Strategies

Knowledge dissemination: education and courses

We started off by completely revamping our in-house education program. We increasingly introduced simulation and developed a blog,[6] an online education and knowledge translation resource to deal with staff on nights, leave, or too busy to attend. The blog is linked to our pre-existing website[7] and available 24/7. Although initially set up for local purposes, the blog's audience is now more than two thirds from overseas, from more than 130 countries, and receives an average of 1,000 hits per week.

Having markedly improved on our mortality and all our key KPIs, being stimulated by the interest shown on our activities and having refined our teaching techniques internally, it was incumbent on us now to share our knowledge with the wider ICU community.

Starting off with just a few, we developed external courses that have now grown to more than 30 individual events per annum. These courses also serve as an impetus for our Intensivists teaching the courses to stay up to date and at the cutting edge of their area of subspecialty and as a result, they are much better clinicians. In order to run the courses, the Intensivists need to work with each other and this further improves team dynamics and performance within the unit. Another spin-off benefit has been the funds generated for the department, which are 100% allocated to research, education, projects, and equipment for the ICU.

From a medical point of view, many of these courses are not restricted to ICU, and are appropriate for other disciplines, thus enhancing further our stakeholder interactions.

There is a clear understanding among the Intensivists of the importance of this aspect of our non-clinical work and of the expectation that all Intensivists will participate and assist. Each course undergoes a formal evaluation on completion and our scores are consistently in the high 80s or higher. As a result, our "branding" is enhanced and we are able to further establish our ICU and the hospital as a centre of excellence in education, research and patient care.

Organizational engagement

Clear expectations were set for the team and individuals with regard to engagement in Hospital activities, involvement with other hospital departments, and participation in internal and external committees.

This has enabled the ICU to become an active partner in achieving hospital-wide goals, which previously were viewed as secondary to the priorities of the department. The silo mentality of the team was diminished, enabling ICU to attain common goals across a wider stakeholder group.

Currently the members of the ICU team sit on 30 internal hospital committees and 67 external committees. This effectively means that we have situational awareness, are actively involved and aware of all plans and activities involving or potentially involving ICU and are able to influence them, and pro-actively position the Unit to maximize opportunities as they arise.

Further, this level of organizational engagement means that the ICU can provide seamless patient care across the organization. Some examples to give context to this include:

1. The "hospital at night", an initiative in which the ICU has taken a key role. The "Clinical Lead", the most senior junior medical role in the hospital at night, responsible for the team work, work-load levelling amongst the junior staff, supervision, teaching, etc. on nights, was given to the ICU senior registrars in addition to their ICU duties. The ICU has built a training course to develop the skills required for this position including leadership, mentoring, negotiation skills, prioritization, etc.

2. The ICU has for years operated at >100% occupancy. The pressure for ICU beds is high and patients are discharged to the wards, often as soon as no longer requiring inotropes or invasive ventilation. This, together with the Hospital's particular case mix, contributes to very high patient acuity in the hospital wards. So the ICU set up an additional team, with no internal responsibilities in ICU, but solely to deal with "external to ICU" issues. These include: a review of all ICU discharges within 24 hours of discharge and continued review as required, attendance at all trauma calls for major trauma arriving to the Emergency Department (ED), attendance at all Medical Emergency team (MET) calls, etc. This has resulted in a high ICU presence throughout the hospital, facilitating new referrals to the ICU, and increasing the interactions with other hospital departments, further breaking down silos. This team consists of an ICU consultant, senior registrar and ICU liaison nurse during the day, and a separate senior registrar overnight liaising with the in-house ICU night Consultant. This has almost certainly contributed to this ICU having different patient survival to Australian and New Zealand ICUs for out of hours discharges. Our mortality is about 2% for both in and out of hours, whereas Australian New Zealand data shows a 78% increase in mortality from 3.6% for in hours to 6.4% for out of hours ICU discharges.[8]
3. In Australia, we have a KPI that requires patients presenting to the ED to be either admitted or discharged within 4 hours. There are financial consequences to not meeting this target. Historically, less than 50% of ICU admissions from the ED were within this target. The ICU proactively worked with the ED to rectify this problem, implementing a number of actions. These included a "Rapid ICU Admission Team" (RIAT) round at 9.30 pm every evening, led by the night ICU consultant, to assess any critically ill patients in the ED and expedite their admission. Our four hour KPI now consistently sits above 75%, leading to positive results for the patients and the hospital.

Financial responsibility and independence

A rigorous approach to hospital funding has meant that, while not able to control who presents and with what problems, we have been able to accommodate an increasing number of patients, with not only an increasing number of beds (36% in 8 years) but more importantly, with an increased efficiency, admitting more patients per bed per annum (27% in 8 years) and remain within budget.

Much of the latter has been due to improved practices and processes and has meant that we have eliminated cancellation of elective surgery due to lack of ICU bed availability, decreased after-hours discharges, eliminated premature discharges and inter-hospital transfers due to lack of ICU bed availability. It also meant that patients previously unable to be admitted to ICU, such as those with oesophagectomies, hemi-hepatectomies, Whipple's and complex vascular surgery, can now be admitted.

On the nursing front, we have become more fiscally viable through implementation of several changes. We have eliminated the expensive use of agency staff from a peak of 18 EFT per month. We have eliminated expensive rostering such as double shifts and reduced our overtime from more than 300 hours per week to less than 25 hours per week. We have also reduced our leave liability from more than 10,000 hours to less than 750. This has been viewed very positively by the hospital as they seek to work within budget constraints. Subsequently, the ICU nurse manager is being accessed as a resource within the hospital to promulgate the ICU success with other units.

A similar rigorous approach to our consumables budget, eliminating unnecessary variation, has resulted in major savings for the unit, and therefore the hospital.

Access to soft monies together with the profits generated from the courses, has allowed the purchase of the latest technologies that may not otherwise have been affordable.

Monitoring processes

We actively seek feedback from all staff. For the ICU team to achieve optimum performance, giving and receiving feedback must become spontaneous, a matter of routine and part of the culture.

In addition to the consultant yearly 360° reviews, at the end of each rotation we seek feedback from all the junior medical staff using the NASA task load index (Figure 4).

	Role	Date

For all questions, place a X on the vertical line that best represents your response.

1. Mental Demand How mentally demanding is your workload in ICU?

Very low Very high

2. Physical Demand How physically demanding is your workload in ICU?

Very low Very high

3. Temporal Demand How hurried or rushed is the pace of your work in ICU?

Very low Very high

4. Performance How successful were you in accomplishing the work you were required to do?

Perfect Failure

5. Effort How hard did you have to work to accomplish your level of performance?

Very low Very high

6. Frustration How insecure, discouraged, irritated, stressed and annoyed were you?

Very low Very high

7. Education Did you learn a lot in ICU, was your term here worthwhile?

Very low Very high

8. Enjoyment Did you enjoy your ICU term?

Very low Very high

9. Recommendation Would you recommend others to do an ICU term here?

Very low Very high

10. Any comments?

Figure 4. NASA task load index.

Additionally, all nursing staff (>400) are invited yearly to participate in a questionnaire from which key issues affecting nursing morale, retention and well-being are identified, strategies developed and implemented to address these.

It was from feedback in these surveys that we developed the program for the advancement of the nursing leadership team. Survey feedback also led to the nursing teams being restructured and rosters and patient allocation reworked.

Annual surveys ensure key issues continue to be addressed and teamwork and communication improved within the Department.

To close the loop on feedback, mechanisms were developed (posters, e-mail, rumour file, quality report, website, blog, meetings, screensavers) to provide staff with feedback on clinical and financial unit performance, KPIs, and updates on achievements and other "good news". Our achievements are also communicated to the wider organization for other areas to replicate where applicable.

We also obtain regular feedback from the families of our critically ill patients via the iPad app available in the reception area which averages more than 1,500 screen views per day. The app has enabled great improvements in our communication with families and hence they are now consistently scoring us as very good/excellent, 98% of the time.

Performance in all aspects of our work is continuously monitored to ensure that our improvements are sustained, and any new issues arising are identified early and targeted for improvement.

The situational awareness of the ICU, fed by the multiple interactions within and external to the hospital arising from the Intensivists involvement in committees, sabbaticals and overseas meetings is routinely discussed at the consultant meetings and assists and guides the future activities and efforts of the group.

An enormous amount of hard work has gone into achieving our excellent patient outcomes and premiere position amongst ICUs. We are proud of our achievements and the team is clear that, the work is not over — we must continuously be improving our performance.

The turn-around was not fast. It took eight years, but now we are "reaping the rewards".[9]

The Future

One of the ICU consultants recently commented that having reached the top of the hill, there was only one way to go: down. I say having gotten to the top of the hill, we now look for a mountain.

References

1. Katzenbach JR and Smith DK (2006). *The Wisdom of Teams, Creating a High-Performance Organization.* Harper Collins, New York.
2. The Intensivist: ANZICS December 2014.
3. Senge PM, Roberts C and Ross RB (1998). *The Fifth Discipline Field book, Strategies for Building a Learning Organization.* Bantam Doubleday Dell Publishing Group, New York.
4. Kouzes JM and Posner BZ (2012). *The Leadership Challenge, How to Make Extraordinary Things Happen in Organizations*, 5th Edition. Jossey-Bass, San Francisco, CA.
5. Kotter J (2012). *Leading Change.* HBR Press, Boston, MA.
6. Available at: http://intensiveblog.com (2014) (Accessed 28 July 2015).
7. Available at: http://www.alfredicu.org.au (2010) (Accessed 21 July 2015).
8. Gantner D, Farley K and Bailey M (2014). Mortality related to after-hours discharge from intensive care in Australia and New Zealand, 2005–2012. *Intens. Care Med.*, 40, 1528–1535.
9. Available at: http://www.alfredicu.org.au/about/awards-and-accomplishments/.

Part III

Decision-Making and Communication

Ethics

Thomas Woodcock
Clinical Ethics and Law at Southampton, University of Southampton

Key Points

1. Awareness of the many ethical issues in critical care (CC) is essential for all practitioners.
2. The ability to conduct an ethics consultation is a skill that can often avoid legal intervention.
3. CC patients are often too ill to exercise their own will or judgment about their treatment or research participation.
4. CC gives practitioners the ability to sustain the body's metabolic processes even after recovery to independent existence has become impossible. This has led to the need to redefine death and futility.
5. Pandemics have created the need to allocate relatively scarce CC beds to dying patients with much discussion about the ethics of choosing one patient over another.

Making Difficult Choices

What ought I to do? It used to be enough to recall what we previously did in a similar situation, or what we had seen respected colleagues do. Such case-based reasoning (casuistry) is probably the way most non-contentious ethical choices are made in modern practice. Philosophers, ethicists and politicians have taken a keen interest in medical ethics in recent years and there is an increasing volume of professional standards, guidelines, national laws and Human Rights legislation attempting to tell us what we must do. Even so, there remain enough hard cases to which we apply a system of reasoning that we trust to be fair, objective, and consistent. We have to be aware some of the ethical strategies that decision-makers can apply.

Moral reasoning

Consider the following scenario:

You have only 5g of resuscitol left, and you are about to administer it to Mr. A to save his life when nurse Goody points out that there are five other patients on the ward whose lives you could save by giving them 1g of resuscitol each. Mr. A's condition is such that 1g would not save him. Will you still give the 5g to Mr. A, or will you give it to five other patients instead?

Functional magnetic resonance imaging studies have provided remarkable images of moral reasoning in biological action.[1] Emotion-related brain regions are engaged when we contemplate abhorrent actions, but regions associated with abstract reasoning and cognitive control (including dorsolateral prefrontal cortex, and anterior cingulate cortex) are recruited to resolve difficult personal moral dilemmas in which utilitarian values require "personal" moral violations. Harvard psychologist Joshua Greene calls this the dual process theory; that moral judgment is influenced by both automatic emotional responses and controlled, conscious reasoning. The scenario above is a variant of the "Trolley problem" proposed by Phillippa Foot in 1967 and used by Greene.[1]

Principlism: A Dominant Approach in Western Moral Philosophy

The Belmont Report[2] was commissioned by the National Commission for the Protection of Human Subjects of Biomedical and Behavioural Research to identify core bioethical principles in the wake of the Tuskegee syphilis experiments. The three principles that emerged were respect for the individual, beneficence and justice. A series of bioethics commissions came and went, leading to Barak Obama's current Presidential Commission for the Study of Bioethical issues. The Kennedy Institute of Ethics, founded in 1971 at Georgetown University, Washington, is one of the older academic ethics centres in the USA. In UK, the Nuffield Council on Bioethics was established in 1991 as an independent body to examine and report on ethical issues in biology and medicine. The World Health Organization maintains a list of National Ethics Committees.

The most commonly quoted set of modern ethical principles is that enumerated by Beauchamp and Childress of Georgetown University in the USA. To the Belmont Report principles of respect for the individual's autonomy, beneficence and justice, they added non-maleficence, which reminds us of the axiom *primum non nocere* (first do no harm). They are so widely quoted, they have been referred to as the Georgetown Mantra. There are other principlist ethicists, other text books, and other sets of principles. The particular emphasis on respect for autonomy, or the right to self-determination, is characteristic of modern (Western Educated Industrial Rich and Democratic (WEIRD) morality. In the WEIRD view, patients are often thought of as consumers.

Pluralism

It is said that respect for the family and the community are generally valued more highly than individual and consumer rights by traditional 'Eastern' cultures. Feminists have claimed that women's values are inadequately addressed by standard ethical approaches, and that women would give greater weight to caring, empathy and the preservation of relationships than male ethicists do. The ethics of justice is thereby challenged by the ethics of care. Faiths and laws tend to embrace rules about the sanctity of life, or at least of human life. The ethics to be applied in any clinical situation will therefore depend upon the religious and moral convictions of the patient and his healthcare professionals, and the culture of the institution in which care is delivered.

Structuring the Problem; Quadrants

Any ethical analysis must proceed from factual analysis, and the four quadrants approach is one useful model. In quadrant 1 we write the clinical facts such as diagnosis, treatment options, and prognosis. Quadrant 2 looks at the patient's position; if she has capacity, is she adequately informed and is her choice freely made? If she lacks capacity, what do we know of her expressed wishes or her values? Quadrant 3 examines the patient's quality of life in terms of her mental, physical and social welfare. Finally, an eclectic mix of contextual influences and ethical perspectives are considered in Quadrant 4; the views and preferences of the patient's friends and family, the possible prejudices and biases of the patients medical advisers and care providers, cultural and religious convictions and institutional traditions may all be relevant.

Keeping the Dialogue Open

Disagreement about the right thing to do eventually leads to break-down in communication and may precipitate recourse to law. Try to provide information to the patient and family in a way that maximizes their understanding of the diagnosis, treatment, and prognosis. Different information providers should take care to avoid giving an impression of disagreement between treating professionals. In tragic circumstances, engage supportive agencies such as spiritual care, social work and religious, or cultural leaders from the family's community. Offer a more formal ethics consultation mediated by a third party where doubts persist. The family may feel the institutions employees are united against them, in which case they should be provided with an opportunity to seek a second/independent opinion and the family should be provided access to the patient's health record to facilitate this process. Failure to notify a patient or family of a treatment limitation decision denies them the opportunity to get second opinions and has been confirmed to be a breach of their Article 8 Human Rights in Europe. If all these avenues are exhausted, the family should be provided with reasonable notice of the intention to treat (or withdraw treatment) unless a court application is brought to prevent it. Where patient capacity is impaired or in doubt, there may be a specific legal pathway such as the Court of Protection in England, and the

Consent and Capacity Board (CCB) in Ontario. If no such application is made, the care team should continue to engage the family in the process and provide support.

Teaching ethical practice

Given the extreme sensitivity of critical care (CC) ethics and communication it makes sense to use simulated situations for teaching and improving the necessary skills.

Issues of Consent

Article 8 of the European Convention of Human Rights requires national laws to protect every person's right to private and family life,[3] while Article 9 of the Oviedo Convention (on Human Rights and Biomedicine) covers the situation in which a patient is no longer able to express his or her will.[4] It stipulates that the previously expressed wishes relating to a medical intervention by a patient who is not, at the time of the intervention, in a state to express his or her wishes "shall be taken into account".

Non-voluntary treatment in an emergency; necessity to treat

The legal purpose of consent is to protect the practitioner from a criminal charge of trespass. The words of Justice Cardozo in a New York State Judgment of 1914 (Cardozo's Dictum) have become classic; "Every human being of adult years and sound mind has the right to determine what shall be done with his own body; and a surgeon who performs an operation without his patient's consent commits an assault, for which he is liable in damages".[5] Morality and the law quite properly make exceptions for emergency medical treatment which can be justified as 'necessary' to restore and preserve his health and well-being when consent cannot be obtained. In fact, we can go further and say that we have ethical and legal duties to administer such treatments in an emergency as we have good reason to believe they are necessary to the patient's eventual recovery. Necessity is not, however, a defence against treating a patient in defiance of an expressed refusal.

Refusal of treatment

Logically, the right to consent to treatment means nothing if the patient may not also refuse treatment. In practice we rarely question a patient's ability to consent, but when the patient refuses a treatment which the doctor sees as important to the preservation of life and health, her consideration will turn to whether the patient is of sound mind. The responsibility for deciding whether a patient is competent to decide lies with a medical practitioner.

Decision-making capacity

Justice Cardozo mentioned 'sound mind'. What do we mean by that today? Across the western world, people who have reached the age of 'majority' are presumed to have the capacity to give or withhold their consent to proposed medical treatment, but this presumption may sometimes be rebutted. When a practitioner has reason to doubt a person's decision-making capacity she should determine whether the person understands and remembers the information he is given about the treatment, and has the ability to weigh the information before making a free choice. Importantly, the practitioner should not decide the patient lacks capacity merely on the grounds that he has a psychiatric illness, is receiving drugs that affect the mind, is mentally distressed, has previously changed his mind, or that the choice he makes is illogical or self-harming. Psychiatrists are regarded as the most expert medical specialists for the ultimate determination of capacity.

Involuntary treatment

When a competent person refuses appropriate medical treatment it would normally be unethical and illegal to administer treatment 'involuntarily'. The law typically makes provision for involuntary medical treatment of mental illnesses that cause inappropriate or dangerous behaviour and, in very rare cases, involuntary hospitalization for patients with contagious disease.

Advance directives (living wills)

It is estimated only a tiny minority of the Council of Europe's 800 million citizens actually have advance directives, living wills and/or continuing powers of attorney — making it difficult, if not impossible, to take their previously expressed wishes into account. The Council of Europe passed Resolution 1859 in 2012 "Protecting human rights and dignity by taking into account previously expressed wishes of patients",[6] to be adopted into National laws. Advance directives, living wills and/or powers of attorney should be promoted. They should be made in writing and be registered, ideally in State registries. They should be respected when they are valid and applicable; prior instructions which are contrary to the law or good medical practice will not be followed. Complicated forms or expensive formalities should be avoided so that people will not be deterred from registering their Directives. They should be encouraged to review their advance directives, living wills and/or continuing powers of attorney at regular intervals to ensure they are up-to-date, and should be able to revoke and/or change them at any time. A system of supervision should be established under which a competent authority is empowered to investigate and, if necessary, intervene, in particular in cases in which an attorney is not acting in accordance with the continuing power of attorney or in the interests of the granter. Surrogate decisions under power of attorney that rely on general rather than personal value judgements should not be admissible and, in case of doubt, the decision must always be pro-life and the prolongation of life.

Life sacrificing directives made by adults on behalf of children are not likely to be accepted by a court which must be responsible for the child's welfare. Though older children may sometimes be empowered to give consent to treatment, it would be rare to allow a minor to refuse lifesaving transfusion.

Non-voluntary treatment for the adult who lacks decision-making capacity

There are essentially two approaches. The first (common in North America) is to identify a proxy or surrogate to give consent on behalf of the patient. The proxy will be someone who was named in the patient's advance directive, or someone who knows the patient and will be expected to exercise a 'substituted judgment', that is, to decide as he believes the patient would decide if he had the capacity. The second (common in England) is to treat in the patient's 'best interests'. The family of the patient are not excluded from this process, as their views as to what they believe the patient would have wanted should be considered by the doctor before he decides. An advance directive might assist the doctor in deciding what the patient would have wanted, and in identifying somebody who will best represent the patient's wishes. Where consensus of the parties cannot be reached a Court can exercise its power to identify a proxy decision-maker or to make a decision on behalf of a patient with incapacity according to the law of the country. Caution must always be exercised that identified surrogates are truly representing the patient's values and likely judgment.

Decision-making; children

For children there is a presumption that the ability to consent to treatment will lie with the parents, and especially with the mother. In the case of parents, it is widely expected that parents should regard themselves as having a duty to act in their child's best interests rather than see themselves as having rights over the child. When a parent appears to be acting other than in the child's best interests (for instance, by refusing medical advice), a Court can be asked to consider the child's welfare. In America, parental authority will usually remain with the parents unless what they decide would be clearly abusive or neglectful of the child. In England, when parental choice is questioned, a Court will weigh best interests and choose for the child the best of the available choices.

Older children have the intellectual maturity to take less weighty decisions for themselves even though they are still minors. Law tends to allow that minors may consent to certain medical treatments, but may be less keen to allow a minor to refuse recommended medical treatment.

The unborn child; treating a pregnant woman

Many people would instinctively say that in the body of the pregnant woman there are two lives whose preservation and interests are to be considered.

AC was just a day or two from death, and carrying a 27 week pregnancy. She was offered a Caesarean Section, which would give her viable fetus a 50:50 chance of survival. She refused, so the Hospital Authority petitioned a judge for declaratory relief. On the judge's order, the Caesarean section was performed against AC's wishes. Her daughter died within a few hours of delivery, and AC died the following day.

Since the tragic case of AC[7] courts have usually refused to accept that the right to self-determination of a woman is in any way compromised by the existence of a pregnancy. A competent woman may refuse any treatments, including those intended for the protection or safe delivery of her fetus. But what if a pregnant patient who comes to the Intensive Care Unit (ICU) is unable to make decisions about treatment? Where there is no reason to believe that the woman would not wish to have her fetus preserved and protected, you may reasonably judge that you would be acting in her best interests to undertake such reasonable interventions as are needed to achieve that end. However, where there is a serious conflict between the interests of the patient and the interests of her fetus, the laws of most countries in the world require that the interests of the patient must be put first. Ireland is a notable European exception. In December 2014 doctors asked a High Court to rule on the case of a brain-dead woman carrying a fetus of 15 weeks gestation. On the facts they found that the prospect for the fetus was "nothing but distress and death" and that to continue life support would be to impose" unimaginable distress in a futile exercise" on her family.

Clinical Research

Patients are benefitting from the knowledge gained by large randomized controlled trials such as the Acute Respiratory Distress Syndrome Network (ARDSNET) program, but they have attracted ethical scrutiny and criticism, especially on the question of consent to participate.[8] In 2008 the Food and Drug Administration of the United States of America formally rejected the World Health Organization's Declaration of Helsinki, and it has largely been replaced by Good Clinical Practice (GCP), an international quality standard written by the International Conference on Harmonisation (ICH) from which national authorities can now formulate national regulations for clinical research, including involuntary research.

The essence of research is that the subject cannot be presumed to benefit from his involvement, and is used for the purpose of gaining information for scientific curiosity. Though there is an undoubted public interest in the advancement of science, the subject is being altruistic if he consents to participate. On this basis Nuremberg principles demand that informed consent precedes research participation. Critically ill patients are almost by definition lacking the capacity to make a choice, so how then can we ever conduct experiments in critical illnesses? The most obvious device is to seek and obtain consent from a proxy or surrogate decision-maker recognized by national law, but evidence suggests that proxies don't always choose as the subject would. Even in the UK, where proxy 'consent' has no legal standing, this method may be approved by ethical review boards.

Obtaining consent from a patient or surrogate when emotions are running high and time is short is obviously difficult. Researchers in France found that most consent-givers had 'therapeutic misconceptions' about the nature of the research they had consented to, most importantly failing to grasp the purpose of randomization. The more acute and severe the disease process under investigation, the higher was the incidence of therapeutic misconception.[9]

Retrospective criticism of the consent process for critically ill children and adults risks the reputations of researchers and the public confidence in clinicians. An ethically approved randomized controlled trial of tidal volume in ventilated adults was stopped after 861 patients had been recruited because of high mortality in the 12 mL/kg control group. Critics pointed out that the true standard of care at the time was to use 10 mL/kg and so the information on which consent was given was misleading.[10] An ethically approved randomized controlled trial of oxygen therapy that enrolled 1,300 babies was published in the New England Journal of Medicine in 2010. In 2013 the Office for Human Research Protections (OHRP) of the US Department of Health and Human Services determined that the Informed Consent documents had failed to adequately explain to parents the reasonably foreseeable risks of death.[11]

For some research, such as 'cardiac arrest' therapies, there is no time to obtain any kind of consent. In such cases Ethical Review Boards may grant a waiver of consent. One way to make such research more acceptable is offer community consultation exercises and to make available wristbands which identify the wearer as someone who consents or refuses.

Goals of Treatment at the End of Life

Preserving life

It is important not to make assumptions about the wishes of the severely disabled, dying patient at the end of life. To do so one may give insufficient weight to the importance of preserving life while attributing too little worth to the comfort, contentment, and dignity that can be experienced even in a limited existence.

Futility; the appropriateness and advisability of treatment

Futile treatment should not be offered to a patient.[12] But is a treatment with only a slim chance of effectiveness also futile? What of a treatment that is effective in prolonging life but is otherwise considered non-beneficial and therefore inappropriate? Some clarification came to English law through the case of Aintree v James in 2013.[13] Critical Care (CC) life support was deemed to be "overly burdensome" for a patient with "no prospect of recovering such a state of health as will avert the looming prospect of death if the life-sustaining treatment is given." Appeal to futility may be less successful in USA and Canada. In Canada in 2013, the Supreme Court ruled in Cuthbertson v Rasouli that withdrawal of life-sustaining treatment will only be lawful with the consent of the patient or his surrogate decision-maker; 'Rasouli Consent'.[14] The physicians' objection that such a principle undermines the professional clinical obligation to provide only those treatments that are effective and beneficial was rejected. On the tragic tale of Ruben Betancourt, Arthur Caplan wrote;

> "Physicians are not waiters, and the options that exist to treat the very sick and dying are not offerings on a menu. True autonomy requires advice and dialogue. Merely doing what the patient or surrogate says is not respecting autonomy but rather permitting preference, fear, guilt, and fantasy to substitute for it."[15]

Accepting death as the inevitable or preferable outcome for a patient is always difficult. The science of predicting death is weak, and survival after forgoing life support therapy may be as high as 5%. The hope that we could know with confidence what our patients' preferences are has proved elusive; changes of hearts and minds are common. We often hold that better communication between staff, patients and surrogates would increase the possibility of consensus, but have no evidence for that. Subjected to controlled trial in a Californian practice, proactive ethics consultation with a trained bioethicist did not reduce the amount of treatment provided which was classed as non-beneficial.[16] There is wide variability in end of life practices both within and between nations, and we can hardly blame the internet savvy relatives of our patients for sometimes having little confidence in our judgments.

Optimal care; to treat for survival or to treat for comfort?

It is important to reflect on factors that have been associated with end of life decision-making so that we can take them into account and ensure that every individual is treated fairly. Decisions to limit care are more frequent in older patients, patients with comorbidities, and patients with limited functional reserve. The race, ethnicity, religion and nationality of doctors and patients all influence the extent of "technological intensity" provided at the end of life. American and Northern European practices have generally been more accepting of less intensive end of life care than Southern European practices, but that may be changing. The confidence to recommend and deliver less technologically intense care near the end of life increases with clinical experience and is greater in specialist intensivists.[17] To gain acceptance of a switch from survival targeted therapy to palliative care practitioners often adopt an intermediate position of setting arbitrary ceilings of care known as "No escalation of care", for example declaring a maximum dose of pressor.

The "Patients' Rights and End of Life Care" Act came into force in France in 2005.[18] It legalized withholding/withdrawal of life support treatment, and allowed for the lawful 'intensification' of medications that may hasten death (double effect). A national survey revealed that there remained widespread dissatisfaction with the processes surrounding death in hospital.[18]

Withhold versus withdraw

To encourage the initiation of life-sustaining treatment where there are unresolved doubts about its appropriateness, we are often advised that such treatments can and should be withdrawn once they are found to have been inappropriate. Withholding and withdrawing are to be regarded as legally and ethically equivalent aspects of forgoing. The reality is that it is much harder, emotionally, practically, and legally, to withdraw a life sustaining treatment (seen as an act to bring about death) than to withhold it (seen as an omission to allow nature to take its course).

Withholding attempts at cardiopulmonary resuscitation

The doctor's duty to decide whether or not to initiate attempts at cardiopulmonary resuscitation (CPR) in the acute situation must balance the modern trend to 'the vicious circle of overtreatment' against 'respect for the human being' at the end of life. Remember that successful resuscitation will often depend on a period of post-resuscitation CC. If attempts at CPR are not likely to be effective, or if they are not likely to be beneficial, or if they are not in accordance with the patient's wishes the attempts should not be made and the doctor should respectfully examine to confirm death. Otherwise, the presumption should be to attempt resuscitation.

Withdrawal of mechanical ventilation

The very close temporal association with death raises concerns that the process is close to active euthanasia, which is illegal in every jurisdiction. Not surprisingly, there are different schools of thought on how withdrawal of mechanical ventilation should be conducted. Perhaps the commonest approach is the 'terminal' or 'one-way' wean, in which a progressive weaning protocol is implemented, but progression is not halted if the patient fails the criteria that would normally indicate restoration of ventilatory support. The rationale is that one cannot be entirely sure the patient is ventilator dependent until one has discontinued support and shown that death is inevitable; but one must consider the potential for harm to the patient if agonal dyspnoea is not extremely well treated with opiates.

An alternative view is to acknowledge that there may remain uncertainty about the question of ventilator dependence, but to focus on the certainty that the decision to withdraw in the clear expectation of death is the correct one. Adherents to this view remove ventilator therapy abruptly once the decision to withdraw is made and the patient and family are prepared. Even amongst proponents of abrupt withdrawal, there is no consensus over whether anaesthesia should be administered, muscle relaxants used prior to cessation of mechanical ventilation, and whether or not the endotracheal tube should be withdrawn.

Acts and omissions at the end of life; the doctrine of double effect

The Catholic doctrine of double effect is often appealed to in law and ethics. An example is the Vatican declaration that narcotics may be used 'at the approach of death' to 'suppress pain and consciousness even if one foresees that it will shorten life'; the intention must be 'to relieve pain effectively, using for this purpose pain killers available to medicine'. Crucially, death must be 'in no way intended or sought, even if the risk of it is reasonably taken'. This distinction between intent to alleviate suffering and intent to shorten life is critical yet fine.[19]

Institutional Admission and Discharge Policies

Responsible ethical, medical, and legal opinion acknowledges that it is necessary in some circumstances to limit access to services such as CC. Healthcare purchasers (governments, healthcare organizations) allocate a finite amount of money each year, and some resources (such as qualified staff or organs for transplant) are limited by factors other than financial considerations. Macro allocation decisions precede rationing or triage decisions (micro-allocation) that are made by physicians on a day-to-day basis. Protocols are recommended so that the process is transparent, and extreme care must be taken to ensure that the criteria are seen to be fair and non-discriminatory.

CC treatment should be offered primarily to those who have a reasonable prospect of benefiting from active treatment, so some judgment about the prognosis is required. Sometimes an ICU bed is not available within the hospital for a patient who needs one. One solution is to transfer a patient to another hospital with spare capacity.

Pandemic diseases arise just a few times in a century, but when they arrive they may threaten the lives of more people than can possibly be treated in our ICUs and force us to turn away patients we might otherwise have been able to save. This offends our impulse to attempt to save those facing avoidable death; the Rule of Rescue.

Providing only the most efficient treatments — those that provide the greatest benefit for the least consumption of resource — is one approach founded in utilitarianism. Another approach is to use a method of selection that gives each candidate an equal chance of being selected for treatment perhaps a lottery, or the first-come, first-served system. Attempts to attribute greater worth or societal usefulness to some individuals over others would generally be disapproved; the dedicated nurse and the convicted murderer must be given equal consideration for the last bed. However, there is a school of thought called prioritarianism that does recognize some morally acceptable distinctions between individuals. For example, the young may be preferred over the elderly because, in cricketing parlance, they are owed a fair innings, or people regarded as socially disadvantaged/vulnerable may be prioritized to level the playing field with those who have never been disadvantaged — the poor man may be preferred to the rich. Chivalry would prioritize women over men, though feminism may reject that notion.

One proposed 'ethical' response to a recent pandemic was to suspend clinical judgment and to delegate decisions to withdraw support from the sickest patients to an arbitrary organ system failure score. It was hoped this would be perceived as objective and therefore fair, achieving the greater good for as many people as possible and minimizing stress on any human decision-maker. An unresolved problem is the fact that post-Nuremberg ethical and legal principles in Europe do not allow a patient to be sacrificed for another, or for the possible benefit of the wider society. Tillyard's proposal is to take a wider view of organizational triage and treatment triage which achieves maximization of treatment provision while respecting the best interests of every patient.[20]

The threat of Ebola virus coming out of Africa led to consideration of refusing CC treatment to infected patients on the grounds that the patient poses too great a risk to health workers. There is an acceptance that potential rescuers are under no moral or legal obligation to risk their own life or health, but when they choose to act we acclaim them heroes. Mortality appears to be reduced when patients are treated with intravenous resuscitation fluids and antibiotics.

Brain Death

Controversial since it was first proposed as a legal solution to the problem of transplanting a beating heart from a cadaver, three concepts of brain death have been debated. While the brain stem formulation has been doggedly retained in the United Kingdom, the whole brain formulation is accepted and practiced most widely. The higher brain or cortical death formulation — that patients in permanent vegetative state be used as heart beating organ donors — was quickly rejected. The conceptual basis for regarding whole brain death as human death is the loss of the organism as a whole.

The diagnosis of brain death requires a meticulous clinical determination, usually by more than one qualified clinician, but confirmatory tests demonstrating the cessation of cerebral electrical activity or cessation of intracranial blood flow can be used in cases in which the necessary examination cannot be fully performed or correctly interpreted. Confirmatory tests also serve a useful purpose in reassuring relatives that there has been no human error in arriving at this momentous diagnosis, and are a way to audit clinical expertise in order to inspire public confidence in the process.

There remain problems of acceptance of the brain death concept among some people of certain ethnic origins or religious persuasion, and this sometimes coexists with a desire to go to paradise with all one's organs in place. Logical flaws in the concept of brain death make for stimulating and sometimes heated philosophical debates, but the sceptics have not persuaded any jurisdictions to abandon brain death statutes and have largely failed to change clinical practice guidelines. There have been calls for the abandonment of brain death as a legal requirement for heart beating organ procurement, but the 'dead-donor' rule has so far survived such challenges. Brain death has been accepted and has formed the basis of successful public policy on donors after brain death (DBD) in diverse societies throughout the world.

Donors after Circulatory Death (DCD)

The traditional triad of death is unresponsiveness, apnoea and absence of cardiac output. It is known that spontaneous recovery of absent circulation can rarely occur up to about a minute after it has ceased. After two minutes it becomes extremely unlikely that spontaneous recovery will occur, even though resuscitative attempts may still restart the circulation and brain function. After five minutes of 'death', even resuscitative efforts are likely to be unsuccessful, and after 10 minutes of absent circulation (at normal body temperature) death is generally to be regarded as irreversible. At what point then is it acceptable to diagnose death and proceed to recovery of organs for transplantation? The Pittsburgh Protocol originally required just two minutes. The so-called No Touch Period in European practices is at least five, or as long as 15–20 minutes.

One of the greatest changes in CC practice in recent years has been the promotion of donation after cardiac death. Spain, Austria, Belgium, and Italy prefer to harvest organs from people who have suffered sudden "uncontrolled" cardiac arrest, often outside a hospital. United States, United Kingdom and Netherlands prefer to identify patients in ICUs who are to have life support withdrawn, so that cardiac arrest is "controlled". Germany, Finland and Poland do not use DCD. The Uniform Anatomic Gift Act was revised in 2006 and has been adopted by many of the States in USA. It permits non-consented intervention to preserve the viability of vital organs while suitability is determined, even in cases where the patient has a clear advance directive against life-sustaining treatment. Similar developments are occurring in Europe. There has been concern that the public policy goals of increasing the availability of donated organs go too far in presuming the potential donor's intention to consent and there is a call for further revisions to protect truly informed and voluntary end of life decisions for patients. The professional integrity of physicians who have legal and ethical fiduciary duties to their dying patients is potentially compromised.

It is reported that "brain death is on the decline" in Canada as advances in neurosurgical care are reducing the number of people who die after acute brain injury.

References

1. Greene J. Research: Moral Cognition. Available at: http://www.joshua-greene.net/research/moral-cognition (Accessed 8 July 2015).
2. Office for Human Research Protections (OHRP) (1979). US Department of Health & Human Services Ethical Principles and Guidelines for the Protection of Human Subjects of Research. Available at: http://www.hhs.gov/ohrp/humansubjects/guidance/belmont.html (Accessed 14 July 2015).
3. European Convention on Human Rights (1950). Available at: http://www.echr.coe.int/Documents/Convention_ENG.pdf (Accessed 6 September 2015).
4. Convention for the Protection of Human Rights and Dignity of the Human Being with regard to the Application of Biology and Medicine (1997): Convention on Human Rights and Biomedicine (1997). Available at: http://conventions.coe.int/Treaty/en/Treaties/Html/164.htm (Accessed 6 September 2015).
5. Schloendorff V (1914). Society of NY Hospital. Available at: http://biotech.law.lsu.edu/cases/consent/Schoendorff.htm (Accessed 6 September 2015).
6. Council of Europe Parliamentary Assembly (2012). Resolution 1859 Protecting Human Rights and Dignity by Taking into Account Previously Expressed Wishes of Patients. Available at: http://assembly.coe.int/nw/xml/XRef/Xref-XML2HTML-en.asp?fileid=18064&lang=en (Accessed 6 September 2015).
7. In re A.C., 533 A. 2d 611 (App D.C. 1989); In re A.C., 573 A. 2d 1235 (App D.C. 1990).
8. Woodcock TE (2010). Research in intensive care. In *Law and Ethics in Intensive Care*, Danbury C, Newdick C, Lawson A and Waldmann C (eds.). Oxford University Press, Oxford.
9. Durand-Zaleski IS, Alberti C and Durieux P (2008). Informed consent in clinical research in France: assessment and factors associated with therapeutic misconception. *J. Med. Ethics.*, 34, 16.
10. Mann H (2005). Controversial choice of a control intervention in a trial of ventilator therapy in ARDS: standard of care arguments in a randomized controlled trial. *J. Med. Ethics.*, 31, 548–553.

11. Drazen JM, Solomon CG and Greene MF (2013). Informed consent and support. *N. Engl. J. Med.*, 368, 1929–1931.
12. Bosslet GT, Pope TM and Rubenfeld GD (2015). An Official ATS/AACN/ACCP/ESICM/SCCM policy statement: responding to requests for potentially inappropriate treatments in intensive care units. *Am. J. Respir. Crit. Care Med.*, 191, 1318–1330.
13. Aintree University Hospitals NHS Foundation Trust v James (2013). Available at: https://www.supremecourt.uk/decided-cases/docs/UKSC_2013_0134_Judgment.pdf (Accessed 6 September 2015).
14. Cuthbertson v Rasouli (2013). Available at: https://scc-csc.lexum.com/scc-csc/scc-csc/en/item/13290/index.do (Accessed 6 September 2015).
15. Caplan AL (2012). Little hope for medical futility. *Mayo Clin. Proc.*, 87, 1040–1041.
16. Andereck WS, McGaughey JW, Schneiderman LJ and Jonsen AR (2014). Seeking to reduce non-beneficial treatment in the ICU: an exploratory trial of proactive ethics intervention. *Crit. Care Med.*, 42, 824–830.
17. Frost DW, Cook DJ, Heyland DK and Fowler RA (2011). Patient and healthcare professional factors influencing end-of-life decision-making during critical illness: a systematic review. *Crit. Care Med.*, 39, 1174–1189.
18. Pennec S, Monnier A, Pontone S and Aubry R (2012). End-of-life medical decisions in France: a death certificate follow-up survey 5 years after the 2005 act of parliament on patients' rights and end of life. *BMC Palliative Care*, 11, 25.
19. Lindblad A, Lynoe N and Juth N (2014). End-of-life decisions and the reinvented Rule of Double Effect: a critical analysis. *Bioethics*, 28, 368–377.
20. Tillyard A (2010). Reorganizing the pandemic triage processes to ethically maximizes individuals' best interests. *Intens. Care Med.*, 36, 1966–1971.

Communication

Peter G. Brindley
Division of Critical Care Medicine, Adjunct Professor Anesthesiology and Pain Medicine Adjunct Professor, Dossetor Ethics Centre University of Alberta, Edmonton, Alberta, Canada

Key Points

1. Communication should be promoted as one of Intensive Care Medicine's (ICM) most important skills.
2. Proficiency in communication need not (and should not) be left to chance.
3. Communication is nuanced and includes verbal, paraverbal, and non-verbal aspects.
4. We should know (and practice) communication tools applicable to (i) medical crisis (ii) handover (iii) talking with patients/families/surrogates.
5. Communication simulations and audits are highly recommended.

Introduction

Journalist Peter Findlay Dunne described Critical Care (CC) when he claimed his job was to "comfort the afflicted and afflict the comfortable". After all, growing evidence suggests that being an expert clinician means becoming an expert communicator, and in multiple arenas.[1–4] Suboptimal communication may be the largest source of preventable medical error during (i) acute clinical crises; (ii) sign over between practitioners and (iii) less acute, but no less critical, conversations with patients and surrogates.[1–7] Accordingly, communication may be 'the most important but least accomplished aspect of quality care'.[6,7] More optimistically, it is one of our greatest opportunities to mitigate the 'care gap' (the distance between optimal care and usual care), the 'expectation gap' (the gulf between what patients expect and receive), and the 'accidental curriculum' (the difference between skills needed by healthcare workers and those usually taught).[3–8] In short, communication is likely our greatest asset, or keenest liability.

If we define communication as "sharing, uniting, or making understanding common"[1–4] then better communication becomes a key strategy to create more reliable, resilient, and patient-focused systems.[1–4] Whereas ICM previously focused on scientific discovery and technology, it is now increasingly understood as a complex social system.[5] Accordingly, ICM should now also make a 'science of reducing complexity' and a 'science of managing uncertainty'.[5] Much of this will be achieved (or squandered) based on how well we address communication as a core non-technical skill. In a similar vein, we should accept that patients come to Intensive Treatment Units (ITUs) as often following bad outcomes and bad decisions: not just bad disease. As such, we are as much a Relationship Repair Unit (RRU) as an ITU. Therefore, communication is one of our most potent 'therapies', and the means by which we coordinate (or fragment) ongoing care, bolster (or impair) teamwork, and enrich (or erode) trust.[1–8]

While communication is an extremely large topic this chapter will limit its focus to strategies in three key arenas: (i) medical crisis communication; (ii) handover between healthcare workers, and (iii) talking with patients and surrogates. This includes strategies for those patients unable to communicate due to knowledge, illness, or language barrier. These ideas are rarely native to medicine (or to this author), but are instead from other high-risk or communication-centric professions: notably aviation and psychology. With the risk of hyperbole, communication may now be the most dangerous 'procedure' in modern medicine. Regardless, it is time for our 'verbal dexterity' to match our manual dexterity and factual know-how.[1–5]

Background

Communication skills are rarely innate, and may not be improved by more unstructured experience.[1–4] Fortunately communication can be taught and mastered: just like any other medical skill. Similar to other medical interventions, communication is not one-size-fits-all, nor is it a panacea. However, deliberate training has been associated with increased confidence, improved patient satisfaction, lower anxiety, decreased depression, and reduced post-traumatic stress.[1,9,10] What we say, how it is communicated, and how it is understood can act as a placebo (good communication can actually reduce pain and anxiety) or a nocebo (bad communication can increase pain and anxiety).[1] Better communication might also decrease litigation and improve hospital reputation.[1] Accordingly, communication is everybody's business: it should be taught to trainees and expected from senior practitioners.[1–4]

As outlined by St Pierre *et al.*[2] communication is more than just what words are said (aka *verbal* communication). This means that we should also address *Paraverbal* communication, namely, how words are said (pitch, volume, pacing, and emphasis). However, communication also includes how words and ideas are understood.[1–4] Therefore, while this review will focus on verbal communication, instruction in *non-verbal* communication may become increasingly widespread. This includes ensuring that clinicians demonstrate appropriate body language, suitable eye contact, response to emotions, active listening, and the use of reflective silence. After all, we really cannot not communicate: failing to make the effort sends its own message.[1–4]

Communication Models

In 1949, Shannon and Weaver (working for Bell Laboratories) developed a technical model for telephone communication.[2] Their model remains relevant to medics over six decades later. Transmitters (i.e. speakers) must encode messages, and receivers (i.e. listeners) must decode them. To be successful, both should be on the same channel (i.e. possess similar situational awareness) and there should be minimal interference or noise (i.e. chaos, stress, or cognitive-bias). They also identified the issue of 'channel overload': not so much 'noise' but overburdened communication (and akin to cognitive overload). Overload occurs unless the receiver filters data into usable and prioritized information (i.e. you receive data, but need to create usable information).[2]

Shannon's model has limitations. After all, complex communication also requires *meaning*: which is harder to encode, transmit and decode.[2] Moreover, this model describes communication as unidirectional (transmitter to receiver), whereas medical communication is often multi-directional, multi-disciplinary, and multi-hierarchical.[2–4] While location should not affect data transmission, it often affects communication quality, impact, and efficiency. When transmitter and receiver are no longer face-to-face (or if facial expressions are obscured by masks) their communication may lose non-verbal cues and shared situational awareness.[2] This is why the medical telephone call (and resuscitation while wearing protective gear) is so important to practice. Non-visual communication (both intra-hospital and inter-hospital) relies only upon verbal and para-verbal cuing. Confirming understanding by routinely summarizing and repeating-back becomes an important fail-safe (*qv*).[1–4]

Psychological models may offer more for medical communicators, especially as they focus on relationships, not just tasks. The 'four mouths and four ears model'[2] has sender and listener separated by a message with four equally relevant sides: (i) content; (ii) relationship; (iii) self-revelation (iv) appeal.[2] Content refers to objective facts and words. However, the relationship aspect means that senders reveal (consciously and unconsciously) how they regard receivers through specific words, intonations, and non-verbal signals. Senders also offer an insight into how they feel about *themselves*, namely a 'self-revelation'. Fourthly, there is an appeal (or request) where each message prompts the receiver to do (or not do) something. These four aspects apply to both talker and listener, namely, we speak with four mouths and listen with four ears. This is done consciously and unconsciously and depends upon mental state, expectation, and previous interactions.[2] Notably, the sender cannot fully force the listener's mind (and vice versa). A practical example follows:

When a surgeon says to an anaesthesiologist: "the blood pressure is low, what are you doing?" the surgeon may presume that he stated objective facts and requested simple feedback. However, his intonation might suggest otherwise. For example, he may have revealed that his relationship is one of low confidence with this anaesthesiologist (i.e. "why must I operate and manage haemodynamics"). Also, the surgeon's self-revelation could be one of either appropriate patient concern or excessive nervousness about his own abilities (i.e. "I daren't have another bad surgical outcome"). His request or appeal (albeit unstated) might be objective: "please consider a fluid bolus or inotrope" or accusatory: "hey; focus on the patient". The anaesthesiologist also listens with four ears, and anyone can be more or less open. For example, a content-based response would deliver objective facts ("I'm bolusing saline; I added norepinephrine"). However, if the anaesthesiologist hears the self-revelation he might reply: "I will manage the blood pressure; you can safely focus on surgery". If the anaesthesiologist is sensitive to relationship aspects, or misreads the appeal, (i.e. "he implied that I was ignoring the patient") then he may be more curt (i.e. "that's my concern, not yours"). This model neatly shows how communication can create a virtuous cycle that bolsters teamwork, or a vicious cycle that destroys it.[2,3]

Communication is modified in both meaning and interpretation by the paraverbal (volume, tone, pitch, pacing) and non-verbal (furrowed brow; angry eyes).[1–3] These, in turn, are greatly affected by subconscious forces such as emotions and attitudes. If verbal and non-verbal communication are incongruent (words say one thing; volume or expressions another) then we typically place less emphasis on verbal communication.[2] In other words, we rely upon tone and body language before words. If there is incongruence then we also default to what we expected (i.e. "he said X, but I believe he usually means Y", or "he sounds calm, but he's usually stressed"). In short, incongruence should be avoided because it invites misinterpretation.[1–3] Accordingly, if someone asks if you need help, do not answer "I'm okay" with a tone suggesting otherwise.[2] Congruent communication is even harder when those involved are unfamiliar, or when the medical situation is novel. Therefore, mature communication means transmitters become dextrous enough to rephrase, and receivers become flexible enough to reinterpret.[1–4] Mature communication also includes active listening (making a conscious effort to hear and understand). This is especially important if communication is incomplete (i.e. from stress) or unidimensional (i.e. when enunciation and non-verbal cues are lost behind a mask).

A familiar debate suggests that Medicine can either be understood as an 'art or a science'. However, several authors have suggested that it should also be understood as 'engineering'.[5] This is because the complexity of modern care means that it exceeds the skill set of any one person. One of the first rules of teamwork is that 'a team of experts is not automatically an expert team".[2] In engineering, complexity and unpredictability are lessened by fail-safes and standard operating procedures. The same rigor can now be applied to communication, along with (sensible) checklists and Global Rating Scores.[11] Strategies to lessen communication errors can also be summarized using an insightful quote from Gaba and Rall: "Meant is not said; said is not heard; heard is not understood; understood is not done".[3] What follows is an attempt to mitigate our communication shortcomings using strategies from high-stakes industries, and applied to our CC reality.

Improving communication during medical crises

A key communication strategy is to create a 'shared mental model' (a common understanding; a sense that "everyone is on the same page").[2] This helps foster task-focused (rather than power focused or ego focused) communication. The 'shared mental model' provides a roadmap to prioritize; manage information; establish roles; stabilize emotions and build confidence.[2] If time allows, leaders should invite members to suggest a mental model ("what do you think? what should we do?"). After all, diverse inputs can provide a more complete understanding.[1–3] Under time pressure, the leader has to rapidly communicate a reasonable mental model that others will support ('I believe it's septic shock, please do the following').[2,3] The best situational awareness and the most adept communication will likely come from practice and prior exposure.[5] As a result, regular simulation is an important 'immunization booster' to improve the speed and strength of the team's response.

The greater the overlap in shared mental model the more team members predict and adapt even when dealing with stress or novelty.[2] Accordingly, teams who are well-practiced frequently work in relative silence (i.e. implicit coordination). However, silence is not always 'golden'[2] and unpracticed teams usually require more explicit (i.e. verbal) coordination.

When coordinating mature teams, task-assignment is often implicit by profession (e.g. anaesthetists intubate; surgeons operate).[2] As such, leaders can focus their verbal communication on other tasks. However, if there is the potential for confusion (both anaesthetists and surgeons can insert central lines) then the skilled communicator knows to be more explicit ("Dr. Smith will intubate, Dr. Jones will insert lines"). It is also important to regularly reinforce or update the mental model ("the airway is now secured; our next priority is…"; "we now have ST elevation: our priority has changed").

In aviation, poor cockpit communication between crew, is one of the commonest reasons why mechanically sound planes crash.[3,5,9,11] Therefore, flight investigators have made flattening the authority gradient a priority.[7] 'Horizontal communication' means all members of the team are authorized (actually, obligated) to speak up.[1–3,6,7] Moreover, aviation has mandated 'transmitter orientated' communication (where it is the speaker's responsibility to be understood), rather than 'receiver orientated' (where it is the listener's responsibility to divine what was meant).[7] Making communication more deliberate also means promoting active listening.[2] This requires that team members confirm understanding or demand clarification.[1–3] All team members take responsibility for how messages are delivered, received, understood and carried out.[1–3] After all, communication is a team sport.

Investigation of aviation crashes often and finds black box silence for minutes before catastrophe.[2–3] Similarly, ask nurses about the last bad resuscitation and it was likely notable for silence despite impending disaster. Physicians may not speak due to stress or uncertainty (the military calls this 'helmet head'), or because we cannot think of what to say in a timely fashion.[1–3] Therefore, team members can be taught how to speak up using standardized responses: "we still have no pulse: what am I missing?" or "I do not know this patient, please summarize?"[2,3] Other members need statements that help them quickly join a team (i.e. "I am from Surgery, is there any job for me?").

The military has promoted Situation, Background, Assessment, Recommendation (SBAR) to provide a recognizable structure to communication.[1–3] While it can be overly formal especially when team members are familiar with each other or the problem is routine it offers a construct for junior staff and unfamiliar situations. A simple example could be: Situation: "this is Dr. X, I need your help now"; Background: "he's a 35 year old with a blunt splenic injury"; Assessment: "he is still hypotensive despite blood"; Recommendation: "You should review him for laparotomy now".[1–3]

In addition to getting aviators to speak up, they are taught how to have their concerns heard. This can be done by teaching how to escalate communication (from least to most insistent) and through levels or grades of assertiveness.[1–3, 9–13] For example, the three step CUS acronym consists of: i am Concerned; i am Uncomfortable; this is a Safety issue … so stop. Robert Besco's four step P.A.C.E acronym progresses from Probing to Alerting to Challenging to Emergency language. Other constructs include up to six steps. This includes the 'hint' (e.g. 'should things look like this?'); 'preference' (e.g. 'I would suggest…'); 'query' (e.g. 'what do you think?'); 'shared suggestion' (e.g. 'you and I should'); 'statement' (e.g. 'we need to') and 'command' (e.g. 'do this now'). Those actively listening should detect escalating urgency, which they mirror with increasing engagement. Once again, these models emphasize that communication is as much about listening as talking.

Without instruction, junior team members may only hint, and, if ignored, fail to escalate.[1–4, 6,7,12,13] Alternatively, senior team members may over-rely upon blunt commands.[1–3] Orders are unequivocal, and are justified when team members repeatedly fail to respond. However, they can destroy teamwork if used as the initial, or only, communication style.[7] Aviation also teaches a five step model of advocacy and confirmation.[13] The following includes aviation examples and medical corollaries: 'Attention Getter' ("Captain/Doctor"); 'State Your Concern' ("We're low on fuel/the patient is hypotensive"); 'State The Problem As You See It' ('I don't think we can land/I think we need to operate now'); 'State a solution' ("Let's re-route to a closer airport/I'll book the OR"); 'Obtain Agreement' (e.g. "Okay, Captain/Doctor?").[13]

Applying the "C's of communication" means we must Cite names (for role clarity); remain Clear and Concise (to avoid confusion) and most importantly, Close the loop (to confirm things have been done).[1–4] The other result of closed-loop communication is that commands are first verified and then amplified. For example, we tell a specific person to intubate but also to tell the whole team when it is done (along with calling out the end tidal CO_2: which is an additional numeric form of closed-loop confirmation). Similarly, we do not just order blood, but instead we state: "Nurse, two packed-cells … and tell me the blood pressure when infused" or: "obtain an arterial blood gas … and bring the result to me". While there are many ways to "close the loop", this strategy confirms instructions were heard, understood and done. A fourth C might be "crowd control". This includes ensuring enough people are present ("I need one person for intubation; one for lines; one to bolus drugs), the right people are present ("I may need a surgical airway; get me Dr. X"), and not too many people are present ("thank you, but I need to remove all but the following").

The 'call out' means alerting the team to important changes (i.e. "he's back into ventricular fibrillation").[2] The 'step back method' means verbally forcing a 'time out' and compelling the team to reassess their assumptions (i.e. "stop chest compressions, are we still in asystole?" The 'repeat back method'[2] provides a safety check: using repetition to confirm mutual understanding (i.e. "so was that one full mg of epinephrine?"). The 'read back method'[2] means confirming a verbal order before processing it (i.e. "so, you want two units of blood? Then repeat the haemoglobin? Then call you?").

Team members must be encouraged to speak up, but also taught how to make those inputs task-focused and appropriately timed. If not then it can further exacerbate the chaos.[1–3] Non-helpful interruptions are such a safety hazard in aviation that they are addressed in standard operating procedures. This 'Sterile Cockpit Rule'[14,15] means that non-operational talk is forbidden during critical phases, i.e. taxi; take-off; landing. Enforcement depends upon all those in the cockpit, not just those currently talking.[2,14,15] We understand the need for microbiologic sterility in surgery, so why not 'communication sterility'.

The 'Sterile Cockpit Rule'[14,15] can be readily adapted to medicine. In non-critical situations we should confirm if others are able to focus their attention (i.e. "I want your opinion, do you have two minutes now or later?"). In more critical situations we can demand attention (i.e. "Please stop your conversation and focus on this patient").[1–3] As pointed out to me by a wise trainee, the anaesthetist is in his/her critical phase during induction and awakening. Therefore, the surgeon must avoid unnecessary noise or distraction. Once the operation is underway the surgeon is now in their critical phase, while the anaesthetist no longer is. It is now as important for the anaesthetist to avoid unnecessary disturbance of the surgeon. Again, all members are responsible for communication.[1–5]

Ambiguous or non-committal speech (aka 'mitigating speech') is common prior to airline crashes, and probably during medical crises.[1–3] This is why we must replace comments like "perhaps we need help", or "we should think about surgery", with "get me a surgeon" and "we need the operating theater, now". Junior members (or those that do not feel safe sharing their opinions) may mitigate speech to show deference, when embarrassed, or if unsure.[1–3] If time permits then 'mitigating language' can be harmless, even desirable for team building (i.e. "perhaps you can help me with this stable patient, when you get a moment?"). However, the wrong communication tool during a crisis is likely no less dangerous than the wrong drug during resuscitation.

Overcautious language is inappropriate during crises, just as overly strident language can be inappropriate at non-critical times. Crisis communication should still be polite, but unambiguous (i.e. "John, intubate now, please"). Communication must also be addressed to a specific person to avoid diffusion of responsibility.[1–3] This is why words like "someone" and "anybody" are inappropriate in a crisis. However, just as we need to control communication during crises, we should loosen the reigns once it has passed. Communication that is less regimented is essential when discussing emotions. Therefore it is appropriate (perhaps preferable) during conflict management, stress relief, and debriefing. In other words, communication is also how we keep each other resilient for the next crisis.[3,4]

Improving communication during handover

Handover (aka handoff, or sign over) is how medical practitioners and medical teams transfer information and responsibility.[15,16] It is akin to the 'baton pass' in a relay race, and is, similarly, one of the key areas where we succeed or fail. Doctors, nurses, and allied health workers all perform handovers. In fact, there are approximately 4,000 daily handovers (by all healthcare providers) in an average large academic hospital, or approximately 1.5 million per hospital per year. Reduced duty hours have increased the number of handovers by approximately 40% — meaning we may have simply replaced the 'tired' with the 'misinformed'.[15,16] Information lost in handovers causes delays in diagnosis and therapy, and is a potential nexus of error. Accordingly, training in handover communication offers a substantial opportunity to increase patient safety and system reliability.

Most handovers errors are 'content omissions': important information is simply not communicated. Omissions occur at a rate of approximately 1 in 100.[15,16] As with all communication, handover communication should be tailored to the recipient and purpose. Generally, however, routine sign overs should prioritize only the top few concerns (otherwise we risk cognitive overload). Sign over to those covering nights usually focuses only on immediate threats ("if bed-5 worsens please intubate") or ensuring that limits are not exceeded ("if bed-5 worsens *do not* intubate"). Sign over back to the day team (who already know the patient) need not belabor the identifying info, but instead briefly reviews overnight concerns and then focuses on new admissions. When senior doctors take over an entire service a more detailed review is required. This includes reviewing medical issues from head to toe; discussing family concerns, and listing all consulting services. Sign over to the senior charge nurse may focus on those ready for transfer, or which are patients that need nurses with specialized skills (i.e. dialysis).

Some prefer sign over at the patient's bedside (in order to associate facts with a visible patient), while others prefer to remain in one spot to minimize distractions. Regardless, sign over should have a recognizable format (to aid recall) and occur at a designated time (to maximize attendance). It is helpful to have those that are taking over repeat back their assigned tasks, and to allow time for discussion. Printed handover sheets supplement a verbal handoff. This allows receivers to focus; as well as providing comprehensive information; bolstering the shared mental model, and providing an aide-memoire. To be meaningful, these sign over forms require regular update and senior oversight.

While communication tools can seem little more than codified common sense, they are supported by the same intuitive rationale as checklists. Supporters argue that checklists provide structure, fail-safes, and a way to quickly address the 'simple things'. Done right and this frees up the brain for complex cognition. Opponents argue that checklists encourage exactly the opposite: reducing our problem solving abilities (when checklists no longer apply), reducing our ability to deliver individualized care, and encouraging 'medicine by menu'. Presumably, the issue is not merely having a communication checklist, but rather having a *good* checklist that is regularly practiced and battle hardened.[5]

Several promising handover acronyms exist.[12,16,17] The anticipate model stands for A: accurate administrative information; N: new information (also a brief history and diagnosis, updated medications, problem list, current baseline status, recent procedures, significant events); T: tasks or 'to-do' lists; I: illness: the primary provider's subjective assessment of the illness severity; C: contingency plans (to help anticipate problems). Identify, situation, background, assessment and recommendation (ISBAR) is closely allied to the SBAR technique (see above) but with a more inclusive Introduction (who, what, and where you are) and ending with a response portion that includes current plans and contingencies.

The appropriately named (and very comprehensive) acronym IPASS BATON stands for: introduction (your job/role) patient (name, age, sex, location); assessment (chief complaint; vital signs; symptoms; diagnosis); situation (current circumstances; code status; level of uncertainty; recent changes; response to treatment); safety (critical lab values/reports; allergies); background (comorbidities; previous episodes; current medications; family history) actions (what was done and why); timing (level of urgency; priorities and timing); ownership (who is responsible; including family members) and finally, next (what is the plan; what is the contingency; what will happen next). The shorter IPASS handover acronym includes I: illness severity (stable, watch; unstable); P: patient summary (demographics; events prior to admission; hospital course; plan); A: action list (to do; timeline and ownership); S: situational awareness and contingency plan (know what is going on now; plan for what might occur); S: synthesis (which is performed by the Receiver and includes summary; questions; and restating the key actions). The IPASS's division of patients into stable (akin to a green traffic light), watcher (orange light), and unstable (red light) is also an especially useful way to summarize patients and prioritize actions.

Improving communication with patients and families

The expression: "people do not care how much you know unless they know how much you care" is usually attributed to Theodore Roosevelt. Regardless, this reminds us what matters most to patients: whether we are delivering news; providing comfort; lessening hostility; combating disbelief, or mitigating denial.[1,4] We should not be surprised that patients and families routinely claim to value clinicians' communication skills as equal or more important than clinical skills.[4,18] Communication tools and bundles are outlined below. The hope is to provide structure and reliability to complex communication but not make these interactions scripted or devoid of personal connection.

The Calgary–Cambridge guide divides the interview between patient and provider into: (1) initiate; (2) gather information; (3) provide structure; (4) build relationships; (5) explain and plan, and (6) close the session. The GREAT acronym consists of (1) greetings/goals; (2) rapport (3) evaluation/expectation/examination/explanation; (4) ask/answer/acknowledge; (5) tacit agreement/thanks), and the LAURS acronym consists of: (1) listening; (2) acceptance; (3) utilization (of appropriate words); (4) reframing, and (5) suggestion. The VALUE acronym divides communication into (1) value statements from family; (2) acknowledge emotions; (3) listen; (4) understand the patient as a person; (5) elicit questions can facilitate shared decision-making. The SPIKES acronym is recommended when delivering bad news, and divides communication into: (1) settings; (2) patient perception; (3) invite to share; (4) Knowledge transmission; (5) emotions and empathy; (6) summarize and strategize).[2,4]

We also have tools to audit communication with patients and surrogates.[19–20] For example, Black *et al.*[19] have promoted a communication bundle (as part of a multi-faceted quality improvement process) with 10 requirements. Six of these are expected within 24 hours: identification of (i) the surrogate decision-maker; (ii) code status; (iii) advance directive; (iv) pain; (v) dyspnoea, and also (vi) distribution of a brochure. Four additional goals are to be met in 72 hours: (i) family meeting; (ii) discuss prognosis; (iii) assess patient-specific goals, and (iv) offer spiritual care. This approach emphasizes that communication is more than just facts transmitted from doctor to patient. The patient is validated as someone with beliefs and values, and as part of a larger 'life support system' that includes family, friends and community.[1,4,19,20]

Patients and families usually only speak up when they feel safe to do so. Pincince and others suggest that families and patients need familiarity (which we may undermine by changing staff too frequently); predictability (which we may undermine when we keep families waiting); support systems (which we erode when families are excluded) and a sense of control (which is threatened by illness and unfamiliar environments). Families who feel safe may be less likely to respond with anger or intransigence (aka "neural hijacking of the rational brain") and use their vagus nerve to engage rather than to fight (aka Stephen Porges' polyvagal theory). Particularly when communicating bad news, providers should remember that while this may be routine for us for families these are seminal moments which they are unlikely to forget.[1,4] Combined with 'active listening', the effort put into communication becomes a key way to demonstrate non-abandonment.[1,4] Investing the time to establish initial 'rapport' (usually defined as 'common perspective'; 'being in sync' or 'on the same page') can facilitate all future interactions.[1,2,4] Good communication may also reinforce the patient's psychological reserves and resilience.[1–3]

These insights apply to those that *cannot* talk (endotracheal tube; tracheostomy; tongue resection), and those that *do not* talk (fear, confusion, respect for authority).[1,4] For patients, already burdened with illness, not being able to verbalize, and not being understood, can accelerate a downward spiral into disengagement. Also, when healthcare workers do speak we may not speak the same way as patients.[1] For example, physicians often use technical language and focus upon gathering information and delivering news. Patient language and family language may be more concerned with beliefs, fears, and hopes. Similarly, patient and family coping strategies may include denial or aggression, whereas caregivers intellectualize to protect their emotions. Communication that is sensitive, but objective, functions as a bridge between the 'natural world' of patients and the 'scientific world' of caregivers.[1,4]

Communication difficulty is compounded when caregivers and care receivers speak not just different words but different languages.[1,4] Even with sufficient time, doctors are less likely to discuss psychosocial issues, or offer lifestyle counselling, to language incongruent patients. Similarly, patients are less likely to ask questions and may find it harder to trust.[1,4] Communicating across the cultural barrier (not just across the language barrier) is beyond this chapter's scope, but likely further exacerbates the situation. This is especially true if there are different ideas about whether autonomy and disclosure are empowering or enfeebling.

Translators can be helpful and may be unavoidable but are also fraught with potential error.[1,4] Firstly, using inexperienced translators family, friends, or staff are probably associated with more errors than using professional translators. Using friends or family also threatens confidentiality, which can increase distress in the short term, and affect relationships later. However, even with professional translators, communication errors are common. In an albeit small study ($n = 10$), of CC family meetings, use of a professional interpreter was associated with a communication alteration in over half, and over three-quarters of these were clinically significant.[1,4]

Acute Medicine is synonymous with inconvenient hours and time pressure. This means translators are not always on-site. Many hospitals now have telephone translation services. In addition, clinicians have long employed speech boards (containing common words or drawings). Just as other types of communication have been altered by technology so has medical communication: portable smartphones (i.e. Google translate™) and tablet applications (i.e. Vidatak™) can translate, and other innovative devices are under development (the 'Eye-Writer' is a prototype communication device for patients with severe strokes). These offer great promise. However, currently all translation strategies impair the natural conversational flow, and take more time. This can mean less information is delivered, less time is reserved for questions, and less emotional support is provided. Accordingly, patients requiring translation may be less satisfied, less informed when providing consent, and less compliant as outpatients.[1,4]

Reasons for translation errors are diverse but include inadequate medical comprehension or the misguided desire to protect patients (some translators see themselves as 'cultural buffers' i.e. not just interpreters but 're-interpreters'). To mitigate this, clinicians are advised to conduct a pre-translation briefing, and emphasize the need for accuracy, not just sensitivity. Briefings should include the diagnosis, its certainty and its gravity. It is also advisable to debrief afterwards. This reviews what went well and how to proceed in future. It also maintains the translator's emotional state.[1,4]

Resources have been produced, for both translators and those that access them, by groups such as the Healthcare Interpretation Network and the International Medical Interpreters Association. Healthcare workers should also familiarize themselves with local translation services, but then practice. Simulations, (with actors, standardized patients or actual translators) are not only risk free but can be immersive, reflective, and allow repetition until right. Despite the apparent simplicity of verbal simulations (all that is needed are telephones and chairs) they may be more realistic than acute care simulations (requiring expensive computer manikins and operators). Verbal simulations (via telephone or face-to-face) should be welcomed as they offer the benefits of high fidelity simulation but without its usual costs or logistics.[5]

Conclusion

Communication is increasingly recognized as acute care medicine's most important non-technical skill. This makes sense once we accept that communication is how we exchange meaning, reduce complexity; address uncertainty; manage emotions; inform, encourage, comfort, and challenge. Communication is central to the human experience of illness, and therefore central to healthcare delivery. It is also nuanced, complex, and error prone. We work in an environment under constant stress and time pressure. Accordingly, patients, families, surrogates, and coworkers, may assume nobody will take time to talk or to listen. To create a robust system that is patient-focused, family-focused, and team based we should seize all opportunities to communicate that we care, and to ensure that we are 'fit for task'.

References

1. Cyna AM, Andrew MI, Tan SGM and Smith AF (2011). *Handbook of Communication in Anaesthesia & Critical Care: A Practical Guide to Exploring the Art.* Oxford University Press, Oxford, New York.
2. St Pierre M, Hofinger G and Buerschaper C (2008). *Crisis Management in Acute Care Settings: Human Factors and Team Psychology in a High Stakes Environment.* Springer, New York.

3. Brindley PG and Reynolds SF (2011). Improving verbal communication in critical care medicine. *J. Crit. Care*, 26(2), 155–159.
4. Brindley PG, Smith KE, Cardinal P and Leblanc F (2014). Improving medical communication: skills for a complex (and multilingual) world. *Can. Respir. J.*, 21(2), 89–91.
5. Brindley PG (2010). Patient safety and acute care medicine: lessons for the future, insights from the past. *Crit. Care*, 14(2), 217–222.
6. Aron D and Headrick L (2002). Educating physicians prepared to improve care and safety is no accident: it requires a systematic approach. *Qual. Saf. Health Care*, 11, 168–173.
7. Azoulay E and Spring CL (2004). Family-physician interactions in the intensive care unit. *Crit. Care Med.*, 32(11), 2323–2328.
8. Azoulay E, Chevret S and Leleu G (2000). Half the families of ICU patients experience inadequate communication with physicians. *Crit. Care Med.* 8, 3044–3049.
9. Dunn EJ, Mills PD and Neily J (2007). Medical team training: applying crew resource management in the veterans health administration. *J. Comm. J. Qual. Patient Saf.*, 33(6), 317–325.
10. Leonard M, Graham S and Bonacum D (2004). The human factor: the critical importance of effective communication in providing safe care. *Qual. Saf. Health Care*, 13, 85–90.
11. Kim J, Neilipovitz D, Cardinal P and Chiu M (2009). A comparison of global rating scale and checklist scores in the validation of an evaluation tool to assess performance in the resuscitation of critically ill patients during simulated emergencies. *Sim Healthcare*, 4, 6–16.
12. US Department of Health and Human Services. Agency for Healthcare Research and Quality (AHRQ). Pocket Guide Team STEPPS. Available at: http://www.ahrq.gov/professionals/education/curriculum-tools/teamstepps/instructor/essentials/pocketguide.html (Accessed January 2015).
13. Canadian Pilot Resource Centre (CanPRC). Available at: http://www.canprc.ca/crm-toolbbox/communication (Accessed January 2015).
14. Airbus Flight Operations Briefing Notes. Human performance: Managing Interruption and Distractions. Available at: http://www.airbus.com/fileadmin/media_gallery/files/safety_library_items/AirbusSafetyLib_-FLT_OPS-HUM_PER-SEQ03.pdf (Accessed January 2015).
15. The Sterile Cockpit Rule Aviation Safety Reporting System (ASRS) (1993). Available at: http://asrs.arc.nasa.gov/publications/directline/dl4_sterile.htm (Accessed January 2015).
16. Starmer AJ, Sectish TC and Simon DW (2013). Rates of medical errors and preventable adverse events among hospitalized children following implementation of a resident handoff bundle. *JAMA* 310(21), 2262–2270.

17. Gordon M and Findley R (2011). Educational interventions to improve handover in health care: a systematic review. *Med. Educ.* 45(11), 1081–1089.
18. Heyland DK, Rocker GM and Dodek PM (2002). Family satisfaction with care in the intensive care unit: results of a multiple centre study. *Crit. Care Med.*, 30(7), 1413–1418.
19. Black MD, Vigorito MC and Curtis JR (2013). A multifaceted intervention to improve compliance with process measures for ICU clinician communication with ICU patients and families. *Crit. Care Med.*, 41, 2275–2283.
20. Davidson JE, Powers K and Hedayat KM (2007). Clinical practice guidelines for support of the family in the patient-centred intensive care unit: American College of Critical Care Medicine task force 2004–2005. *Crit. Care Med.*, 35(2), 605–622.

Part IV
Performance

Performance Standards and Measurement

Andre Carlos Kajdacsy-Balla Amaral and
Brian H. Cuthbertson
Chief of Critical Care Medicine,
Interdepartmental Division of Critical Care Medicine,
University of Toronto, Sunnybrook Health Sciences Centre

Key Points

1. Performance standards in healthcare use evidence to improve outcomes.
2. The ideal standard should be relevant, reliable and actionable.
3. Metrics should be carefully interpreted with rigorous methodological concepts.
4. Local quality improvement should rely on processes of care.
5. Public reporting of performance standards may have important unintended consequences.

What is a Performance Standard?

Interest in improving quality of care has increased in recent times. In the past few decades we borrowed ideas from the industry and other sectors and adapted them to our needs. We have embraced the industrial concept of measuring the quality of a product and comparing it to a certain standard.

In industry these standards and the factors that can be manipulated to determine them are obvious, such as delivering a shoe without defects, or the cost that it takes to produce a specific number of microprocessors. However, in healthcare it is not as simple, due to decreased availability of data on the product and processes, and the existence of a large number of variables outside of our control. For example, while the automobile industry is able to measure defects in every car that is produced, we struggle to even agree on what an important "defect" in healthcare means. Therefore we are still learning the best approaches to selecting, acquiring, and interpreting performance standards in healthcare.

Quality is defined by the International Organization for Standardization as "the totality of features and characteristics of a product or service that bears its ability to satisfy stated or implied needs" (ISO 8402:1986 standard).[1] Healthcare defines quality as "the degree to which health services for individuals and populations increase the likelihood of desired health outcomes and are consistent with current professional knowledge"[2] Therefore adherence to performance standards (current professional knowledge) should increase the likelihood of desired outcomes. Although necessarily vague, this definition emphasizes two fundamental aspects of measuring performance standards in healthcare: (1) the need to improve outcomes; and (2) the importance of evidence. Throughout this chapter we will focus on these two concepts to discuss measuring performance standards through evidence-based processes of care that should ultimately lead to improved outcomes.

Why measure performance standards?

"Count what is countable, measure what is measurable, and what is not measurable, make measurable" is frequently attributed to Galileo.[3] The ability to improve outcomes or processes of care is tied to the ability to measure them. This is not to say that all important determinants of quality can be measured, or that those that cannot be measured should be ignored. Deming, the grandfather of quality metrics, stated that "running a company on visible figures alone" is one of the seven deadly sins of management[4], and a good manager will constantly look at qualitative information, either from surveys or from informal conversations with stakeholders, to further improve their unit. However, metrics are required to demonstrate improvement or to detect deviations from expectations. Thus, performance standards include only those processes or outcomes that are measurable, while the totality of quality of care may also include other less tangible, but equally important processes and outcomes.

Governments, regulators, clinicians, insurance companies, and patients may be interested in different performance standards and these should reflect their relevance and validity to each stakeholder. Unfortunately, quality indicators are often selected based on convenience, feasibility, or politics rather than validity. In this chapter, we will try to define what the ideal characteristics of quality metrics should be and apply these principles to the current metrics proposed for intensive care medicine (ICM).

Characteristics of an Ideal Metric

An ideal performance standard should have three key characteristics: (1) it needs to be *relevant* to stakeholders; (2) it should be *reliable* when measured over time and in different facilities; and (3) clinicians and organizations must be able to *act in a timely manner on the standard* by changing behaviour or improving processes of care.

Relevance

Performance standards should measure outcomes that are relevant to some or all stakeholders, or processes of care and structure that are associated with these outcomes. Healthcare providers are frequently sceptical of standards not based on available scientific evidence. Standards not considered relevant by stakeholders are received with resistance and disregarded or subjected to data manipulation in conscious or unconscious ways.

While for most outcomes, such as mortality, the relevance is implicit, for processes of care and organizational structure it is mandatory to judge the level of the evidence before recommending a new performance standard. For example, one study demonstrated an association of night-time discharges with mortality in the intensive care unit (ICU),[5] however external validity was threatened by differences in healthcare systems, and the internal validity due to lack of risk adjustment for severity of illness at the time of discharge, a fact later confirmed in a multi-centred study.[6] In this situation it would be difficult to convince stakeholders that night time discharges is a good performance indicator. Another caveat is the use of performance standards that "make sense" and are not derived from empirical data. One such example outside ICU is the recommendation for select quality measures of skilled nursing facilities. While it "makes sense" to consider quality metrics such as "star rating" systems of staffing, independent inspection ratings and the proportion of residents with new or worsening pressure ulcers, investigators found no difference in the rates of hospital readmission or death when comparing more than 1,000,000 residents in "better" and "worse" facilities according to these standards.[7]

Reliability

A good performance standard should deliver the same results on repeated measurements. This is called reliability of a test. An unreliable performance standard should not be proposed to evaluate quality of care. An example of a reliable standard is the measurement of time to reach target cooling temperature after cardiac arrest. The time zero (hospital arrival) and the time of goal temperature are clearly defined and abstracted from charts. On the other hand, ventilator-associated pneumonia (VAP) rates are less reliable. A study comparing the identification of VAPs by two experienced providers, using the older Centres for Disease Control and Prevention (CDC) VAP definition observed a twofold variation in the total numbers of VAP. Based on these data, increases or decreases in VAP rates could be simply due to variation in interpretations of the CDC VAP definition.[8] For this reason the new definitions emphasize reliability[9]; however, this is offset by the apparent loss of relevance, as it seems that many clinically defined events are missed with the new metric.

Another important metric that passes the test for relevance, but fails on reliability is the measurement of risk adjusted mortality. While administrators and clinicians rate mortality as a highly relevant metric, they also understand that different units are difficult to compare, due to differences in severity of illness or case mix. What most fail to realize is that risk adjustment does not solve this problem for benchmarking, due to problems with (1) residual confounding and (2) differences in data sampling. Residual confounding is a term frequently used in observational studies to refer to the lack of complete adjustment for variables that are associated with mortality and the unit of interest, but are not measured. The lack of adjustment for these confounders makes it impossible to compare units. An interesting example of this is the fact that when multiple risk adjustment systems are used in a cohort of different ICUs, some units may be rated as high performer using one of the standards and as a low performer in another standard.[10] This obviously doesn't make any sense, and it relates to the different variables entered for risk adjustment in each system. Furthermore, many units collect data for risk adjustment directly from monitors, while others rely on the charted data. As the electronic data are more granular, more extreme variations of physiologic data may be captured and may suggest patients are "sicker" when compared to manual data collection,[11] which results in a 10% decrease in the standardized mortality ratio.

Actionable

Users and managers must be able to act on the performance metrics of interest directly and with timeliness. For example, although long-term quality of life in ICU survivors is a relevant outcome, it is a poorly actionable quality measure as its determinants are not yet fully understood, and may not be primarily determined by ICU processes of care. Also, indicators that are not under direct control of the providers are difficult to improve. For example, some experts recommend delayed ICU discharges as performance standards.[12] However, the main factor leading to delayed discharges, bed availability on the wards, is not under control of the ICU team and cannot be immediately managed.

On the other hand, indicators that measure compliance with evidence-based best practices are powerful tools for ICU managers, as gaps in quality can be immediately addressed with the team. Examples include use of deep venous thrombosis prophylaxis, use of lung protective ventilation for patients with acute respiratory distress syndrome, use of sedation minimization strategies and spontaneous breathing trials.

Relevant Epidemiological Concepts

Stakeholders address quality of care based on a panel of different performance standards. This is, in essence, drawing a causal inference between observed data, specifically the chosen performance standards, and "quality of care". Therefore, users should approach this problem with the same rigor used to address causality in research data, including assessment of chance, bias, regression to the mean, confounding and secular trends. Incorrect conclusions about quality are possible if these are ignored.

Chance

Consider comparing VAP rates in two different ICUs. Assume that, in reality, VAP rates are the same between units. At any given time period, it is plausible that unit A has a VAP rate of 10/1,000 mechanical ventilation days, while the unit B has a VAP rate of 4/1,000 mechanical ventilation days. This could be due to chance. To avoid this type of random error, quality indicators should be formally compared with statistical tests, to quantify the magnitude of the association that could be due to chance alone. This is usually demonstrated with ***p*-values** or **confidence intervals**, which gives us a sense of the probability that chance explains the results. In the example above, one unit could have 5 VAPs over 500 mechanical ventilation days and the other one over 250 days. Although the rates seem to be 2.5 times higher in the poorly performing ICU, the *p*-value in this case would be 0.12 and the 95% confidence interval of the relative risk would be from 0.39 to 16. These results would therefore be expected to occur by chance alone 1 out of every 8 measurements and the 2.5 times increase in VAP rates would also be compatible with an actual decrease in VAP of 60%. Analyses of rates are particularly unstable when studying rare events over short periods where a single event can lead to apparently large differences in rates.

Strategies to decrease chance include sampling a larger number of patients, choosing processes and outcomes that are more frequent and increasing the precision of measurements. For example, a continuous variable that measures the time to delivery of antibiotics is a more precise measure of quality than the proportion of patients that receive antibiotics in less than one hour and would require fewer patients to demonstrate differences in quality.

Bias

Bias is as a **systematic deviation** from the truth. While there are many sources of bias, there are fundamentally two types: non-differential and differential. Non-differential bias introduces noise but not a deviation into the measurement. For example, using physician documentation as the measure of VAP presumably would both over- and under-diagnose VAP depending on a variety of physician factors. The major problem with non-differential bias is that the noise introduced will obscure actual quality differences. To solve this problem, a protocol with objective parameters for detecting VAPs should be used.

Measuring performance standards in different ways is more problematic, as it may introduce differential biases. These are worse than non-differential biases because they create differences in the performance standards that are unrelated to quality of care. Differential biases can be subtle. If a standardized definition requires detection of bacteria in sputum, an ICU that has a policy of ordering sputum cultures for every febrile patient will have a higher VAP rate due to colonization than an ICU that has a protocol for selective ordering of sputum cultures.

Regression to the mean

Regression to the mean is a statistical phenomenon with important implications for the interpretation of changes in performance standards.[13] A typical example is to screen patients for high blood pressure and offer treatment to those with elevated values. Regardless of the efficacy of this treatment, the next set of blood pressures will be lower (and this is why we perform *placebo* controlled studies). The same phenomenon occurs in quality; however, there isn't a *placebo* group to control for the intervention, which creates a dilemma when selecting outcomes to improve or even hospitals with a perceived poor performance. Since the labeled outliers may not be real outliers, their ratings will improve in the next measurement regardless of the presence of a quality issue or the efficacy of the quality improvement project.

Many before–after quality improvement projects suffer from this potential error. One of the solutions to this problem is the use of serial measurements of performance standards as opposed to random audits. With serial measurements trends can be observed over time, either demonstrating consistently poor performance prior to an intervention or a real and sustained improvement after implementation.

Confounding

Confounders are variables associated both with the ICU and the performance standard of interest. For example, if it is known that patients with post-cardiovascular surgery are less prone to develop a VAP compared to patients intubated for shock, the comparison between units could be confounded if the patient demographics in the ICUs are very different (the cardiovascular unit will look "better" than the shock unit). Obviously, this is less of an issue when following a unit over time; however, changes in the case mix of an ICU over time could lead to the same problem. There are several approaches to deal with confounding. In quality the most common ones would be: (1) **restriction**, the exclusion of certain subsets of patients where the quality measure is known to be more or less common; and (2) **adjustment**, using mathematical models to "balance" confounding variables. The most common approach is the use a severity of illness measure to adjust the risk of death in analyzing mortality differences between ICUs. However, as we discussed before, there is always the possibility of residual confounding, making interpretation of risk adjusted performance standards very difficult.

Secular trends

Performance standards change over time for reasons other than quality improvement projects. These secular trends are not a problem when trying to demonstrate that quality is improving over time; but may be misleading when used to attribute improvements to a specific intervention. An excellent example of this problem can be seen from the original description of the central line bundle to decrease central line infections (CLI).[14] The study showed a significant decrease in CLI rates, from 2.7 to 0 per 1,000 catheter-days. The data are probably correct, but at the same time CLIs were decreasing in other units that were not implementing this bundle.[15] Therefore, there is a real decrease in CLI rates over time, but the intervention may not be the cause, as rates were declining due to secular trends. To solve this problem when trying to infer causality, different models of analysis, beyond the scope of this chapter, should be used, such as an interrupted time series or controlled interrupted time series.

Performance Standards to Improve Healthcare

Standards may be used to monitor and improve quality for a single organization or for more than one organization, such as in integrated healthcare systems. Reporting may be regional or national.

Local performance standards

Individual organizations should focus on processes of care. These items are relevant and actionable at the local level. The decision to monitor, measure and improve should be based on mission and vision of the organization, the patient population and informally identified gaps by stakeholders. Organizations can and should focus on a limited number of relevant processes of care per period, to avoid conflicting messages and wasted efforts. Individual organizations can define the best metric for their processes based on data availability. Examples of processes of care that may be useful for improvement include use of lung protective ventilation, minimization of sedation, compliance with targeted temperature management post-cardiac arrest, early mobility, deep venous thrombosis (DVT) prophylaxis, pain assessment and management, initiation of end-of-life discussions, amongst others.

Systems reporting of performance standards

There is a growing interest in using performance standards to identify high and low quality performers at a systems level, which would prompt actions to help low performers to improve. However, the relationship between public reporting and improved outcomes is not very clear. There are reports of decreased mortality after cardiac surgery since the introduction of the New York State public reporting system in 1991.[16] However, concurrent data from other states without public reporting, demonstrated a similar improvement, questioning the benefits of the state wide reporting system.[17]

Public reporting may create incentives to improve performance, but does not necessarily direct providers on how to improve. Standards can improve through the implementation of evidence-based practices, data manipulation or avoidance high-risk patients.

Other unintended consequences include improperly diagnosing and treating patients to improve a standard. For example, the Infectious Diseases Society of America recommended the administration of antimicrobials within four hours of admission for patients with pneumonia, a standard that was public reported in the US. The recommendation and reporting led to bizarre consequences, such as antimicrobials being administered before obtaining imaging,[18] and an increase in antimicrobial utilization for patients without pneumonia.[19]

Furthermore, standards can also be seen as diagnostic tests for how "healthy" a system is. In this framework, performance is a "test" used to diagnose whether an ICU has high quality or not. We can apply the same criteria of validity, reliability, chance, confounding and bias to see if the application of performance standards can be used to identify quality. Unfortunately, using simulations Hofer demonstrated that both sensitivities and positive predictive values are inadequate. Depending on the case mix, sensitivities would range from 8% to 10% (that is approximately 90% of low performers would not be detected) and positive predictive values would range from 16% to 24% (which means that 76–84% of units classified as low performers would actually be average or high performers).[20]

It is still unclear whether there is value in public reporting of performance standards either in driving the market to use high quality centres or in motivating quality improvement. However, it is clear that payers, governments, and consumers are likely to demand these reports in the future.

References

1. Quality management and quality assurance — Vocabulary. ISO 8402:1994 (2015). Available at: http://www.iso.org/iso/catalogue_detail.htm?csnumber=20115 (Accessed 17 July 2015).
2. Lohr KN and Schroeder SA (1990). A strategy for quality assurance in medicare. *N. Engl. J. Med.*, 322(10), 707–712.
3. Kaydos WJ (1999). *Operational Performance Measurement: Increasing Total Productivity.* St Lucile Press, Boca Raton, FL.
4. Deming WE (2000). *Out of the Crisis*, 1st Edition. MIT Press, Cambridge, MA.
5. Laupland KB, Shahpori R, Kirkpatrick AW and Stelfox HT (2008). Hospital mortality among adults admitted to and discharged from intensive care on weekends and evenings. *J. Crit. Care*, 23(3), 317–324.
6. Santamaria JD, Duke GJ and Pilcher DV (2015). The timing of discharge from the intensive care unit and subsequent mortality. A prospective, multicenter study. *Am. J. Respir. Crit. Care Med.*, 191(9), 1033–1039.
7. Neuman MD, Wirtalla C and Werner RM (2014). Association between skilled nursing facility quality indicators and hospital readmissions. *JAMA*, 312(15), 1542–1551.
8. Klompas M (2010). Interobserver variability in ventilator-associated pneumonia surveillance. *Am. J. Infect. Control*, 38(3), 237–239.
9. Klompas M, Magill S and Robicsek A (2012). Objective surveillance definitions for ventilator-associated pneumonia. *Crit. Care Med.*, 40(12), 3154–3161.
10. Glance LG, Osler TM and Dick A (2002). Rating the quality of intensive care units: is it a function of the intensive care unit scoring system? *Crit. Care Med.*, 30(9), 1976–1982.
11. Suistomaa M, Kari A, Ruokonen E and Takala J (2000). Sampling rate causes bias in APACHE II and SAPS II scores. *Intens. Care Med.*, 26(12), 1773–1778.
12. de Vos M, Graafmans W and Keesman E, (2007). Quality measurement at intensive care units: which indicators should we use? *J. Crit. Care*, 22(4), 267–274.
13. Morton V and Torgerson DJ (2003). Effect of regression to the mean on decision-making in health care. *BMJ*, 326(7398), 1083–1084.
14. Pronovost P, Needham D and Berenholtz S (2006). An intervention to decrease catheter-related bloodstream infections in the ICU. *N. Engl. J. Med.*, 355, 2725–2732.
15. Zuschneid I, Schwab F and Geffers C (2003). Reducing central venous catheter-associated primary bloodstream infections in intensive care units is possible: data from the German nosocomial infection surveillance system. *Infect Control Hosp. Epidemiol*, 24(7), 501–505.

16. Hannan EL, Kumar D and Racz M (1994). New York state's cardiac surgery reporting system: four years later. *Ann. Thorac. Surg.*, 58(6), 1852–1857.
17. Ghali WA, Ash AS, Hall RE and Moskowitz MA (1997). Statewide quality improvement initiatives and mortality after cardiac surgery. *JAMA*, 277(5), 379–382.
18. Pines JM, Isserman JA and Hinfey PB (2009). The measurement of time to first antibiotic dose for pneumonia in the emergency department: a white paper and position statement prepared for the american academy of emergency medicine. *J. Emerg. Med.*, 37(3), 335–340.
19. Welker JA, Huston M and McCue JD (2008). Antibiotic timing and errors in diagnosing pneumonia. *Arch. Intern. Med.*, 168(4), 351–356.
20. Hofer TP and Hayward RA (1996). Identifying poor-quality hospitals. Can hospital mortality rates detect quality problems for medical diagnoses? *Med. Care.*, 34(8), 737–753.

Methods of Control

Robert C. McDermid
Clinical Professor, Division of Critical Care, Department of Medicine, Faculty of Medicine and Dentistry, University of British Columbia
Yvonne I. Csanyi-Fritz
Associate Clinical Professor, Division of Pediatric Anesthesia, Department of Anesthesiology, Pharmacology and Therapeutics, Faculty of Medicine and Dentistry, University of British Columbia

Key Points

1. Healthcare must be radically redesigned with a focus on delivery of systematically integrated high-quality care.
2. The Structure–Process–Outcome framework allows the components of care within the intensive care unit (ICU) to be analyzed in order to develop control over the quality of healthcare delivery.
3. The organization of the ICU in terms of composition, staffing and leadership provides the foundation for consistency of high-quality care.
4. The time-dependent nature of critical care (CC) therapy requires a hospital wide integrated approach to the flow of patients into and out of the ICU in order to ensure capacity and optimal use of resources.
5. The three phases of care — *resuscitation, support, and liberation* require different tools and approaches to ensure consistent performance.

Introduction

"Fifteen years ago, Israeli scientists published a study in which engineers observed patient care in ICUs for 24 hour stretches. They found that the average patient required 178 individual actions per day, ranging from administering a drug to suctioning the lungs, and every one of them posed risks. Remarkably, the nurses and doctors were observed to make an error in just 1% of these actions but that still amounted to an average of two errors a day with every patient. Critical Care (CC) succeeds only when we hold the odds of doing harm low enough for the odds of doing good to prevail."

"The volume and complexity of what we know has exceeded our individual ability to deliver its benefits correctly, safely, or reliably".

These excerpts from Gawande's, 'The Checklist Manifesto: How To Get Things Right[1] identify one of the greatest challenges facing modern medicine, that is the complexity and interdependency of the many processes that are required for the delivery of effective care. The pathway to the medical successes of the past, which were predicated on the autonomy, courage and self-sufficiency of physicians, will no longer lead to success in the 21st century. Healthcare delivery must be radically redesigned in the face of exponentially increasing knowledge and costs.

Societal expectations in developed nations also create challenges for the healthcare systems of these countries. In an interview with the Harvard Public Health Review, Weinstein[2] stated that 90% of people in the US:

- Want the best available medical care regardless of cost.
- Think that healthcare is too expensive.
- Think healthcare should be available for everyone.

These ostensibly conflicting beliefs require reconciliation. In response to these conflicts, the Institute for Health Innovation (IHI) has developed its "Triple Aim" framework, which addresses three critical dimensions of healthcare: (1) improving the patient experience of care (including quality and satisfaction); (2) improving the health of populations; and (3) reducing the per capita cost of healthcare. Fortunately, as demonstrated by some notable case studies, high-quality care also results in reduced costs. Regardless of whether the economic model under which a healthcare system operates is socialized, universal healthcare or for profit medicine, the finite nature of the resources that are available for healthcare requires fiscal awareness and responsibility, if the model is to be sustainable. As expressed by Cassel in 1982, it is the duty of a physician to focus jointly on cure of disease and relief of suffering — ignoring this latter component can compound suffering.[3] It is perhaps by focusing on the patient experience of care through an exploration of a multi-dimensional model of suffering that the "best" care (rather than interpreting this as equivalent to the "most expensive") can actually be delivered.

In critical care medicine (CCM), complexity and interdependence of processes coexist with two additional challenges: (1) many therapies in ICU are time-dependent for their efficacy, and (2) many patients in the ICU are extremely vulnerable, and their ability to tolerate the adverse consequences of errors is low. When Peter Safar established the first ICU in North America in 1958, his expressed mandate was to "save the hearts and minds of those too young to die" through timely and appropriate institution of cardiopulmonary resuscitation and advanced life support.[4] Today, the primary goal of advanced life support in ICU is "to prevent unnecessary suffering and premature death by treating reversible illnesses for an appropriate period of time".[5] In comparison to its much more humble beginnings, advanced life support has now become extremely sophisticated, allowing physicians to prolong life in circumstances that were not possible in the recent past. Unfortunately, the ability to predict outcome and hence allocate resources in concrete and accountable ways has not kept pace with technological advancements and their exponentially growing costs.

What is clear is that high-quality CCM in the modern era demands processes that consistently deliver accurate therapy rapidly to every bedside, every time. As previously mentioned, the business aspect of CCM also demands rapidity and accuracy of the processes that deliver effective care to patients if it is to be sustainable.

What is Quality?

Quality has been described as being comprised of five different dimensions: (1) excellence, (2) perfection or consistency, (3) value for money,

(4) fitness for purpose, and (5) transformative potential.[6] In the context of medicine, the first three described static features of quality related to the output and fiscal accountability of specific processes, and are captured by the recently appearing references to quality as "Right First Time" that have begun to appear in medicine journals.[7] The concept of "fitness for purpose" suggests a different expression of quality: one that reflects the importance of ensuring that the healthcare system is designed to meet societal needs, and requires a conscious ongoing re-evaluation of the healthcare system's deliverables with respect to societal expectations and demands. Together, these four dimensions are related to quality control and quality assurance in medicine.

The last dimension — transformative potential — is related to identifying and realizing opportunities for improvement in processes. This is perhaps the most important, transcendent dimension, in that it captures the dynamic, changing nature of medicine, and its modern foundational principles of innovation, discovery and continuous quality improvement. While quality control, assurance and quality improvement are inextricably linked and necessary in modern medicine, quality improvement is outside the scope of this chapter.

Quality Control and Quality Assurance

While CC services commonly generate a tremendous amount of data, it can be very difficult to measure the quality of care that an individual ICU provides. Clinicians have traditionally been most concerned with outcomes of care. However, making these outcome measures useful in terms of guiding daily practice is challenging. As an example, standardized mortality rates are commonly used to compare performance across ICUs, but death statistics are influenced by many factors, including patient volume, admission diagnosis, severity of illness, and as such may be misleading. Adjustments are made to control for variables that are known to have consistent effects on the outcomes of patients, but many other variables, such as lead time, emergency status and referral source, as well as many unmeasured factors, contribute to outcome for an individual patient. When examining the impact of interventions or changes in practice within the ICU, the relatively low frequency and complex nature of mortality in the ICU implies that a time delay will necessarily exist before the effect of the change on mortality can be recognized. While standardized mortality rates are crucial markers to follow to ensure overall quality of care, the numbers of patients admitted and deaths that subsequently occur in most ICUs do not lend themselves to data streams that will be useful in guiding process management. In fact, simulation models have suggested that standard mortality rates take upwards of two years to reach statistically detectable levels of change with an acceptable false positive rate for average size ICUs.[8,9] For these reasons, it may be more useful to track these sorts of data on a regional level to obtain the volume of admissions and outcomes required for meaningful analysis. While there is no question if it is essential to follow outcome measures, we must look to other techniques and metrics if we are to create actionable data within an individual ICU.

The Structure–Process–Outcome framework, described in the seminal medical quality article by Avedis Donabedian in 1966, provides an approach to this task.[10] This framework first considers the elements that are required to deliver high-quality care. These are termed the *structural components* of quality, such as full body drapes and chlorhexidine cleaning solution for the prevention of central line infections. The framework then examines the circumstances and methods through which these structural components are applied, which are termed the *process components.* The objective is to make these structural components of high-quality care systematically, consistently and immediately available during the tasks for which they are required. Finally, the framework requires establishing of *outcome components.* In contrast to clinical outcomes (such as rate of central line associated blood stream infections and deep vein thrombosis (DVT) in critically ill patients), events related to process measures (like adherence with central line insertion protocols, and utilization of DVT prophylaxis) occur much more frequently. Furthermore, while there is often a time delay between the adverse event and the specific clinical outcome, process measures can be followed in real time. This provides foundation for continuous quality improvement by creating the opportunity for frontline staff to measure and act upon live data that are associated with desired clinical outcomes.

In the manufacturing industry, it is critical to ensure that products created by the various manufacturing processes meet required standards.

There are two subtly different yet complementary approaches to this problem: quality control, which focuses on detection and rejection of defective products that do not meet the standards; and quality assurance, which emphasizes the importance of error detection early in the process to avoid wasted materials and effort. In the past, there has been significant emphasis on quality control measures in medicine, such as using two client identifiers prior to providing any service or procedure, as a "final check". However, with the growing awareness of the costs of medicine, interest in avoidance of waste is rising, and focus is beginning to shift towards quality assurance metrics and techniques and the concept of *process control.*

Process Control

In the early part of the 20th century, academics developed interest and knowledge regarding methods to improve efficiency and accuracy of manufacturing processes. Mathematical physicist W. Edwards Deming believed that the management of a system of processes determined far more of the overall quality of the output than the individual processes themselves. Together with his mentor, the engineer, statistician and physicist Walter A Shewhart, he examined the effects of variation on manufacturing quality through mathematical modeling and statistics, and pioneered the field of process control.

Modern process control is an engineering discipline that deals with maintaining the output of a specific process within a desired range. It is the foundation of modern quality assurance and quality control, and involves monitoring the components of a process for variability to decide whether the process is stable. Once stable, a process can be modified to optimize its output in terms of quality and efficiency. Process control is very useful in the practice of acute care medicine, as it is important to ensure processes are appropriately activated and sequenced if timely and accurate delivery of the intended therapies is to occur in a fiscally responsible manner.

Prerequisites for process control

Process control has several prerequisites with respect to its applicability to the practice of medicine. Similar to the Structure–Process–Outcome framework, the current processes must be (1) mapped, (2) standardized and (3) measured. Process mapping is essential in order to understand exactly what is being done currently to create the outcome of interest. The value of careful examination of the details of the processes in question should not be underestimated. Tremendous opportunities for waste reduction, efficiency improvement and quality assurance and/or control are often evident through process mapping, even at an early stage.

Following process mapping, standardization of appropriate processes should be undertaken. For any given output, a standardized process that is well designed will facilitate monitoring, evaluation and modification of the process more easily than one that is not standardized. However, enthusiasm should be tempered for universal standardization. One must not forget the importance of avoiding the standardization of deleterious care, as was demonstrated by the adverse outcomes associated with worldwide acceptance and generalization of the positive results of Van den Berghe's paper on tight glycemic control in post-operative cardiac surgical patients, which were later refuted for general CC in the Normoglycemia in Intensive Care Evaluation and Surviving Using Glucose Algorithm Regulation (NICE-SUGAR) study.[11,12]

Tasks that benefit from standardization include those requiring a narrow range of skills or equipment, and lend themselves to structured work. An example in the ICU would be the process to obtain daily laboratory investigations. By standardizing the timing of phlebotomy, the required investigations, and the process of sample delivery, savings both in term of human and economic resources could be realized. However, an attempt to standardize the mode of mechanical ventilation for all patients in an ICU would sacrifice the necessary individualization of care for those patients who respond poorly to the standard mode or method of ventilation, potentially resulting in worsened outcomes. The ICU of the future may do well to define explicitly a model under which "flow" tasks (where a narrow range of tasks are standardized and efficiency is the key) coexist with but are distinct from "job" tasks (where individualization, creativity and flexibility are required).

Finally, appropriate and meaningful metrics must be chosen. There is a management truism with respect to quality in healthcare: "you can't manage what you don't measure".

What are some useful tools to guide process control?

In keeping with the approach mentioned above, three of the seven basic tools of quality initially popularized by Ishikawa in 1985[13] are very useful in process control: fishbone charts, Pareto charts, and control charts. *Fishbone charts*, also known as Ishikawa diagrams, are often used to deconstruct processes (Figure 1). With this tool, the various components of a task are categorized and mapped under headings such as equipment, materials, people, environment, processes, and management.

Pareto charts are based upon the concept of the Pareto principle, also known as the "80/20 rule" or the "rule of the vital few and the trivial many". This principle is essential to understanding both quality and error in medicine. Simply put, the Pareto principle holds that 80% of effects are due to 20% of the causes and understanding that 20% will reduce error and improve quality. In medicine, Pareto charts are useful to prioritize the causes of process failure such as the reasons underlying delayed or missed diagnostic tests. In the prior example of early defibrillation for ventricular fibrillation, applying the Pareto principle would allow one to focus attention of those sources of error that are maximally contributing to the undesired outcome. Once the errors are categorized and root causes of single or multiple events are determined through techniques such as fishbone charts, Six Sigma or Lean methodologies, the Pareto principle is then

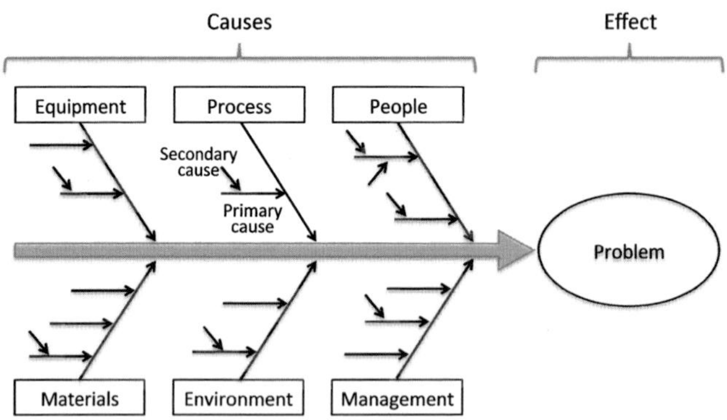

Figure 1. Fishbone (or Ishikawa) diagram.[13]

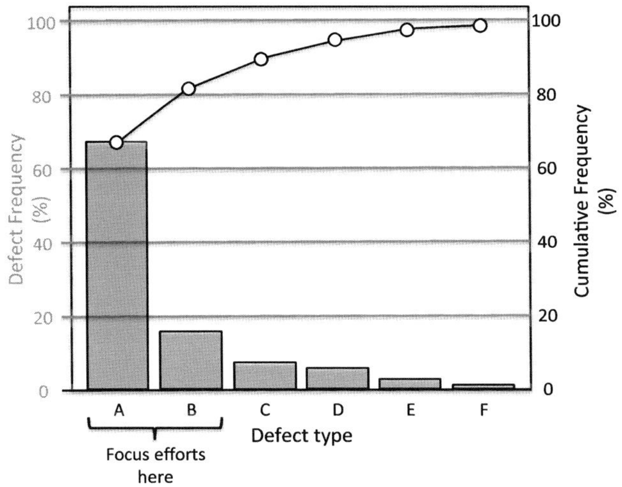

Figure 2. Pareto chart.

applied to quantify the categories of error and narrow the suite of possible interventions (Figure 2).

Control charts are used in a subset of process control, termed *statistical process control*, where statistical analysis is used to separate common cause (or inherent) variability of a process from special cause (or extrinsic) variability imposed upon a process by outside influences. These charts typically have a centreline (mean) and control limits (usually set at three times the standard error above and below the mean). Data points outside of these control limits suggest a special cause. The utility of this approach lies within the fact that different actions are required to deal with the two kinds of variability. Common cause variation is addressed through modification of the process under consideration, whereas special cause variation requires that the extrinsic cause be identified and altered. A recent systematic review identified anaesthesiology and CC as the fields with the highest number of citations related to statistical process control in healthcare emphasizing the importance of this particular tool for ICU management.[14] Commonly used metrics that use control charts are plots of glycemic control and ventilator-associated pneumonia (VAP) rates over time that include upper and lower confidence error lines.

Factors to consider in developing effective process control

To develop effective care processes, two main components must be considered: human factors and engineering factors. While these factors have often been considered independently, a recent shift in theory regarding organizational development suggests that both factors are inextricably interrelated. The traditional perspective, termed *diagnostic organizational development*, ascribes to the principle that change management can be accomplished through an evaluation of the present state of an organization, along with the creation of a future state vision, followed by the development of an algorithmic plan to affect the necessary change. A new theory, termed *dialogic organizational development*, begins from the perspective that an institution is a socially co-created reality; an institution cannot be separated from the people who comprise it. This theory invokes three principles necessary for wide scale change: (1) the past state is no longer possible or acceptable, (2) the institutional narrative has changed, and (3) a generative image has emerged.

These theories provide complementary frameworks under which change management can be analyzed. However, the dialogic theory emphasizes the importance of the people and human agency associated with the processes. Within the context of medicine, dialogic theory provides for new, emergent processes to develop out of widescale organizational change. While it is beyond the scope of this chapter to discuss change management strategies and human factor analysis in detail, the topic warrants a brief discussion. It is crucial to recognize that process control measures will not be effective in the practice of CCM if the desired outputs cannot be altered in response to the changing nature of medicine and the changing context in which the treatments are being delivered.

Human factors

Human factors analysis is a growing discipline with roots in the applied engineering and refinements in the field of aviation. Applied human factors analysis shows great promise within medicine in the design of technological features of modern equipment and the communication and interaction among healthcare team members. As disparate as these two attributes of human factors analysis may sound, they have strong analogues in aviation; human factor principles are integral to the design of cockpits and instrumentation (including warning systems and alarms), and crew resource management, the latter having developing into its own subspecialty of analysis. In medicine, human factor analysis has only recently received attention in the design of equipment, such as infusion pumps and anesthesia machines. It has also been applied to the communication and interaction in operating rooms necessary to complete a surgical safety checklist. For some years, human factor analysis has been incorporated into simulation training, such as mock codes, to evaluate team functioning and situational awareness.

Perhaps the most important and relevant contribution of human factor analysis is the development of the Hierarchy of Intervention Effectiveness. In brief, the Hierarchy of Intervention Effectiveness posits that all interventions can be ranked in a gradient of outcome effectiveness, with education and training being the least effective and force functioning the most effective intervention modality and occupying the apex of the hierarchy. Understanding and utilizing the Hierarchy of Intervention Effectiveness enables the design of better interventions to improvement outcomes, with force functioning (where you are forced to do it the right way every time) being the best of all designs.

Most of our historical interventions in healthcare have been people-focused, with the attendant vulnerabilities that accompany all human dependent systems. As all of medicine becomes increasingly more reliant on technology to perform routine, repetitive, and complex tasks, we run the risk of the technology outpacing our ability to communicate effectively in situations requiring complex human interaction and teamwork. Human factor analysis can help to structure the communication, aid in its sequencing and script the responses needed to produce the desired outcome.

Prevalence/consequence framework

One framework that allows a determination of the kinds of process control measures that are necessary for a given circumstance considers two factors: the *prevalence* with which the process is activated, and the *consequences* of having an error occur during the process.

Consider a time-dependent, high consequence process such as early defibrillation for ventricular fibrillation. Ensuring the arrival of a highly skilled team with a defibrillator and other appropriate equipment required to resuscitate a patient suffering an in-hospital cardiac arrest within 3 minutes of the call demands a very high fidelity, efficient process. The consequences of errors in the process are severe — death of the patient is virtually certain if the initial process fails. Hence, a large investment of human and capital resources to ensure this process works every time without error is substantial.

On the other hand, delivery of the appropriate routine medications to each patient in an ICU is extremely complex and requires many steps. Fortunately, although this is very common, these processes are able to tolerate multiple checks and balances to ensure the correct medication is delivered to each patient — often the consequences of the wrong medication being dispensed outweigh those of slight delays in actual time of administration. Furthermore, the costs of designing sequential and redundant, moderately high fidelity processes are often much lower than designing a single process with the required ultra high fidelity necessary to achieve the desired outcome (Figure 3).

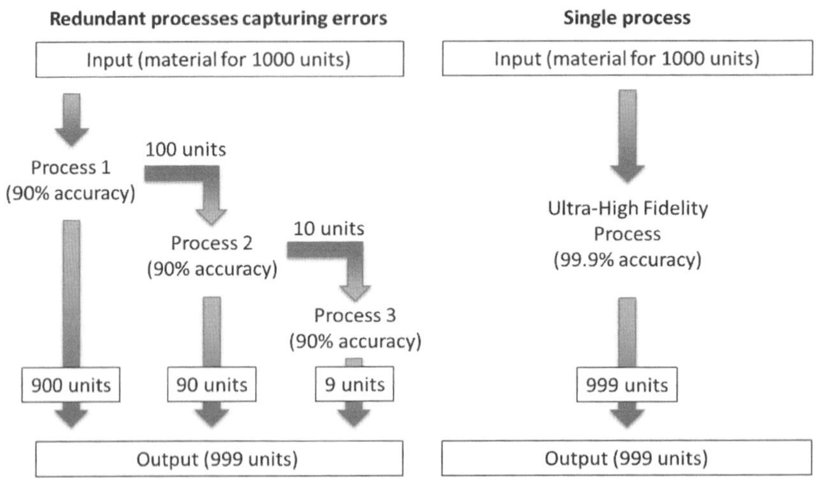

Figure 3. Single versus redundant processes.

ICU organization and integration as the foundation for control of performance

Despite its cross-disciplinary beginnings, CCM has evolved over the past 50 years into a distinct specialty in many countries, including those in Europe, North America, and Australia. Within the CC environment, the shift from individual practitioners caring for patients in an open ICU model to intensivist-led, multi-disciplinary team-based coordinated bedside rounds in a closed-unit model has been shown to improve outcomes and reduce mortality in critically ill patients.[15] Many international societies, including the European Society for Intensive Care Medicine, the Society for Critical Care Medicine and the Canadian Critical Care Society, now actively support the closed unit model of care within the ICU. Given the high dependence of care process initiation on physician orders, the presence of qualified and certified CC physicians forming the core of the CC service of a hospital is an essential cornerstone of ICU performance.

Although there is not complete consistency, many CC societies support standards with respect to CC physician availability, work patterns, continuity of care, physician/patient ratios, and leadership. Standards for nursing care also exist with respect to training, education, nurse/patient ratios, contingency planning for surge capacity, nursing leadership presence and availability, and utilization of agency (non-staff) nurses. Additionally, despite the identification of the CC physician as the leader of the multi-disciplinary team, the membership of the team is also critically important. The presence of the bedside nurse as a facilitator of patient- and family-centred care has been recognized. The inclusion of pharmacist as part of the multi-disciplinary team has been shown to avoid drug interactions and errors and reduce medication expenditures. Complications such as critical illness neuropathy/myopathy are reduced, with a concomitant reduction in ICU length of stay when physiotherapist-guided early mobilization strategies are employed. Daily input from medical microbiology provides a framework for empiric therapy of sepsis, and adds the content expertise for antimicrobial stewardship initiatives. Given the importance of nutritional support with respect to recovery from critical illness, the presence of dietitians on rounds is also advocated.

Finally, due to the previously mentioned time-dependent nature of CC therapies, patient flow is a crucial aspect of care that must be considered in an approach to control of performance. Both admission and discharge from the ICU should occur in a timely fashion once the decision to transfer into or out of the ICU is made. Further to admission, the need for a hospital-wide standardized approach to the deteriorating inpatient is crucial, as failure to rescue patients from complications (rather than the incidence of complications themselves) has been identified as a primary difference separating high-performing hospitals from those with low performance.[16] And lastly, as timely admission is crucial, timely and standardized transfer out of CC permits efficient use of existing CC capacity. Nonetheless, processes must be designed to avoid nocturnal discharge from ICU, as care fragmentation and adverse outcomes result from transfers that occur after hours.

Phases of Care as a Framework for Achieving Control of Performance

There are three philosophically distinct but functionally overlapping phases of care in the management of the critically ill patient: the resuscitative phase, the maintenance phase and the liberation phase. With respect to process control, each of the phases requires different tools and different approaches. The resuscitative phase, during which patients who suffer acute, catastrophic deterioration are rescued from imminent death, requires the arrival of a skilled team armed with the necessary equipment to deliver the specific and necessary time-dependent therapies to prevent adverse outcomes. The support phase, during which patients receive ongoing somatic support to allow time for healing, demands frequent and systematic review of the patients' status to titrate and modify therapies to optimize physiologic function. The liberation phase, during which patients' readiness for discontinuation of somatic support is tested, benefits from protocols to avoid unnecessary delays in removal of life supportive technology.

Process control: resuscitative phase

The early resuscitative phase of care for critically illness requires timely intervention and close attention to the rapidly changing status of the patient. The immediate availability of specialized acute care teams, such as rapid response teams and trauma teams, has beneficial effects on the care of deteriorating in-patients and multiply injured patients respectively, although the magnitude of benefit, associated costs and unintended consequences of these teams is debated.

Consistently, the resuscitative process involves concurrent assessment and institution of treatment prior to obtaining complete clarity regarding patient diagnosis, and clear, structured communication in this setting is necessary. The Situation — Background — Assessment — Recommendation (SBAR) tool has been promoted by the IHI to improve the quality and efficiency of information transfer between members of the healthcare team. This includes the rapid institution of supportive therapy based upon patterns of clinical presentation rather than upon diagnostic certainty. Standardized order sets reduce unnecessary variation in care, and have the potential to improve outcomes if properly designed. These should be developed for commonly encountered clinical problems such as hospital or community acquired pneumonia, sepsis, exacerbations of chronic obstructive airways disease, and respiratory failure requiring mechanical ventilation, and should include recommendations for empiric antimicrobial therapy based upon knowledge of local patterns of microbial resistance.

Finally, standardized handovers are important. Transitions in care are commonly associated with errors and loss of information. Structured communication during transfer of care, either from a resuscitating team to a management team, or from the treating team to the on-call team, builds consistency and reliability into this period of patient vulnerability.

Process control: support phase

Once the early resuscitative phase ends, the majority of care decisions are made during intensivist-led multi-disciplinary patient care rounds. This is due to the need for frequent but systematic reassessment of all developing and ongoing care requirements during the support phase. Facilitators of high quality bedside rounds were identified in a systematic review of best practices as: (1) standardizing the structure of rounds, and (2) utilizing quality checklists that focused on the discussion and documentation of daily goals of therapy. On the other hand, poor documentation and inconsistent information retrieval, long rounding times and interruptions in addition to team fragmentation are significant barriers to effective rounding.

The concept of checklists in medicine have been emphasized by Gawande[1] and Peter Pronovost'.[17] The use of carefully designed checklists in CC has been shown to reduce central line associated blood stream infections, prevent nosocomial Methicillin-resistant *Staphylococcus aureus* transmission, reduce the incidence of nosocomial *Clostridium difficile* infection, and improve ICU mortality.[17,18] The mechanism of benefit is felt to be due to the reduction in unnecessary variability by deconstructing a process into its component tasks and standardizing those that are amenable to standardization.

Process control: liberation phase

Once patients have been resuscitated and stabilized, the somatic support needs require re-evaluation on a regular basis, if complications related to unnecessary support are to be avoided. Life supportive therapy is dangerous for those who do not require it, and attention should be paid to rapid de-escalation of therapy. For example, nurse-driven analgesia and sedation protocols, daily sedation interruption, and spontaneous breathing trials with standardized application of objective tests of readiness for liberation from mechanical ventilation all contribute to reductions in duration of ventilatory support and ICU length of stay. Given the linkage between duration of mechanical ventilation, the incidence of VAP, ICU length of stay and mortality, interventions that prevent the introduction of unnecessary variability in the duration of mechanical ventilation are very important both from a quality of care and economic perspective.

The Future, and CC as a "State of Mind"

In a presentation in 2012 entitled "How do we heal medicine?" Atul Gawande described the fundamental shift in philosophy that is demanded of practitioners of medicine.[19]

In every field, knowledge has exploded, but it has brought complexity, it has brought specialization and we have come to a place where we have no choice but to recognize, as individualistic as we want to be, complexity requires group success.

The radical redesign that is required involves the integration of care processes into a comprehensive, seamless and individualized care plan that guides a patient's journey from presentation to convalescence and reintegration into the community. The CC patient experiences the greatest departure from health, and consequently, requires the most inclusive and broad reaching care plan. This integration of services and processes requires stability and predictability of its component parts. By extension, attention must be placed upon developing robust mechanisms to ensure that quality of care is maintained in the face of ever-shifting demands and increasing knowledge. Continuous quality improvement demands inquisitiveness along with the willingness and ability to adapt to changing circumstances and change our way of working. However, change is not necessarily synonymous with improvement. Through the aforementioned approaches to control of performance in ICU, it is possible to understand the component tasks that comprise care processes, discriminate between those that are effective and those that are unstable, and focus attention on the aspects of care where change is likely to provide the greatest positive impact.

The future of healthcare will place new demands upon healthcare providers and will require different skills. This is being recognized and addressed in the shift towards competency-based medical education, which strives to create physicians who will be responsive to changing face of healthcare and will have the skills necessary to maintain competence throughout their career. This involves providing a standardized foundation for learning, while identifying the needs of individual trainees as they prepare for independent practice. Ultimately, the CC physicians of tomorrow must be also skilled communicators, capable of working in multi-disciplinary teams; they must be fluent in the language required to communicate effectively with boards of trustees, senior executives and administrators, clinical chairs and chiefs, patients, and staff; they must be excel in the all aspects of the cross-disciplinary time-dependent care that is required. As eloquently stated by Dr. Ashish Khanna and Dr. Lewis Kaplan in an opinion piece published on the Society of Critical Care website[20]:

A good intensivist must have the keen observation of a pediatrician, the patience of an obstetrician, the thoughtfulness of a physician, the rapid reflexes of an anesthesiologist, the aggressiveness of a surgeon, and the communication skills of a psychiatrist. Synthesizing all of these skills is the intensivist, who crosses specialty boundaries and knowledge lines and provides dedicated team direction, while offering emotional support, empathy and compassion throughout critical illness and injury management. It is clear that individuals with various backgrounds may embody such attributes. While the future holds the promise of expanding the number of intensivists, our current deficit compels us to explore and embrace all who may serve patients by driving team-based care in the ICU. Truly, CC is more than a medical or surgical specialty — it is a state of mind.

References

1. Gawande A (2009). *The Checklist Manifesto: How to Get Things Right.* Metropolitan Books, New York.
2. Weinstein M (2010). *Can Cost-Effective Health Care = Better Health Care?* Available at: http://www.hsph.harvard.edu/news/magazine/winter10assessment/.
3. Cassel EJ (1982). The nature of suffering and the goals of medicine. *N. Engl. J. Med.*, 306, 639–645.
4. Lenzer J (2003). Peter Josef Safar: the father of cardiopulmonary resuscitation. *Brit. Med.*, 327, 624–625.
5. Singer PA, Barker G and Bowman KW (2001). Hospital policy on appropriate use of life-sustaining treatment. University of Toronto Joint Centre for bioethics/critical care medicine program task force. *Crit. Care Med.*, 29, 187–191.
6. Harvey L (2006). Understanding quality. In *EUA Bologna Handbook: Making Bologna Work*, Froment E, Kohler J, Purser L and Wilson L (eds.). Raabe Academic Publishers, Berlin.
7. Gulliford S (2010). Harmless cuts in health care. Right first time, every time. *BMJ*, 340, 1846.
8. Koetsier A, de Keizer NF and de Jonge E (2012). Performance of risk-adjusted control charts to monitor in-hospital mortality of intensive care unit patients: A simulation study. *Crit. Care Med.*, 40, 1799–1807.
9. Foltran F, Baldi I and Bertolini G (2009). Monitoring the performance of intensive care units using the variable life-adjusted display: a simulation study to explore its applicability and efficiency. *J. Eval. Clin. Pract.*, 15, 506–513.

10. Donabedian A (1966). Evaluating the quality of medical care. *Milbank Memorial Fund Q.*, 44, 166–203.
11. Van den Berghe G, Wouters P and Weekers F (2001). Intensive insulin therapy in critically ill patients. *N. Engl. J. Med.*, 345, 1359–1367.
12. Finfer S, Chittock DR, Su SY and NICE–SUGAR Study Investigators (2009). Intensive versus conventional glucose control in critically ill patients. *N. Engl. J. Med.*, 360(13), 1283–1297.
13. Ishikawa K (1985). *What is Total Quality Control? The Japanese Way.* Prentice-Hall, New Jersey.
14. Thor J, Lundberg J and Ask J, (2007). Application of statistical process control in healthcare improvement: systematic review. *Qual. Saf. Health Care*, 16, 387–399.
15. Pronovost PJ, Angus DC and Dorman T (2002). Physician staffing patterns and clinical outcomes in critically ill patients: a systematic review. *JAMA*, 288, 2151–2162.
16. Reddy HG, Shih T and Englesbe MJ (2013). Analyzing "failure to rescue": is this an opportunity for outcome improvement in cardiac surgery? *Ann. Thorac. Surg.*, 95, 1976–1981.
17. Pronovost P, Needham D and Berenholtz S (2006). An intervention to decrease catheter-related bloodstream infections in the ICU. *N. Engl. J. Med.*, 355, 2725–2732.
18. Abbett SK, Yokoe DS and Lipsitz SR (2009). Proposed checklist of hospital interventions to decrease the incidence of healthcare-associated clostridium difficile infection. *Infect Control Hosp. Epidemiol.*, 30, 1062–1069.
19. Available at: http://www.ted.com/talks/atul_gawande_how_do_we_heal_medicine?language=en (Accessed 30 August 2015).
20. Available at: http://www.sccm.org/Communications/Critical-Connections/Archives/Pages/A-Critical-Care-State-of-Mind.aspx (Accessed 30 August 2015).

Human Factors

Frank A. Drews* and Jonathan R. Zadra
Department of Psychology, University of Utah, Salt Lake City
VA Centre for Human Factors in Patient Safety,
VA Health Care System, 390 E. 1530 S, Salt Lake City,
UT 84112, USA
* *drews@psych.utah.edu*

Key Points

1. A socio-technical perspective can improve our understanding of human performance in Critical Care (CC) and lead to more successful interventions.
2. More effective communication as an essential, non-technical skill is required to reduce the frequency of human error.
3. Increased levels of coordination of care and a reduction of variability can improve the quality of care.
4. Technology can support clinicians but its development needs to be guided by Human Factors (HFs) to succeed.
5. Methods exist that can help to systematically analyze safety issues in CC and support the development of safety solutions.

Introduction

HF contribute to improvements in the CC Environment. Interaction between the human and technology is one of the biggest areas where improvements in patient safety can occur. In addition, to implement technology successfully in the intensive care unit (ICU), realistic perspectives of what technology can and cannot accomplish are necessary. HF can provide this perspective.

The ICU: Yesterday and Today

The first CC units opened in Europe in the late 1950s and spread rapidly to the US. Five decades later there are more than 5,000 ICUs in US hospitals. Among the reasons the ICU evolved was the development of new technology and more effective organizational structures.

Organizationally, critical care (CC) evolved from having numerous parties provide independent care, into an open organization where primary physicians were supported by a team of consulting specialists with the intensivist playing the central role in each ICU patient's care.

Interdisciplinary work between many medical professions is essential in an ICU to deliver high quality patient care. Members of the ICU team include physicians, nurses, technicians, therapists, nutritionists, pharmacists, and other support staff making effective management an important element of a highly functioning ICU.

Currently, healthcare delivery has far lower levels of reliability than that achieved in other industries (e.g. aviation). Despite intrinsic limitations on how reliable healthcare can be[1] there is a need for improvement. In the ICU, this translates to improving the usability of technology, improving coordination of care and reducing variability in care, minimizing human error, and reducing the gap between current and desired outcomes.

A Socio-Technical Perspective of the ICU

Successful improvement of CC requires a perspective that treats the ICU as a complex, socio-technical system. Failure to take this perspective will ultimately result in interventions that fail to improve patient safety and the ICU work environment.

People

Physicians

Numerous physician specialties are present in the typical ICU. Typical operational tasks intensivists perform include prescribing orders, documenting, performing daily patient assessments, carrying out endotracheal intubations, or placement of central venous catheters. A cognitive task analysis[2] described the five most frequent cognitive activities required in the ICU: pattern recognition, management of uncertainty, strategic and tactical thinking, team coordination and maintenance of common ground, and the creation and communication of meaning.

Given the highly specialized skills involved in CC, there is a move towards increasing the proportion of ICUs staffed with intensivists.

Nurses

Critical care nurses (CNNs) provide care for acutely and critically ill patients. CCNs face numerous challenges. Typical problems include: noisy work environment, distractions from patients' relatives, hectic and crowded work environments, delay in getting medications from the pharmacy, spending considerable time teaching families, equipment not available, patient rooms not well-stocked, insufficient workspace for completing paperwork, time spent locating supplies or patients' charts, delay in seeing new medical orders, and misplaced equipment. Given these working conditions, it is no surprise that stress levels and burn-out rates among ICU nurses are high.

Other staff

Other staff providing support to the ICU includes pharmacists, respiratory therapists, radiology technicians, dieticians, and social workers.

The Organization of the ICU

Currently there are three models of ICU organization. In the *open ICU model* patients remain under the care of the primary attending physician, with the intensivist being available for elective consultation "as needed". The *intensivist co-management* model is also an open ICU, but consultation by the intensivist is mandatory. In the *closed ICU model* patients are admitted under the care of an intensivist. Patient admission requires intensivist evaluation and approval. Intensivists in this model have primary responsibility for ICU patients and no other concurrent responsibilities. Variants of the models exist.

It is estimated that intensivist staffing reduces both mortality and length of stay, which could translate into savings in an 18-bed ICU ranging from $1.3–4.2 million annually.[3]

The integration of advanced technology and improved organizational structures into clinical processes allows the high level of patient care provided in the ICU. HF can contribute to further gains in improvement of the quality of care by creating more user-friendly technology and more efficient organizational structures.

Human Skills and Human Error

Acquisition of technical skills

The acquisition of technical skills for ICU workers is regulated by certification and exam processes. One less formalized but highly relevant aspect in the context of HF is the acquisition of non-technical skills.

Non-technical skills

Non-technical skills have been the focus of attention of aviation researchers since the 1950s. Any skill not related to technical expertise is considered a non-technical skill including interpersonal skills (communication, teamwork, and leadership) and cognitive skills (task management, situation awareness and decision-making). Both interpersonal and cognitive skills are important for members of the CC team yet, despite their contribution to break-downs and error, these skills are often not formally taught.[4]

Unfortunately, relatively little work has been performed on non-technical skills in the ICU with the exception of work that emphasized the importance of teamwork and communication skills.[5]

ICU non-technical skills

Reader *et al.*[4] identified four core ICU non-technical skills: task management, teamwork, situation awareness, and decision-making. In this context, task management involved managing available resources and organizing required steps to achieve a goal. Teamwork was defined as skills for working in a group, to ensure task completion and team member satisfaction. Situation awareness at the individual and team level involved developing and maintaining an overall awareness based on the interplay of elements in the environment, an understanding of their meaning and the projection of their state into the future. Finally, decision-making involved reaching a judgment or diagnosis, or selecting a course of action based on experience or new information.

In analyzing 2,677 incidents Reader *et al.*[4] found that 50% of the incidents were due to non-technical skill deficits with task management being the largest contributing factor.

Methods to identify and group non-technical skills required in the ICU include simulator-based or real life observational studies, studies of cognition, survey based methods, and root cause analyses (*qv*).

Leadership and team skills

Strong team leadership is critical for effective teamwork. Strong leadership involves the team leader ensuring that the goals and the needs of the team are met. Previous work established the importance of effective team leadership in the ICU to maintain and improve patient safety.[6] Team leadership is most often associated with senior ICU physicians. However, other team members may display team leadership behaviour as well. Reader *et al.*[7] analyzed ICU team leadership behaviour. They distinguished between context-specific functional leadership behaviour and team development behaviour as preconditions for high levels of team performance. Elements of functional leadership behaviour were identified as information gathering, planning and decision-making, managing team members, and managing materials. Behaviours such as providing team direction, establishing team norms, coaching and providing organizational support were classified as team development behaviours. In 25 semi-structured interviews with senior ICU physicians they applied the critical incident technique to elicit behaviours displayed by experts during complex tasks. The most frequent among the four functional leadership behaviours was managing team members, followed by information gathering, and planning and decision-making. Among the team development behaviours, establishing team norms and coaching were mentioned most frequently, followed by providing team direction. An important finding was that the borders between the medical team (senior and junior physicians) and the nursing team (senior and bedside nurses) were often not clearly defined, potentially resulting in diffusion of responsibility due to a lack of senior leadership behaviours.

Clearly, the collaboration between ICU nurses and physicians is important. Successful collaboration with physicians is positively correlated with patient outcomes. Knaus *et al.*[8] report that poor collaborative communication among nurses and physicians resulted in a 1.8-fold increase in risk-adjusted patient mortality and length of patient stay. In addition, ICUs with higher collaborative interaction have higher job satisfaction and higher retention rates of nurses.

Miller[9] examined the perspectives of nurses and physicians concerning collaborative interaction in the ICU. In this study physicians reported more collaboration in communication (openness, timeliness, and satisfaction), problem solving, physician expertise, and quality of care than nurses, a disparity which is potentially due to the status differential between physicians and nurses. Overall, the findings imply that the more traditional, hierarchical structure found in many ICUs negatively affects staff perceptions and could potentially be associated with lower patient safety. Several training programs aim to reduce this status differential with the goal to improve patient outcomes.

Models of shared nurse leadership have been implemented in some ICUs, where a single nurse manager is replaced by two nurse managers. The implementation of a shared leadership model led to increasingly positive views of organizational culture, social interactions between members, work satisfaction and leadership. In addition, staff confidence levels were higher with shared leadership model implementation. However, one potential problem with this approach could be a diffusion of responsibility between the nurse managers.

Based on their literature review of health team effectiveness, Lemieux-Charles and McGuire[10] proposed the Integrated Team Effectiveness Model (ITEM). The most important findings of their review concerned the contribution of diverse clinical expertise to both improvements in patient care and changes in organizational effectiveness. Having a diverse ICU team contributing expertise is a critical component for patient safety improvement. In addition, the authors found several factors that improved staff satisfaction and team effectiveness including collaboration, conflict resolution, participation, and cohesion.

Members proficient in team development skills have a positive impact on the performance of other ICU staff and help to improve clinical outcomes. To better understand the breakdowns that can result from poor team development, it is important to also focus on human error in CC.

Human error in CC

Studies have found that errors reported by ICU staff are split roughly equally between physicians (46%) and nurses (54%), with a greater proportion occurring during the day between 10 am and noon when staff activities peak or during shift changes. Importantly, 37% of the errors included nurse–physician communication as a contributing factor.[5] The lack of good communication and transfer of information between nurses and physicians can be partly attributed to the fact that nurses were excluded from participation in rounds.

Rothschild *et al.*[11] investigated the incidence and nature of adverse events and errors in a medical ICU and a Coronary Care Unit (CCU). The authors observed mostly action-based slips and memory-based lapses that contributed to the presence of medical error. More errors were related to the execution of plans rather than decisions about which course of action to follow.

Graf *et al.*[12] analyzed self-reported ICU errors and incidents finding that patients who experienced error were more severely ill than patients who did not experience error. Also, those patients who experienced more than one error were significantly more ill than those who experienced a single error. As contributing factors to error, the authors identified disregard of standards, rules, and orders and poor staff communication. In this study, the large majority of error was preventable and controllable as opposed to chance based events, indicating significant potential for improvement.

Overall, human error in the ICU is common and has a significant clinical impact, and it is often preventable. The performance of all CC workers is prone to error and is often associated with monitoring and daily care tasks like ordering of medication or execution of patient treatment. One effective approach to reduce human error involves establishing more effective communication between staff members (e.g. use of interdisciplinary rounds).

Coordination and Variability of Care in the ICU

Among the most important coordination of care events in the ICU are handovers and rounds. Often these are treated as part of teamwork in healthcare.

Coordination of care

Handover

The goal of an effective handover is to transfer patient-relevant information that will allow the newly responsible nurse to make appropriate clinical decisions, help develop a work plan, and prioritize tasks for the upcoming shift. A well performed handover supports mutual understanding of the patient's condition and can improve clinical decision-making. Handovers have been studied using different indicators of quality and breakdown, e.g. investigating sentinel events, critical incidents, errors, and near misses.

Frequently handovers are informal and unstructured. Handovers often are performed quickly because they occur at the end of a shift, so the inclusion of all aspects of the above items represents an ideal. The omission of information during handover can result in consequences ranging from failure to treat problems to adverse patient events.

Cognitive tools have been developed to support the handover and the medical record should serve in this function. Verbal handovers are often accompanied by a printed or a computerized tool that helps to structure the handover process. The use of paper is persistent in the ICU and in particular in the context of handovers, and still has many benefits when used in parallel with an Electronic Health Record System (EHR), such as enhancing communication, maintaining situation awareness, and serving as a reminder of things to do in the future. Also, unless specifically designed and optimized by application of HF design principles, paper can provide better data presentation than an electronic version of the same document.

Rounds

Rounds in the ICU provide the healthcare team with a formal opportunity to discuss patient care on a daily basis (increasingly, rounds are performed twice a day). Often rounds are intensivist led, and include ICU attending physicians and fellows, anaesthesia and surgical residents, nurse practitioners, nurses and a pharmacist.

Similar to patient handovers, rounds often fail to develop explicit patient goals, and instead focus on a patient's physiology, pharmacology or other aspects of disease progression. In one study, after implementing a daily goals form that included questions related to patient safety risk, interventions to reduce these risks, and activities to be performed prior to ICU discharge, care provider's understanding of patient goals of care improved from 10% to more than 95% and the average patient length of stay decreased from 2.2 to 1.1 days.[13]

Inconsistencies, repetition, and omission of important information during daily ICU rounds are common. A flowchart guiding communication during rounds may improve effective dissemination of knowledge regarding patient care goals.

Some evidence suggests that interdisciplinary rounds improve clinical outcomes and communication between CC workers. For example, the inclusion of ICU pharmacists in rounds reduced the preventable adverse drug event rate by 66% in one ICU, and the inclusion of ICU nurses increased the perception of teamwork and collaboration. Increasingly, family members are being asked to participate in rounds.

One newer type of round that focuses on safety is the Comprehensive Unit-based Safety Program (CUSP). An important element of this program is monthly safety rounds that involve senior leadership and unit staff to discuss safety issues, and one result of these rounds has been an increase in the perceived culture of safety.

Reducing variability: checklists and protocols

Variability in care delivery poses a problem when a procedure is not performed correctly. Checklists and protocols increase the consistency of behaviour while decreasing variability in performance. Checklists structure items and tasks in a list, support cognitive organization of items in chunks, and simplify the conceptualization and recall of information. In addition, checklists are used as cognitive aids to support task completion or decision-making (e.g. for differential diagnosis). Application of checklists can also decrease the omission of steps in a procedure. Checklists have been demonstrated to be effective in various aspects of performance and error prevention and management. Advocates of checklists and protocols in healthcare cite their ability to decrease hospital acquired infections, and checklist use is considered best practice, since non-adherence to task protocols is not uncommon. Recently, a strong case has been made for a broad application of checklists to enhance patient safety. However, the successful implementation of checklists requires addressing substantial logistical, social, and cultural barriers.

There are other challenges associated with checklists. Checklists do not always eliminate omission of task steps as initially expected. For example, high memory load increases the probability of omissions when using a checklist. Another factor that contributes to omissions is low item conspicuity. The position of steps in a task sequence predicts the likelihood of omissions: mid- and end-sequence steps are more vulnerable to being skipped. In addition, checklist elements may create ambiguity, leaving room for interpretation and potential error. Finally, lack of local cueing can contribute to omissions. Often, many steps are cued logically by a previous step; however, if steps are functionally isolated, their omission is likely.

The requirement to follow a checklist or a protocol introduces an additional task for the clinician and attention has to be divided. Consequently, a clinician has to either perform the task at hand while simultaneously monitoring the checklist or switch between tasks, which increases the likelihood of a performance breakdown. Checklists may be implemented in such a way that the individual elements are "prompted" by a non-care providing person. Thus, implementation considerations of checklists are of great importance for their success.

Implementation considerations are related to the implementation of individual checklists, but also related to the issue concerning the overall number of checklists being used in a particular context. Being required to follow overly long or too many checklists may lead to a negative attitude towards checklists and an increase in checklist violations (checklist fatigue).

Alternatives to checklists

Drews[14] proposed an alternative approach to the traditional checklist in the context of procedures such as central line insertions and maintenance. The conceptual framework of Adherence Engineering[14] provides guidance on how to develop equipment that increases adherence to best practices.

Technology in the ICU

The introduction of new technologies into the ICU can significantly improve quality of care and patient safety. However, more recently there has been evidence that new technologies also introduce significant challenges. New technology is often associated with unintended consequences. In addition, many current healthcare devices are suboptimal from a HF perspective, increasing the risks of device-related errors.

Clinical information systems: patient monitors

In the ICU patients receive continuous physiological monitoring. On traditional patient monitors, the vital signs are presented numerically in real time with graphical data limited to pressure waveform morphology (e.g. arterial blood pressure).

Nurses perform the majority of patient monitoring tasks in the ICU and check physiological parameters on a regular basis to assure patient stability. However, changes in physiological parameters are common, and the timely detection of trends or acute events is important. It is necessary to process all of the individual's parameters simultaneously, put them in the context of that patient's disease history, and compare current parameters with those in the recent past. Thus, providing information about the status of a patient in a manner that is easier and faster to interpret should reduce the time required to detect a meaningful change. Unfortunately, currently available monitors are not designed to be the most effective diagnostic aids.

Current monitors do not display an integrated assessment of the patient's status. To support high levels of situation awareness data should be displayed in a way that takes underlying relationships into account. Traditional monitor designs provide sequential, piecemeal data making it difficult and time-consuming to develop a coherent understanding of the underlying physiology of the displayed parameters. Yet, such an understanding is a necessary precondition for high diagnostic performance and situation awareness.

Alternatives to current monitor design, which may help improve ICU physiological displays for the ICU, are available. These approaches focus on clinicians' needs and follow HF design principles. For example, Agutter *et al.*[15] used an iterative, user-centred design strategy to develop graphical physiological displays. In most of the laboratory-based studies, clinicians' performance when using these graphical displays improved significantly.

These displays are often object-based with variables depicted as rectangles, polygons or more complex geometrical objects (see Figure 1 for an example). Changes in monitored variables create deviations in the normally symmetric shape of the graphical elements facilitating the detection of changes in physiology.

While most novel patient monitoring displays have been developed for anaesthesiologists, the majority of patient-related activities in the ICU are performed by nurses. Recently, Anders *et al.*[17] developed an ICU graphical information display, which integrates a comprehensive array of clinical variables onto one screen. The display organizes variables by physiological system so that related variables are shown in close proximity.

There are clear limitations in directly transferring graphical cardiovascular monitoring displays from the operating room (OR) to the ICU.

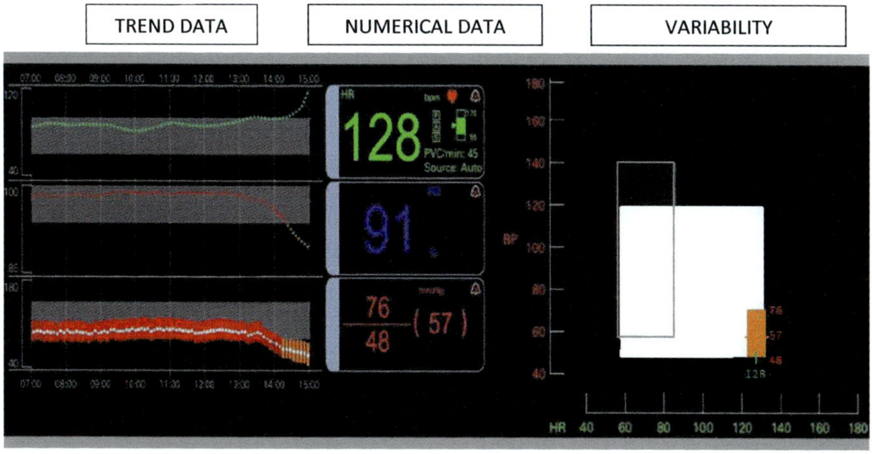

Figure 1. Drews and Doig[16] display. The left panel displays color-coded trend data, the centre panel displays these data in a numerical format, and the right panel displays the current state of the patient with regard to previous data (white reference frame illustrates the variability of this patient's previous heart rate and blood pressure measurements) and a normal patient (gray reference frame).

In one study, ICU nurses using a graphical display had on average 5% lower diagnostic accuracy than when using a traditional display while anaesthesiologists demonstrated improved performance when using the same graphical display. Given the interdisciplinary nature of the CC team, information displays for the ICU present a significant challenge compared to patient monitors used by providers from a single specialty.

ICU nurses pursue multiple simultaneous patient-related goals, e.g. monitoring and maintaining blood oxygenation and tissue perfusion. Processing information from multiple data sources requires considerable cognitive effort as each variable is examined, selected, and integrated into an assessment. Coherent understanding of the relationships between variables and their underlying mechanisms can be time-consuming and difficult. Consequentially, traditional non-integrated displays potentially increase cognitive demand, thereby reducing cognitive resources available for other tasks.

The pathophysiology of many complications in the ICU often presents with small incremental and sometimes fluctuating changes apparent only over time. The presentation of variables can aid the recognition of life threatening events and support other tasks, e.g. vasoactive medication titration. The integration of related variables into configural and contextual trend displays can provide additional decision support. Although there is substantial evidence for improved performance after providing graphical and trend data, in the clinical context many obstacles, some of them cultural, some based on conventions, are in place to delay the implementation of these information displays.

Electronic Health Record Systems

The use of EHR and computerized provider order entry (CPOE) systems is standard in US hospitals. One of the effects of the implementation of EHRs in the ICU are changes in the nursing workflow. An effective ICU EHR system can decrease the time nurses spend on documentation while increasing time available to spend on patient care. In one study a newly implemented ICU information system reduced the time nurses spent on documentation by more than 30%, while it increased time spent on direct patient care such as patient assessments. Consequently, many believe that modern EHRs will improve the quality and safety of ICU care. Unfortunately, the results of implementations are mixed and neither the impact on documentation nor the impact on patient care is consistent. One particular challenge is that effectiveness of EHR systems and their clinical success is a function of usability and user interface design. Only the proper application of HF design principles and processes to EHR systems will help these systems to become sufficiently user friendly so that potential negative side-effects are minimized.

CPOEs were introduced with the intention to reduce prescription errors and reducing annual costs by eliminating potential problems associated with paper based systems (e.g. handwriting identification problems, faster electronic transmission of information, identification of drug-drug interactions). Currently, there is strong support for the implementation of CPOEs from such diverse groups as physicians, hospital administrators, business councils, legislators, and patients. However, empirical support for the effectiveness of CPOEs despite being initially positive is limited because of the relatively young technology and the constant evolution of the systems.[18] In addition, when studying the impact of CPOEs a clear emphasis is given to the positive impact of the systems without also investigating the problems and unintended consequence of their implementation.

Device alarms in the ICU

One solution to support clinicians in the ICU is the use of alarms. Unfortunately, many alarms in the ICU environment are not integrated, with the consequence that multiple alarms may be active simultaneously, potentially confusing the healthcare worker as to how to prioritize the alarms. Alarms in the ICU may be less effective due to frequent false positive notifications, and difficulties identifying the alarm source or alarm type.

Alarms and alerting systems can disrupt workflow. Korniewicz *et al.*[19] evaluated the effectiveness of alarms. Most respondents (94%) agreed that the large number of false alarms leads to clinicians mistrusting alarms and disabling them as much as possible. Most participants supported statements concerning the need for alarms to be prioritized and easier to differentiate.

Overall, improving alarms and alarm management in the ICU is a HF problem. Better alarm design provides support for clinicians in using equipment (and alarm functionality) safely and across its full range of capabilities, which is a usability and interface design challenge. Hospitals need to recognize the complexities of alarm management, which can be addressed only by taking a socio-technical systems perspective rather than the traditional technology centred view.

Methods to Enhance Safety in the ICU

Root cause analysis

Several alternative approaches have been proposed and applied to improve our understanding of human error in healthcare. Among these approaches is Root Cause Analysis (RCA). RCA represents a standard approach for the analysis and assessment of processes in the clinical environment. The Joint Commission for Accreditation of Healthcare Organizations requires this technique as a method to study serious and sentinel events after their occurrence. The goal of this resource intense method is to identify the aberrant processes that have contributed to a particular adverse event. The root causes represent the fundamental reasons for the occurrence of the event and are investigated by analyzing how and why an adverse event occurred. RCA has been criticized for several reasons. One issue with RCA is, as its name suggests, that there is a single cause leading to an error, which is often thought of as an oversimplification. In most cases there is a complex chain of events and a number of contributing factors that lead to an incident or accident. Another criticism is related to the fact that RCA often focuses only on the reconstruction of a particular event, but not on systematically understanding what the event reveals about systemic problems in the healthcare organization in which the investigated case occurred. The consequence of this focus is that the RCA may help prevent only the repetition of highly similar events in the future while failing to prevent events that, although they have a common root cause, are dissimilar in other ways, and even for similar events, it is not quite clear if the risk of a similar event is actually reduced. Finally, RCA often directs its focus only on events that are among the most serious but not on events that are considered less serious. The problem with this limited perspective is that it underestimates the importance of events of lower seriousness, which have the potential to reveal equal or even more insight into the systemic causes for error. As a result of these shortcomings, approaches that aim at improving patient safety in healthcare have to go beyond a RCA and even more importantly, they have to incorporate a psychologically founded theory of human error in organizational settings.

Failure mode and effect analysis

Failure mode and effect analysis and provide (FMEA) originates from Systems Engineering and focuses on improving system reliability. The basic assumption is that it is possible improve system operation by calculating a priority score for risks that allows the quantification of the risk of potential breakdowns of the system, subsystem, or its components. A risk priority score is calculated by including the severity, the frequency of occurrence and the detectability of process breakdowns. The numbers can be used to provide guidance for ranking potential failures in terms of their priority and need of being addressed.

One of the challenges in healthcare is that the individual numbers have potentially a lower variation than in non-healthcare industries. For example, if focusing on severity, in the context of patient care the score is most likely 10 since the most severe consequences are either injury or death to the patient. However, despite its limitations, there were several attempts to apply FMEA in the context of healthcare and the Veterans Health Administration is using one of these instruments widely.[20] Despite the challenges, the main advantage of the FMEA is that unlike the RCA it provides guidance on potential breakdowns, which makes it a proactive rather than a reactive approach.

Conclusions

One of the goals of applying HF Engineering to CC is to increase the performance and resilience of this complex, socio-technical system. This paper reviewed important HF contributions to CC and how HF research can contribute to increase the quality of care delivery, productivity, and patient safety. The work reviewed ranges from device safety and usability, to organizational factors and the safety climate.

The review of HF in CC emphasized the importance of a systems perspective by contrasting this perspective with a reductionist (e.g. device centred) approach. It should be no surprise that the ICU is a socio-technical, or perhaps a socio-natural system and as such, the introduction of new processes, devices, technologies and organizational structures needs to be planned carefully. In addition, diligent monitoring of these changes after implementation is necessary. Only the application of a rigorous planning approach that includes a long-term impact assessment will help avoid surprises and unintended consequences.

In addition, this paper identified important areas of work where HF contributions can help. First, usability evaluations of technologies need to include assessment of the interaction with existing and new technology in the clinical context, assessment of the fit of new devices or technology into the existing clinical workflow, and worst-case assumptions about clinicians operating the devices or technology. Only by taking such a comprehensive system-based approach will it be possible to introduce new devices and technology in a fashion that minimizes disruption and that maximizes their benefit. As described above, this approach is currently not the standard.

Secondly, this review identified a continued need to improve the effectiveness of non-technical skills of ICU staff. Communication issues, either as part of handovers, or as part of clarifying the availability of resources for patient care, continue to be a significant contributor to breakdowns in ICU care delivery.

Thirdly, this review identified the need for a better calibrated perspective on what improvements and changes can be realistically expected after the introduction of new technology in the ICU, and what expectations are unrealistic. Abandoning the simplistic perspective that a single device or technology can provide the solution to a problem in isolation is a first step toward the development of a more realistic perspective that is necessary for successful technology adoption.

Fourthly, another HF topic relates to the goal of reducing variability in care delivery, and minimizing violations and error. HF provides the theories and the tools to make significant steps toward this goal. A selective and appropriate adoption of the lessons learned in other domains is one critical step forward. In addition, the development of specific healthcare centred approaches will be another steps. There is great promise in evidence-based standardization of clinical practice.

Fifthly, a result of the emphasis of the socio-technical systems perspective is the focus on safety climate inside and outside the ICU. This involves active monitoring, management, and improvement of the safety climate. Programs towards improvement of the safety climate involve healthcare workers at all organizational levels. In addition, safety cannot be treated in isolation such as being located in a technology, a person, or a unit only. Safety is an emergent phenomenon and its active management is a continuous effort.

At this time, we are still at the beginning of efforts to re-engineer healthcare in general, and CC in particular, to attain the quality and value society deserves and expects. This endeavor will benefit significantly from the contributions HF Engineering offers.

References

1. Durso FT and Drews FA (2010). Health Care, aviation, and ecosystems: a socio-natural systems perspective. *Curr. Dir. Psychol. Sci.*, 19(2), 71–75.
2. Fackler JC, Watts C and Grome A (2009). Critical care physician cognitive task analysis: an exploratory study. *Crit. Care.*, 3, 33.
3. Pronovost PJ, Needham DM and Waters H (2006). Intensive care unit physician staffing: financial modeling of the leapfrog standard. *Crit. Care Med.*, 34, 18–24.
4. Reader T, Flin R, Lauche K and Cuthbertson BH (2006). Non-technical skills in the intensive care unit. *Brit. J. Anaesth.*, 96, 551–559.
5. Donchin Y, Gopher D and Olin M (1995). A look into the nature and causes of human errors in the intensive care unit. *Crit. Care Med.*, 23, 294–300.
6. Manser T (2009). Teamwork and patient safety in dynamic domains of health-care: a review of the literature. *Acta Anaesth. Scand.*, 53(2), 43–51.
7. Reader TW, Flin R and Cuthbertson BH (2011). Team leadership in the intensive care unit: the perspective of specialists. *Crit. Care Med.*, 39, 1683–1691.
8. Knaus WA, Draper EA, Wagner DP and Zimmerman JE (1986). An evaluation of outcome from intensive care in major medical centres. *Ann. Intern. Med.*, 104, 410–418.
9. Miller PA (2001). Nurse–physician collaboration in an intensive care unit. *Am. J Crit. Care*, 10, 341–350.
10. Lemieux-Charles L and McGuire WL (2006). What do we know about health care team effectiveness? A review of the literature. *Med. Care Res. Rev.*, 63(3), 263–300.
11. Rothschild JM, Landrigan CP and Cronin JW (2005). The critical care safety study: the incidence and nature of adverse events and serious medical errors in intensive care. *Crit. Care Med.*, 33(8), 1694–1700.
12. Graf J, von den Driesch A, Koch KC and Janssens U (2005). Identification and characterization of errors and incidents in a medical intensive care unit. *Acta Anaesth. Scand.*, 49(7), 930–939.
13. Pronovost PJ, Berenholtz S and Dorman T (2003). Improving communication in the ICU using daily goals. *J. Crit. Care*, 18, 71–75.
14. Drews FA (2013). Adherence engineering. Ergonomics in Design: a new approach to increasing adherence to protocols. *Q. Hum. Factors Appl.*, 21(4), 19–25.
15. Agutter J, Drews F and Syroid N (2003). Evaluation of graphic cardiovascular display in a high-fidelity simulator. *Anesth. Analg.*, 97, 1403–1413.
16. Drews FA and Doig A (2014). Evaluation of a configural vital signs display for intensive care unit nurses. *Hum. Factors*, 6, 569–580.

17. Anders S, Albert R and Miller A (2012). Evaluation of an integrated graphical display to promote acute change detection in ICU patients. *Int. J. Med. Inform.*, 81, 842–851.
18. Kaushal R, Shojania KG and Bates DW (2003). Effects of computerized physician order entry and clinical decision support systems on medication safety: a systematic review. *Arch. Intern. Med.*, 163, 1409–1416.
19. Korniewicz DM, Clark T and David Y (2008). A national online survey on the effectiveness of clinical alarms. *Am. J. Crit. Care*, 17, 36–41.
20. DeRosier J, Stalhandske E, Bagian JP and Nudell T (2002). Using health care failure mode and effect analysis: the VA National Centre for Patient Safety prospective risk analysis system. *Jt. Comm. J. Qual. Improvement*, 28(5), 248–267.

Part V
Quality and Safety

Quality Improvement

Carol J. Peden

Associate Medical Director for Quality Improvement and a Consultant in Anaesthesia and Intensive Care at the Royal United Hospitals, Bath, UK

Kevin D. Rooney

Consultant in Anaesthesia and Intensive Care Medicine Royal Alexandra Hospital, Paisley Professor of Care Improvement University of the West of Scotland

Key Points

1. Quality is defined in healthcare as care that is safe, effective, person-centred, timely, efficient, and equitable.
2. The principles of improvement science in healthcare are based on the work of Deming using the concepts of "profound knowledge" and "plan, do, study, act" or PDSA cycles for improvement.
3. The use of run charts and control charts provide a way to display data to make process performance visible over time and to observe whether changes made result in improvement.
4. Bundles and checklists are useful tools in the intensive care unit (ICU) to increase the reliable delivery of key components of care, but to be truly effective, teamwork, and organizational culture must also be addressed.

5. Audit, morbidity and mortality reviews, incident reporting, and screening for harm with tools such as the global trigger tool should be used to collate data and themes for improvement in a systematic way. Themes for improvement should then form part of QI projects with regular and timely feedback to all staff.

Background to Quality Improvement

What is quality?

It is important to ensure that we share a common understanding of what the concept of "quality" means when it is applied to healthcare. In the seminal report "Crossing the Quality Chasm" the Institute of Medicine defined six dimensions of quality in healthcare.[1] These dimensions define healthcare quality as care that is "safe, efficient, effective, patient-centred, timely, and equitable". Don Berwick, the former Chief Executive Officer of the Institute for Healthcare Improvement (IHI), simplified the concept further, seeing quality through the eyes of the patient and stating simply "*Help me, do not harm me, be nice to me*".

Quality improvement (QI) is a formal approach to the analysis of performance, and then the use of systematic efforts to improve it. QI is driven by measurement and constant re-examination of data about where we are now, compared to where we were, and where we want to be. Improvement comes from the application of knowledge and a thorough understanding of the system being improved.

Intensivists, highly trained in medical research based on the testing of hypotheses with randomized controlled trials, but unfamiliar with the tools and concepts of QI, may question the scientific basis behind it. However, there is a science to improvement and many of the improvement and measurement techniques now being introduced into healthcare have been widely used in Industry, Agriculture and Aviation for decades.

Deming and Improvement Science

The "father" of improvement science was Deming (1900–1993), an American mathematician, statistician and business consultant. He is credited with improving industrial production in the US during the Second World War, although perhaps better known internationally for his work in

Japan from the 1950s onwards. He taught Japanese top management how to improve service, quality, product testing, and sales with a variety of methods including the application of statistical process control (SPC) methods. Deming was mentored by Shewhart (a statistician at Bell laboratories) who had developed the concept of statistical control of processes using control charts.[2] Deming *et al.* (another founder of the QI movement) worked together at the General Electric Company in Hawthorne, Illinois after which the Hawthorne effect (individuals improve their performance in response to their awareness of being observed) is named. Deming is regarded as having had more impact upon Japanese industry than any other individual of non-Japanese heritage. Later in his career in the mid 1980s he was credited for transforming the US Ford Motor Company, from failure to the most profitable American car manufacturer at that time. Deming's work shows that the processes used in improvement science are not only firmly based on statistical science, but have also been tested and shown to work successfully to improve many different complex processes.

Profound knowledge

In addition to SPC methods, Deming described a concept that he called "profound knowledge".[3] Profound knowledge is used to examine a system to see where it can be improved. This involves examining four components:

1. Appreciation of a "system", where the system is defined as an interdependent group of items, people or processes working together towards a common purpose. The common purpose aligns the parts of the system; while interdependence considers the relationships and interactions among them[3] Interaction is amongst people, processes, and equipment. Interdependence means that multiple measures are needed to understand the performance of a system to improve the outcome and care of critically ill patients. The system around an ICU is complex and involves multiple interactions with other system components both larger and smaller. To understand the ICU system we must consider how wider hospital issues impact the ICU (the macro-system) and how the behaviour of smaller team units within the ICU (micro-systems) affect the overall performance.

2. Knowledge of variation: a key to understanding how processes vary under normal (e.g. time of day) and unusual circumstances (e.g. a major incident), which can be illustrated with the use of run charts and control charts (*qv*).
3. Building knowledge: to improve the ICU we need to build our knowledge and create hypotheses based on this knowledge in order to understand what might work and how we might successfully implement change.
4. Knowledge of psychology: to create effective improvement we need to have an understanding of how to influence change through individuals.

We cannot improve something until we really understand it. To understand how we can make critical care (CC) safer, more effective and more person-centred, we should closely examine the ICU systems using the components of "profound knowledge" discussed above. All of the components interact much like a Venn diagram within a lens with which to examine the system (Figure 1). A system cannot be fully improved to achieve its potential without consideration of each part. For instance, how the individuals in an ICU behave, different professional teams interact and the culture of that unit is integral to understanding how to improve its care. The first step, therefore to improving a system is to examine it closely, by defining boundaries, including temporal components and to understand successes and defects within the system and the individuals who interact with it.

The science of improvement should not threaten evidence-based medicine. To the contrary, it should complement it, making it easier to make changes that will result in safer and more effective, efficient, equitable, timely, and person-centred care.

The Gap between What We Know and What We Do, and Getting to High Reliability in the ICU

There is a consistent gap in healthcare between the arrival of new evidence and its effective implementation.[4] This gap can be as long as 17 years. An example is the 2,000 acute respiratory distress syndrome (ARDS) network study[5] that demonstrated limiting tidal volume to <6 mL/kg predicted body weight and end inspiratory pressure to not more than 30 cm

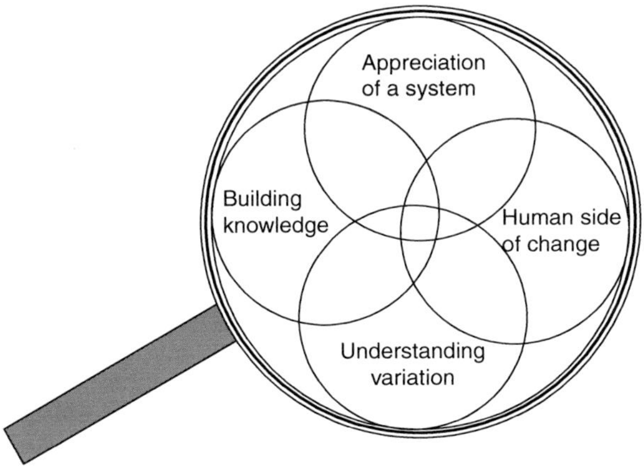

Figure 1. The lens of profound knowledge.

H_2O in ventilated patients significantly reduced mortality in patients with acute lung injury (ALI) and ARDS. Despite the fact that this study provided high-level evidence for a change in management and at little cost to implement, subsequent studies have shown a failure to adopt and deliver this practice reliably. Healthcare is not only slow to adopt change, but once that change is adopted, it is commonly delivered unreliably. A good operational definition of reliability in healthcare is "*failure-free operation over time*".[6]

The IHI has a three step model for applying principles of reliability to healthcare systems[6]:

1. Prevent initial failure using intent and standardization (e.g. use of bundles).
2. Identify failure when it occurs and intervenes before harm is caused (e.g. detection of missed safety steps with the World Health Organization (WHO) Surgical Safety Checklist). Mitigating the harm caused by failures that are not intercepted with a back-up plan or contingency function (e.g. plan B in a failed intubation).
3. Measure and then communicate learning from defects back into the design process; i.e. ensure when things go wrong that we learn from them, have mechanisms to capture that learning and then change our systems to make harm less likely to occur, namely critical incident reporting.

A recent study[7] demonstrates how measurement and system design using alerts displayed on large screens configured to show information routinely collected from a Clinical Information System and to identify breaches of preset tidal volume limits in ventilated patients, led to a significant increase in the time spent with tidal volumes < 6 mL/kg. Although the actual improvement was not insignificant, 17.5–28.6%, the majority of patients remained above the tidal volume limit. Therefore, even with attention and prompts, performance was well below that of a high reliability system and demonstrates how difficult it is to achieve the type of performance we aim to deliver to our ICU patients.

Bundles

A "bundle" is a group of interventions for a given process that, when implemented together, may result in better outcomes for the underlying problem than if each component was implemented individually.[8] The bundle concept is designed to provide reliable delivery (i.e. 90–95% of the time) of key components of care. A bundle does not have to include every process related to that area of care — it is designed to improve delivery of related aspects of care to the patient. The use of a small number of evidence based interventions and the collection of data based on their delivery, leads to the recognition that it is really hard to deliver 3–5 components of care 95% of the time. Most teams when they start measuring will find their performance for bundle delivery is between 20 and 60%. If each component of a five element bundle is delivered at 90%, that means that each component succeeds 9 times out of 10 or alternatively fails 1 out of 10 times. So in a five step bundle like the ventilator bundle with a 90% compliance or 10% failure rate for each element, the final all-or-none delivery rate may be 59% or in other words a 41% failure rate ($0.9 \times 0.9 \times 0.9 \times 0.9 \times 0.9$). This is one of the reasons why it is hard to get to high performance with complex bundles such as the sepsis bundle, although of course the principal problem is the complexity of identifying and managing sepsis.[9]

Use of a bundle promotes awareness that the team must work together to get all the components delivered reliably, and to use improvement methods to redesign care processes. A key component of the success of a bundle is the empowerment of all team members to act independently in the best interest of patients to ensure delivery of bundle components. Examples are: the use of multi-disciplinary rounds and daily goals to reinforce bundle compliance, e.g. planning the sedation hold for a ventilated patient.

The features of bundle design include[8]:

- The bundle ideally has 3–5 evidence-based actions agreed upon by clinicians.
- The steps are all necessary and each step must be performed to achieve success.
- The multi-disciplinary team develops the bundle.
- Elements should be descriptive rather than prescriptive, e.g. deep vein thrombosis (DVT) prophylaxis in the ventilator bundle does not define what the prophylaxis should be.
- Each individual step should be based on level one evidence if at all possible.
- Each step should be clear-cut and all-or-nothing. The answer to completion of the step can only be 'yes' or 'no'. For example in the ventilator bundle: Was the sedation stopped this morning? The answer has to be yes or no.
- The bundle must take place in the same time and space continuum; for example, the central line bundle takes place during a single episode of line insertion, and assessment of the ventilator bundle is made during the ward round.
- There should be no controversy about each step. The bundle is about *how* to deliver best care not *what* the care should be.

As delivery of the bundle components reaches more than 95% reliability, teams can consider what other components would improve care. As delivery of the care bundle improves teams should see a parallel improvement in related outcomes, e.g. increased reliable implementation of the central line insertion bundle should correspond with a decrease in central line associated blood stream infections (CLABSI).[10]

Studies[9,10] indicate using care bundles as part of a comprehensive improvement strategy improve clinical outcomes. Part of the problem with the adoption of care bundles can be the lack of agreement on which measures to monitor. This does not detract from the value of a bundle if it is accepted that bundles are not the 'answer' to the problem, they are just one tool that can be used in the design of services within an environment of continual improvement. The goal is to ensure evidence-based care is reliably delivered every time to every patient.

The success of the central line bundle in the US, after Pronovost and colleagues demonstrated that an intervention including care bundles used in 103 ICUs decreased infection rates by up to 66%,[10] led to the state-wide implementation of the bundle in Michigan and then further across the US and internationally. Key to the success of the Michigan program was a normative pressure to join the programme and conform to its requirements through a networked community, the reframing of central line associated blood stream infection as a social problem, cultural change, team-working and the use of data for improvement.[11] The "Matching Michigan" study in the UK failed to deliver such impressive results as there had already been significant improvement in infection rates. The ethnographic study of the intervention highlighted the importance of distinguishing between technical interventions and implementation strategies when running improvement programmes, and makes interesting reading.[12]

The use of bundles is now wide spread and established in the ICU and has been applied to many aspects of patient care including delirium, weaning and extubation, sepsis, care of the ventilated patient, central line insertion and management of rehabilitation.

Checklists

When multiple steps in a pathway need to be implemented a bundle is not appropriate; a checklist is the tool that should be used. Checklists are now widely used in healthcare, for example, implementation of the WHO checklist has been shown to reduce surgical morbidity and mortality by ensuring adherence to evidence-based practices and reducing preventable error. Checklists are only valuable when there is corresponding change in culture and teamwork. Checklists are designed for clinicians to use to help guide them in situations where steps may be missed or rare emergencies may occur. Checklists may fail because clear implementation strategies are not carried out. They require leadership, data collection and training in teamwork to ensure all team members feel respected and accountable; the way in which checklists are implemented is of great importance in the care and management of the critically ill patient.[13]

The Model for Improvement

Background

The model for improvement (MFI) is an important tool used in improvement science developed by the Associates in Process Improvement[3] and derived from the work of Shewhart and Deming[2] (Figure 2). Other improvement models exist such as Lean, Six Sigma, DMAIC (define, measure, analyze, improve, control) and derive from the same principles based on the work of Shewhart and Deming. It is more important to understand that it is the use of a structured approach that will help to drive improvement, rather than which model is used, although some models may be better suited to one type of improvement than other. Improving reliable care delivery and new ways of working may be better suited to the MFI, whereas reducing waste in a patient pathway, which can include waiting, unnecessary tests and duplication of effort may be better suited to a "Lean" approach. If a QI department exists within a hospital they may be able to assist in choosing the best approach for a particular problem and help with the implementation. Many intensivists may be familiar with the MFI, as it has been widely used in ICU QI programs worldwide such as the IHI Breakthrough Series Collaboratives, the Scottish Patient Safety program and the Patient Safety First Campaign.

The three questions central to applying the MFI method are:

- What are we trying to accomplish?
- How will we know that a change is an improvement?
- What changes can we make that will result in an improvement?

The first question "what are we trying to accomplish" gives an aim; for effective improvement the aim statement should be measurable and time

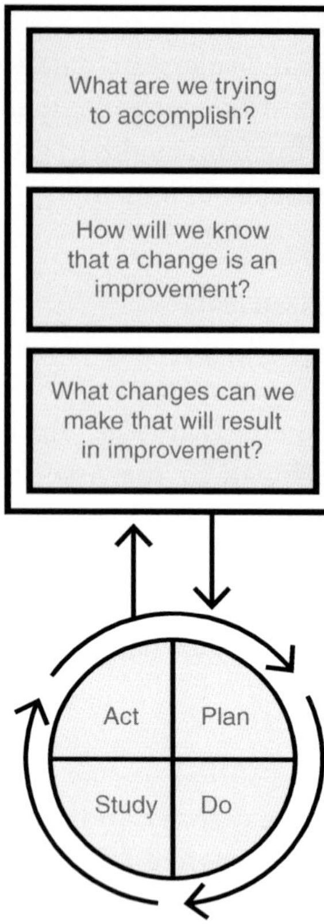

Figure 2. The model for improvement. Reproduced from Langley *et al.* The improvement guide: a practical approach to enhancing organizational performance. Jossey-Bass, San Francisco, CA, 2009.[3] This material is reproduced with permission of (Wiley-Liss Inc, Wiley Publishing Inc, a subsidiary of John Wiley and Sons, Inc.).

focused, e.g. reduce CLABSI to zero by December 1 2015. A clear aim statement will provide an idea of how much and by when.

The second question is "how will we know that a change is an improvement" — here we are referring to the changes we will make as part of an improvement project, as not all changes will lead to improvement. To answer this question **measures** are required. In this example we have a clear **outcome measure** a reduction in CLABSI to zero. As the aim is to reduce to zero we must know our baseline data that should have been recorded frequently enough to give us a median or mean as our starting point; if rates are low, data for the previous six months may be required

If an improvement project is focused on a problem that occurs more frequently, e.g. discharges from an ICU between 10 pm and 8 am, then daily or weekly data can be used for baseline and measurement.

Measurement for improvement

To achieve improvement, we will need some **process measures**. Process measures will measure what we believe we can do to improve outcome, e.g. with central line insertion, our aim is to ensure that we have 100% compliance with all elements of the bundle being used during insertion (process measure — number of line inserted where all bundle components were applied). In addition we could ensure every CLABSI that occurs has a root cause analysis performed to discover defects and consequently the areas required for improvement (process measure: percentage of infections where a Root Cause Analysis (RCA) was performed). Whenever a system is changed we must consider how our changes impact on other parts of the system, namely the unintended consequences. We therefore need **balancing measures**. For example, if we focus on CLABSI prevention do we reduce performance in other key safety processes (e.g. discharges from an ICU between 10 pm and 8 am)?

Once measures are established, then the multi-disciplinary team can start to develop ideas for change. Evidence about what has worked elsewhere and guidelines and research evidence should be gathered. Think critically about the system that impacts the problem (e.g. discharges from an ICU between 10 pm and 8 am) you want to improve. Consider getting a group of stakeholders into the room to process map the patient pathway from the time of the decision to discharge to the time of arrival on the ward. Stakeholders should be multi-professional including ward nurses and porters as well as the ICU team. Where in that pathway might change be most effective? What does it feel like to be a patient in this process — what would make their experience better? With ideas generated in this way you can then start to develop some change concepts.

Plan to Study Act

Once ideas are developed they require testing as "all improvement will require change, but not all change will result in improvement". Start on the

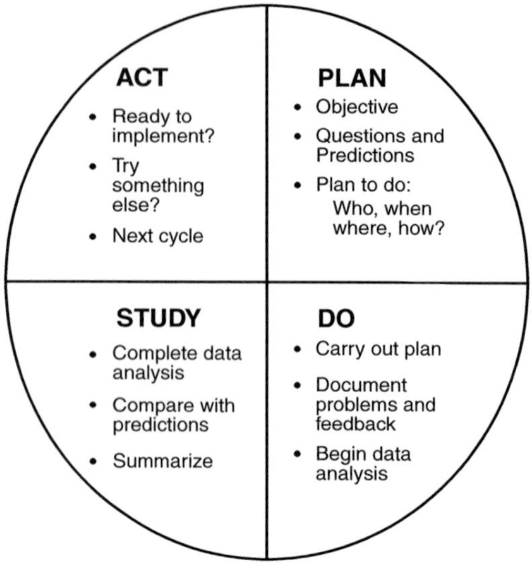

Figure 3. Developing and testing a change within the PDSA cycle, these cycles should be rapid, it is the doing and testing that leads to learning.

plan, do, study and act (PDSA cycle) Figure 3.[3] **Plan** your first test of change, e.g. phone the appropriate ward about the patient discharge immediately at the end of the evening round. **Do** this and study what happens. Start the test on a small scale, e.g. make calls after one round on one day. **Study**: what happened, could you find a nurse on the ward to talk to, how much time did this save on the normal referral process? What was learned about the change idea? **Act**: develop the idea further based on any learning to and test again. The cycle goes on, testing theories about what will work and learning from what does not work (Figure 3). If this idea helps discharge times during a weekday night, does it work on a weekend night? The process is not reliable until it works with different teams and at different times of the day and night. PDSA cycle therefore uses small, rapid cycle changes designed to test, measure impact and test again. Learning from what does not work is as important as learning what works. Ideas should be tested at various times of the day and week and with different teams to ensure they are as robust as possible before full implementation. This is a very different way of change compared with writing a new guideline or policy and circulating it. With the MFI the application and context of the guideline needs to have been considered and tested.

Data for improvement

In order to be able to understand the impact of change we need data collected over time. In many countries ICUs have high quality data for benchmarking outcomes and activity through participation in registries or national audits such as the Intensive Care National Audit and Research Centre (ICNARC) and the Scottish Intensive Care Society Audit Group (SICSAG) programs in the UK. While these centres provide excellent high level data for outcome and resource use, to accomplish rapid cycle change lower level data such as process measures which contribute to outcome must be analyzed and reviewed more frequently.

If a process is not measured in some fashion any change cannot be determined to be an improvement. Key measures are needed to assess a team's progress towards their aim or goal while specific measures can be used for learning during PDSA cycles. Having established baseline data (that can be collected over days or weeks for most QI projects) with initial measurement, we then need to ask the second question in the MFI: how will I know that the change made is an improvement?

Statistical Process Control charts

QI projects commonly use very simple run charts but they can be more sophisticated SPC charts. In healthcare, we have historically relied on aggregated data and summary statistics. Aggregated data (average before and after) presented in tabular formats or with summary statistics do not help measure the impact of process improvement. If we rely on aggregated data to make decisions or comparisons we are concentrating purely on the difference between two numbers rather than what happens to the numbers over time. QI and changes in the ICU happen on a moment-to-moment basis, and as a result, need to be measured over time as a dynamic process (we need to understand how the process is affected by alterations in the system) rather than a single static measurement (see Figure 4).

SPC charts are simple graphical representations of current performance.[14] They are relatively easy to construct, easy to interpret and designed to identify the type of variation that exists within a system. There are two types of variation: 'common cause' and 'special cause' variation. 'Common cause' variation is due to regular, natural or ordinary causes.

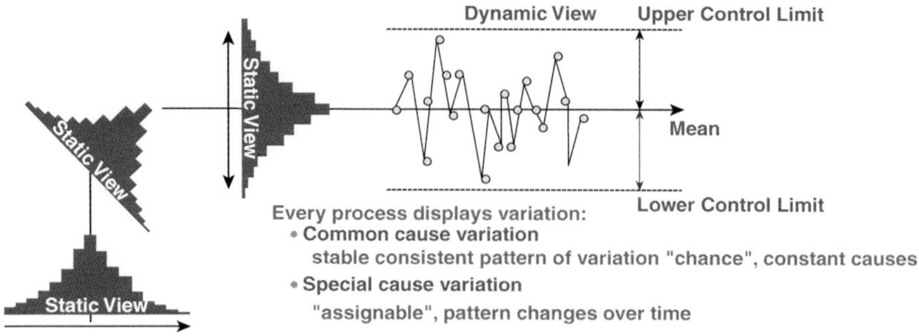

Figure 4. Dynamic SPC chart.

It results in a 'stable' process that, although variable, is predictable (e.g. the variable but regular patterns of admissions to an ICU vary throughout the day but are commoner in the early evening and may increase on a Friday in a pattern we may all recognize). 'Special cause' variation is due to irregular or unnatural causes that are not inherent in the normal variation resulting in an 'unstable' process that is not predictable (e.g. ICU admissions during an influenza epidemic). Two of the most commonly used SPC charts are the run chart and the control chart.

A run chart is a plot of data over time with the unit of time always plotted on the *x*-axis and the indicator (the key quality characteristic) always plotted on the *y*-axis. The data are arranged in chronological order and the centre line of the chart is the median value.

Control charts, like run charts, are graphic dynamic displays of process variation over time. However, there are two key distinctions between run charts and control charts: the run chart is not as sensitive to special cause variation as the control chart. This is because the run chart is not sensitive to extreme values in the data, as the centre line on the run chart is the median in comparison to the mean on a control chart. Although less sensitive than control charts, run charts are generally useful, simple ways of collecting data. Control charts have upper and lower control limits (UCL, LCL) that define the boundaries of the variation around the mean. If all possible data are collected and analyzed, do we really need to look at the data over time; can we not compare the average before and after? Figure 5 shows an example of a hypothetical test of change in three different units. The bar graph shows the same average change for all

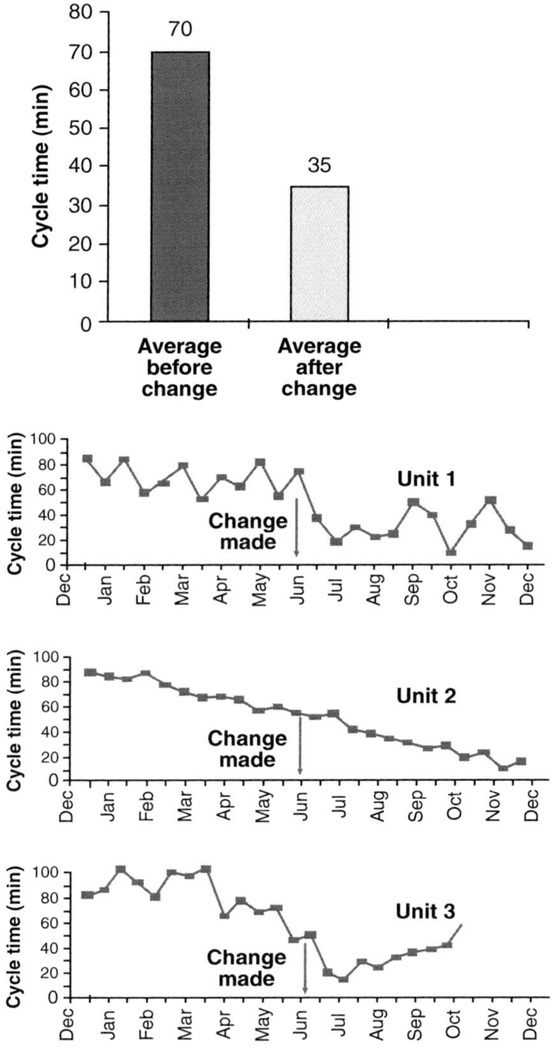

Figure 5. Cycle time results for units 1, 2, and 3. Reproduced from Langley *et al.* The improvement guide: a practical approach to enhancing organizational performance. Jossey-Bass, San Francisco, CA, 2009.[3] This material is reproduced with permission of (Wiley-Liss Inc, Wiley Publishing Inc, a subsidiary of John Wiley and Sons, Inc.).

three units. However, on closer examination, in unit one the run chart suggests that the improvement indicated in the bar graph is genuine and sustained. In units two and three, with the identical bar graph change, there is no evidence from the run chart that the change had any real impact; unit two was improving anyway and unit three improved and then started to deteriorate. Looking at data over time is important to prevent misinterpretation and also allows patterns to emerge, e.g. discharges from ICU after midnight are associated with increased mortality but we would not know that if unit data were recorded only on a daily or weekly basis.

Run charts offer the following advantages over static data displays[14] by

- Displaying data in a way to make process performance visible.
- Determining if changes tested resulted in improvement.
- Determining if gains made by our improvement work are sustained.
- Allowing for a temporal (analytic) view of data versus a static (enumerative) view.

The construction and display of such run charts should form an integral part of a QI process. Results should be made available to staff, patients, and carers. For more in-depth information on SPC charts and the sophisticated statistical analyses that can be made with them read the article by Perla and colleagues.[14]

Audit and QI in the ICU

Principles of audit

In order to support audit and QI, ICUs require robust data collection systems. Data collection systems should be easy to use, secure and resilient. It is important that resources are identified to employ staff to facilitate data collection and input. Recognized national audits, together with collection of national mandated datasets can provide information for both quality assurance and QI but it is important that units review and analyze these data regularly.

Audit is recognized as the cornerstone of clinical governance strengthened by acceptance of the value of systematic critical and objective examination of practice by clinicians and management alike. The quality of delivery of healthcare can be divided into three domains defined by Donabedian[15]:

- Structure: e.g. how many critical care beds are available 24 hours per day for acute admissions?
- Process: e.g. % of delirium assessment correctly performed on at risk patients in the ICU.
- Outcome: e.g. standardized mortality rate of the unit at 30 days.

Much audit has been process based but with an increasing emphasis for patient or person centred care there should be greater focus on what matters to patients, outcomes, and experience. There is also a need for good long term follow up perhaps using telephone evaluation as well as clinics. The use of longer term ICU follow up is leading to a much greater understanding of the link between what happens to the patient in ICU and future health, for example the links between hypoglycaemia and subsequent depressive symptoms and the use of ICU diaries and reduction in post-traumatic stress disorder.[16]

Linking audit to QI

One of the criticisms of traditional audit is that it has often failed to lead to genuine change; therefore, a clear plan to integrate audit with QI is necessary to:

- Know why or what you need to improve (audit provides this information).
- Have a feedback mechanism to identify if improvement has happened (close the audit loop).
- Develop a change that will lead to improvement.
- Test a change before implementation; this may lead to multiple cycles of further change.
- Know when you have an effective change that will lead to an improvement and then implement more widely and aim for sustained change.

Morbidity and mortality meetings

The UK Guidelines for Provision of Intensive Care Services (GPICS) document[17] makes the following recommendations for Morbidity and Mortality meetings in the ICU.

- All unit deaths should be discussed at a Morbidity and Mortality meeting. Morbidity and mortality reviews should use a structured approach so that themes for improvement can be developed.
- Questions such as "how could we have done better?" should be asked rather than "was death predictable?" Deficiencies in care should lead to measurable change.
- Patient and family experience data should be included in audit.
- Reported incidents should be reviewed regularly with a record of actions taken and lessons learnt. There should be clear structures in place for disseminating findings to staff.
- Risks should be recorded and regularly reviewed and updated.

Pro-actively search for harm

ICUs should also consider other screening methods to detect harm in addition to formal structured review of deaths and reporting of incidents. ICUs are high risk settings for patients; it is recognized that only a small proportion of harm to patients is actually reported, both in ICU and throughout the hospital. Therefore, in order to improve care and outcomes we need to have screening systems in place for detecting harm. One such system is the Global Trigger Tool, which is the most widely used validated tool for detecting harm. It has not been widely used in ICU but one Scandinavian study[18] found that almost 20% of patients who died in the ICU were subjected to harmful events. This tool could be used as a review tool on a random selection of all ICU patients each month or to examine care in the period preceding ICU admission in addition to reviewing care in those who die.

In improving care for our ICU patients in what is a high-risk environment we should consider new ways of thinking about safety and harm, how we detect risks, how we act to mitigate them, and how we ensure our unit is safe today and in the future. Vincent's concept of a framework[19] for safety measurement and monitoring asks five questions:

- Has patient care been safe in the past? The answers to this come from audit and screening for harm as well as review of outcome data.
- Are clinical systems and processes reliable? Tools for improving reliability such as bundles and checklists have been described above, and audit and QI should monitor delivery of processes and seek to continually improve.
- Is care safe today? This encompasses review of some of the structural components of an ICU such as staffing and the impact of sickness, which may be affected by the current culture of the unit. This question deals with the capacity of the ICU and teams to respond to changing need.
- Will care be safe in the future? Simulation and team training are techniques that can be used to improve performance against high-risk situations such as accidental extubation. Proactive examination of recognized high-risk areas such as handover and medication safety may also provide projects and ideas for improvement.
- Are we responding and improving? How we integrate, learn, and feedback that learning from our ICU audit and governance systems is critical to ensure that we continue to improve.

Psychology of Change and Sustaining Change

Improving the way we work and deliver care to improve outcomes for ICU patients will require change. This can be challenging and it is helpful to understand some of the concepts of how to deal with barriers to change in order for improvement work to be successful and sustainable. The Harvard Business Professor, John Kotter, described eight steps to sustainable change,[20] which are as relevant to healthcare as they are to business. The eight steps are:

1. Create urgency — does using audit data show that outcome could be better, or incident reports and mortality reviews. Do not let benchmarking

inhibit the drive for improvement. If you are already the best in your network, start asking what are the best units in the world doing?

2. Create a coalition — get the key members of the multi-disciplinary team together to create change.
3. Develop a vision and strategy — state a clear aim such as "by the 1st of December 2015 we will reduce our central line infection rate to zero"
4. Communicate the vision — ensure everyone on the unit knows the aim and the plan to achieve it.
5. Empower action — the PDSA cycle can be used to empower frontline staff to make quick small changes, which they can review for effect.
6. Get quick wins — always start with the easy things and work with people who want to be engaged, once there are a few quick wins momentum and belief in change accelerates.
7. Leverage wins to drive change — use the wins to start to embed the changes into the unit, do not however, try to embed changes until they have been tested and refined under different conditions such as nights and weekends.
8. Embed the culture — use the learning from the project to make the changes sustainable — why did some test work and others did not and celebrate success?

Conclusion

CC teams have been central to development and delivery of some of the modern concepts used in QI such as the use of bundles to provide highly reliable care. ICU patients are at high risk of harm and we should use data for improvement, not only from large national audits or registries, but also from small regular samples to monitor performance and the effect of improvement. Use of the MFI and PDSA cycles can empower front line staff to test small changes that can be developed into sustainable improvement. Change is not easy and any improvement work should take into account the interaction of system issues including the psychology of change. Audit and governance should seek to examine practice in a structured consistent manner so that themes for improvement can be developed.

References

1. Institute of Medicine (1990). *Crossing the Quality Chasm: a New Health System for the 21st Century*. National Academy Press, Washington DC.
2. Best M, Neuhauser D and Shewhart WA (2006). 1924 and the Hawthorne factory. *Qual. Saf. HeathCare*, 15, 142–143.
3. Langley GJ, Moen R, Nolan KM and Nolan TW (2009). *The Improvement Guide: a Practical Approach to Enhancing Organizational Performance*. Jossey-Bass, San Francisco.
4. Sundaram R and Rooney KD (2015). Reliable critical care: making it easy to do the right thing. *Brit. J. Anaesth.*, 115(2), 161–163.
5. The Acute Respiratory Distress Syndrome network (2000). Ventilation with lower tidal volumes as compared with traditional tidal volumes for acute lung injury and the acute respiratory distress syndrome. *N. Engl. J. Med.*, 342, 1301–1308.
6. Nolan T, Resar R and Haraden C (2004). Improving the Reliability of Health Care. IHI Innovation Series white paper. Institute for Healthcare Improvement, Boston. Available at: www.ihi.org/IHI/Results/WhitePapers/ImprovingtheReliabilityofHealthCare.htm (Accessed 7 July 2015).
7. Bordeaux C, Birnie K and Trickey A (2015). Evaluation of an intervention to reduce tidal volumes in ventilated patients on the ICU. *Brit. J. Anaesth.*, 115(2), 244–251.
8. Resar R, Griffin FA, Haraden C and Nolan TW (2012). Using Care Bundles to Improve Health Care Quality. IHI Innovation Series white paper. Institute for Healthcare Improvement, Cambridge, MA. Available at: http://www.IHI.org.
9. Miller RR, Dong L and Nelson NC (2013). Multicenter implementation of a severe sepsis and septic shock treatment bundle. *Am. J. Respir. Crit. Care, Med.*, 188(1), 77–82.
10. Pronovost P, Needham D and Berenholtz S (2006). An intervention to decrease catheter-related bloodstream infections in the ICU. *N. Engl. J. Med.*, 355, 2725–2732.
11. Dixon-Woods M, Bosk CL and Aveling EL (2011). Explaining Michigan: developing an ex post theory of a quality improvement program. *Milbank Q.*, 89(2), 167–205.
12. Dixon-Woods M, Myles L, Tarrant C and Bion J (2013). Explaining matching Michigan: an ethnographic study of a patient safety program. *Implement. Sci.*, 8, 70.
13. Weiss CH, Moazed F and McEvoy CA (2011). Prompting physicians to address a daily checklist and process of care and clinical outcomes: a single-site study. *Am. J. Respir. Crit. Care Med.*, 184(6), 680–686.

14. Perla RJ, Provost LP and Murray SK (2011). The run chart: a simple analytical tool for learning from variation in healthcare processes. *BMJ Qual. Saf.*, 20, 46–51.
15. Donabedian A (1966). Evaluating the quality of medical care. *Milbank Mem. Fund Q. Suppl.*, 44(3), 166–206.
16. Herridge M and Cox C (2012). Linking ICU practice to long-term outcome. Fostering a longitudinal vision for ICU-acquired morbidity. *Am. J. Respir. Crit. Care Med.*, 186, 299–305.
17. Peden CJ and Groves J (2015). Faculty of Intensive Care Medicine and Intensive Care Society. Guidelines for Provision of ICU Services. Quality Improvement, audit and peer review. Section 5.3.4. Available at: http://www.ficm.ac.uk/sites/default/files/GPICS%20-%20Ed.1%20%282015%29.pdf (Accessed 7 July 2015).
18. Nilsson L, Pihl A, Tagsjo M and Ericsson E (2012). Adverse events are common on the intensive care unit: results from a structured record review. *Acta Anaesth. Scand.*, 56, 959–965.
19. Vincent C, Burnett S and Carthey J (2014). The measurement and monitoring of safety. The Health Foundation. Available at: www.health.org.uk (Accessed 7 July 2015).
20. Kotter JP (2007). *Leading Change: Why Transformation Efforts Fail.* Harvard Business Review. Available at: https://hbr.org/2007/01/leading-change-why-transformation-efforts-fail (Accessed 7 July 2015).

Patient and Staff Safety

Gavin Lavery
HSC Safety Forum, Public Health Agency,
Belfast Critical Care Consultant,
Regional Intensive Care Unit, Belfast HSC Trust, Belfast, UK

Key Points

1. Patient safety incidents are common, are usually caused by system failures and are often preventable.
2. Patient safety incidents that do not reach the patient (near misses) are valuable opportunities for change before harm occurs. We should remove barriers that impede the reporting of near misses.
3. We should ask ourselves — was our care safe in the past? Is it safe today? Will it be safe in the future? Are we responding and improving.
4. The intensive care unit (ICU) environment exposes staff to stressful and emotionally demanding situations, which places them at high risk for burnout.
5. Caring for the welfare of staff and engaging them in change improves morale, reduces the risk of burnout and improves the quality and safety of care for patients. Staff engagement is emerging as the antithesis of burnout.

What is Patient Safety?

Patient safety is a discipline in the healthcare sector that applies scientific methods with the aim of building a trustworthy system of healthcare delivery. Patient safety is also an attribute of healthcare systems; it minimizes the incidence and impact of, and maximizes recovery from, adverse events. More simply, patient safety is avoiding harm from care or treatment that is intended to help or cure. The World Alliance for Safer Healthcare has defined a patient safety incident is an event or circumstance that could have resulted, or did result, in unnecessary harm to a patient.[1] Wherever possible we should use this phrase or the term "incident" in place of numerous interchangeable terms — adverse events, critical incidents, unplanned incidents or events.

The scale of the problem

In 1999, To Err is Human[2] highlighted adverse events in healthcare, estimating that they were responsible for 44,000–98,000 deaths annually in the US. Medication errors alone, often estimated to be around 25% of all adverse events accounted for 7,000 deaths. Reports from the UK, Australia, New Zealand, and Canada paint a similar picture.

While much of the data above are 10–20 years old, more recent data are of limited value since patterns of reporting vary significantly in both "mandatory" and voluntary reporting systems. There is no agreement on how we define an "adverse event" (patient safety incident) or what represents patient harm.

In an international study of safety incidents in ICU that sampled 1,913 adult patients in 205 ICUs over a 24 hour period, 584 incidents affecting 391 patients (20%) were reported.[3] The incidents included medication errors in 136 patients (36% of all patients experiencing a patient safety incident); 158 patients had dislodgement or inappropriate disconnection of lines, catheters, and drains; equipment failure affected 112 patients; there was loss, obstruction, or leakage of an artificial airway in 47 patients. The adverse event rate was almost 40 per 100 patient days with organ failure and increasing complexity of care increasing the risk of an incident.

Patient safety — the context

To many clinicians, patient safety is based on delivering the best direct clinical care (CC) possible to patients. This will be achieved by becoming the best-informed and best "hands-on" clinician they can be. For previous generations, this was a reasonable assumption, as CC in hospital was delivered or controlled by key individuals — the senior doctor (attending/consultant) and the senior ward nurse. While individual excellence is still important, in isolation it will not deliver safety in healthcare.

Today, all healthcare systems face increasing complexity on many fronts. The success of a longer-lived population means patients living decades with long-term conditions (including cancer) whose treatment is challenging, due to their chronic health problems and superimposed acute illnesses. Our response to this complexity has been the growth in numbers of highly specialized individuals and teams who deliver very high quality care but in a relatively narrow clinical area. Medicine (and CC generally) has changed from one in which a doctor crafted a clinical solution ("cure") specifically for an individual patient to a quasi-industrial system of processes in which different elements of the solution are supplied by different specialist teams and professions.

Our thinking and approaches to delivering care have not changed in parallel with these changes. Many think improvements in care are based on new technologies or the skill and diligence of individual practitioners. These will help but will not unite what are often fragmented approaches. Some still believe that safety will be advanced by a new policy, guideline or protocol. Such strategies consume much time and energy but often fail to change clinical practice. Increasingly we recognize a culture of learning (from error and success), human factors and designing reliable processes as the path to patient safety.

Care delivered by multiple teams sometimes results in the loss of the compassion in healthcare — the human face of caring often termed person-centredness. Today, some patients in hospital will not know which clinician has overall responsibility for their care. Clinical teams sometimes do not have the same sense of ownership and this can lead to loss of situational awareness in terms of the patient's clinical progress. In turn this can result in "transactional care" in which patients receive treatments or interventions that may not be coordinated and may not be in their best interest.

Improved patient safety needs skills and behaviours that reflect the distributive nature of healthcare delivery — applying human factors, focusing on teamwork, better communication and handovers, learning from adverse events and from examples of excellent practice. We need to redesign processes for reliability, reduce variation in care and, above all, put the patient at the centre of all we do.

Why Do Things Go Wrong?

Patient safety incidents usually occur when a number of defects and errors align to leave a "hole" in the defences which normally prevent harm to patients. This is often termed the Swiss Cheese model[4] first described by James Reason (Figure 1).

Some of these "holes" are present in our processes all the time (latent failures) and some occur sporadically (active failures). Even when one or more active failures occur in a system with pre-existing related latent

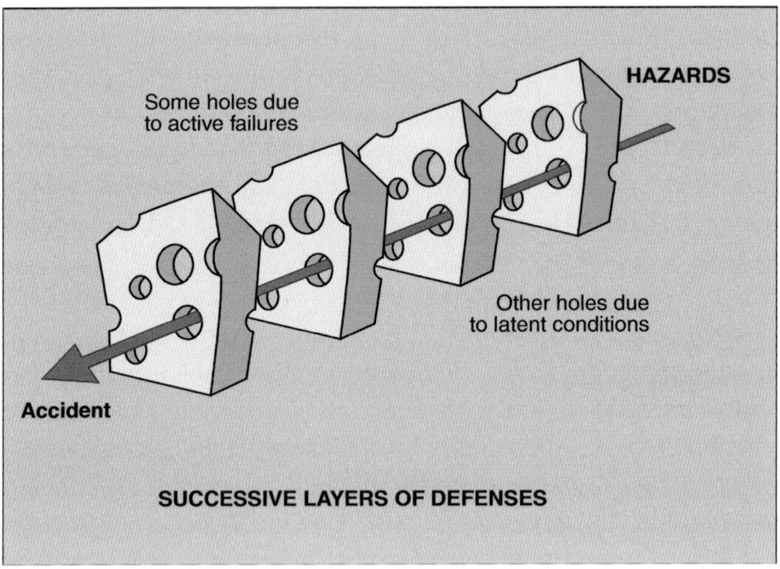

Figure 1. The Swiss cheese model.[4]

failures, the patient usually suffers no harm because other defences are intact — this is what is often termed a "near miss" — a patient safety incident which did not reach the patient.[1] Rarely, a number of failures at different levels within a process combine to breach all defences. This equates to a "hole" penetrating every layer of defence, resulting in patient harm. Decisions and behaviours by humans are involved in most adverse events, contributing either as active or latent failures.

Active failures

Active failures are unsafe acts (or omissions) by those whose actions can have immediate adverse impact. In CC this would include nurses, doctors, technical staff, dieticians, and physiotherapists.

Active failures include:

- Actions — picking up the wrong syringe.
- Thinking errors — memory lapses or misreading a situation.
- Violations — deviating from safe procedure, standards, or rules.[1]

The factors increasing the likelihood of error or active failures are shown in Table 1.

Latent failures

Latent failures are defects and faults that lie within a system. They may be relatively difficult to detect until a near miss occurs. They arise due to decisions, often taken a long time before an incident occurs, often by people not directly involved in the workplace. In the ICU, latent failures would be primarily due to decisions effecting the work and activity of the unit by local or organizational managers and senior clinical staff. Latent failures provide the "fertile soil" from which active failures and unsafe acts arise by impairing staff performance and precipitating errors.

Latent failures in an ICU would include:

- An unsustainable workload.
- Inadequate numbers of appropriately trained staff.
- Inadequate supervision.

Table 1. Factors associated with error/active failures.

Environmental
• Noise, Interruptions, Distractions.
• Poor lighting, temperature control, ventilation.
Team
• Lack of supervision, unsupportive culture.
• Tolerance of violations.
Individual
• Limited knowledge, inexperience.
• Poor insight.
• Isolation.
Task
• Repetitious, poorly designed/absent adjuncts.
• Perception of unimportance.
Patient
• Complex conditions(s).
• Communication difficulties.
• Barriers (isolation/perception) of "difficult" patient.

- Excessive stress or unresolved team conflict.
- Poor communication between clinical teams.
- Poor clinical leadership.
- Rapid staff turnover particularly at senior level.
- Prolonged, excessive or repeated restructuring.

Violations

A violation is a deliberate deviation from an operating procedure, standard or rule.[1] These are more frequent in situations where there is (i) low morale (ii) poor role modeling by seniors, and (iii) poor management.[5] They can be categorized as follows:

Routine violation

Omitting appropriate hand hygiene between patients due to workload is a routine violation. Other examples are habitually poor handovers, not attending patients in a timely fashion and only partially following an ICU protocol. These are common and frequently go unchallenged.

Optimizing violation

An ICU resident allowing an inexperienced doctor to perform a procedure without supervision (e.g. insert a central line) while the resident performs another task in order to appear ultra-efficient is an example of an optimizing violation. Optimizing violations are motivated by personal gain — acquiring praise, advantage, money or occasionally the thrill of taking risks.

Necessary violation

These occur because staff perceive that there is not enough time to follow procedure fully, e.g. omitting some steps in checking before the administration of medication. Even though they are aware that they are not following procedure, staff usually do not view this as risky ("we all do this and nothing bad happens") and certainly do not intend harm to the patient. This type of behaviour is often associated with staff who lack insight regarding risk, have poor understanding of their professional obligations and are poorly managed.

Reporting systems

Patient safety incident reporting systems differ in design and therefore in their ability to define, count, and track adverse events.[6] Reporting systems have disparate data fields, conflicting patient safety terminologies, classifications and characteristics that make standardization difficult. Differing use of terminology by researchers, presenters, and the media contributes to widespread misunderstandings about the language of patient safety.

Reporting systems are local (institutional) or central (external) mechanisms that receive, classify, store, and use patient safety incidents that could, or did, lead to patient harm. Such systems can be anonymous and use voluntary reporting or they can be mandatory. Stakeholders disagree on whether the goal of reporting systems is to improve patient safety or to ensure individual and institutional accountability. To date, most reporting systems focus their attention and resources more on collecting events than analyzing reports and assessing how to use the data to improve patient safety. Reporting systems would be much more useful if they used the information received to identify threats to safety and to prioritize safety efforts. Reporting could aid the development and evaluation of interventions to mitigate safety threats.

Key challenges for reporting systems are the following: what to report, how to minimize burden and cost, how best to conduct expert reviews and prioritize safety efforts, classification — how to place incidents into taxonomies.[8]

In United Kingdom, the National Reporting and Learning System (NRLS) was established in 2003. It has collected over 4 million incidents from both secondary and primary care and has been described as perhaps the most mature, country-level reporting system in existence.[8] However, the volume of reports received, their variable quality and the relevance for system learning creates problems in prioritization. The NRLS has not been successful in designing, testing or evaluating interventions.

In 2003 the Institute of Medicine recommended that standardization and better management of information on patient safety (including near misses and adverse events) were needed to inform the development of strategies to reduce the risk of preventable medical incidents. By 2005, in response 22 US States had passed legislation requiring reporting systems. The Joint Commission requires that hospitals report errors in care. However, there is still no single overarching system within the US for collecting, classifying and analyzing patient safety incidents.

Critical care (CC) Medicine pioneered reporting patient safety incidents in the 1990s with the Australian Incident Monitoring Study in CC.[9] In 2002, the ICU at Johns Hopkins developed and led a web-based electronic reporting system (ICUSRS) involving 30 ICUs.[10] ICUs continue to develop systems to capture patient safety incidents with the intention of identifying threats and improving safety.

What would the ideal incident reporting system look like? It would capture all relevant events in a form that could be analyzed as needed and would result in timely feedback of lessons/necessary changes to a system which welcomed the information. Such a system would have three elements — input, analysis, and feedback.

Input

Input needs to be simple and many feel it should be anonymous if possible. The latter is known to increase the volume of reporting and thus opportunities to learn. Anonymity does produce challenges when additional information is required or when behaviours reported have infringed professional standards.

It may be important to allow reporters to "tell their story" rather than be confined by a rigid structure. This not only promotes reporting but increases quality of data for analysis.[11]

Analysis

Strong analysis of adverse incidents is only possible if sufficient accurate information has been submitted (input) and requires experts in the medical discipline(s) involved and safety or human factors experts jointly interrogating data to generate clinically relevant learning outcomes. This is the most time-consuming step and involves linking the actions or errors that produced the event with defects or failures in the supporting systems. Such analysis should use a standard methodology.

Feedback

The aim is to learn from error and to improve processes and systems leading to safer patient care. This requires all receiving feedback to be open and avoid attributing blame. Feedback is relevant to all staff at all levels not just those at the front-line. To grow a culture of reporting, all staff must view the process as having something positive for them. Feedback and change, should happen in a time-frame that all feel is as rapid as can be managed, mindful that until change occurs patients continue to be at potential risk.

Since feedback is easier to achieve than change, it may be useful to have the following staged feedback; first an acknowledgement to the reporter of the incident that their information has been received — along with a provisional timeline; second, following analysis, distribute the learning report on the incident. The organization (hospital) should then involve front-line staff in designing the changes which are required to prevent repetition of similar incidents. This will improve the impact of the changes and help embed them in routine practice. Finally, the organization should inform all staff of the changes and how/why they have been adopted.

Mandated high-level reporting systems can analyze the frequencies and type of events occurring across a system and distribute this information. This will help the system focus on areas for improvement (e.g. tracheostomy care, nasogastric tube insertion, medication errors) as well as stimulating research, training and curriculum change. This approach, however, is not enough to improve safety at a unit level. This requires local activity — reporting and analyzing local incidents to uncover their root cause and prevent repetition.

In 2002 Lucian Leape wrote "current reporting systems are neither widely used nor highly effective. Reporting systems work best when they are confidential and easy to use, provide expert analysis of reports, and give timely feedback".[7] In 2015, reporting systems are still struggling to fulfill that remit.

Patient Safety Incidents

A patient safety incident can be a reportable circumstance, a near miss, an incident with no harm or an incident with harm (often termed an adverse incident or event). A reportable circumstance is a situation with significant potential for harm, but where no incident occurred (e.g. an ICU severely understaffed for current workload for a shift/day, or bringing a defibrillator to the bedside of a very unstable ICU patient and finding it faulty although it was not needed). A near miss is an incident which did not reach the patient (e.g. a unit of blood checked incorrectly against the wrong patient with the error detected before infusion). A no harm incident is one in which an event reached a patient but no discernible harm resulted (e.g. if the above blood was infused, but, fortunately, was not incompatible). A harmful incident (adverse event) results in harm to a patient (e.g. the wrong unit of blood was infused and the patient died from a haemolytic reaction; the wrong side of the body was operated on; the wrong joint prosthesis was inserted).

The terms near miss, (serious) adverse incident and similar, e.g. adverse event, critical incident are deeply ingrained in our systems. Earlier we defined a near miss as a patient safety incident that did not reach the patient. Using the International Classification for Patient Safety (ICPS) conceptual framework[1] a serious adverse incident might be termed a patient safety incident causing moderate or serious harm or death. Serious adverse incidents have also been defined as events in healthcare where the potential for learning is so great, or the consequences to patients, families and carers, staff or organizations are so significant, that they warrant using additional resources to mount a comprehensive response. Serious incidents can extend beyond incidents which affect patients directly and include incidents which may indirectly impact patient safety or an organization's ability to deliver on-going healthcare.

Patient safety incident without harm — near miss

This can be viewed as the dress-rehearsal for an incident causing harm (adverse incident). To stop the latter happening we must study what nearly happened. We can then change the context by removing latent failures and work to avoid repetition of the active failures precipitating the near miss. In a learning culture, near-misses are reported and used to improve the process before harm occurs. However, in some health systems or organizations this opportunity is lost. Near misses may not be reported,[12] or reported and ignored and, possibly after repeated near misses, a patient may be harmed by the same latent and active failures. Even then, when the incident with harm is reported, the organization concerned may apologize but still do nothing to change the system, with the probability that one or more future patients will be harmed.

Near misses have been described as a "free lesson on your weaknesses". It gives us an opportunity to fix the system without anyone being harmed. The ability to report, analyze and learn from near-misses is one of the most important tools to improve patient safety. Since no harm occurs in a near miss, it can frequently remain invisible to the system, unless staff choose to report it, i.e. reporting cannot be mandated. Thus removing the barriers to reporting is crucial.

The main barriers to reporting are time, fear, and blame. A reporting mechanism that is complex or time-consuming is a barrier, as is fear of being viewed as disloyal or a trouble-maker. A culture of blame will obviously prevent self-reporting and may also reduce the reporting of incidents involving colleagues. This can be overcome by a system allowing anonymous confidential reporting. Such systems have been demonstrated to increase reporting but have the disadvantage that no further information can be obtained from the (anonymous) reporter.

Patient safety incident with harm — adverse incident

Serious adverse incidents are usually reported via a mandatory reporting system to an external entity. They (usually) cause significant harm and so are highly visible. Examples include maternal deaths; deaths or serious harm associated with use of new drug, technology or technique; unexpected deaths in any healthcare setting but often following surgery, anaesthesia or other intervention; abuse. In many health systems, other specific events have been designated as "never events" (e.g. wrong site surgery, events involving high-risk medications, blood transfusion errors) which must be reported. Often significant events, designated as reportable locally may go unreported.[12]

Blame and Just Culture

Our tendency to blame when things go wrong is driven by a belief, sometimes subliminal, that the staff member involved wasn't being careful enough or even chose to do the wrong thing intentionally. With this mindset, it seems appropriate to attribute responsibility for an adverse incident to the mistakes or misconduct of those in operational control of events (active failures — the smoking gun close to the incident) rather than consider the system or those with managerial control of the system (latent failures). It might also seem logical to think that, since individuals are trained to perform various tasks, a failure of one of "their" tasks must relate to failure of that individual — who therefore deserves punishment.

This approach was challenged by Perrow[13] who observed that up to 80% of system failures were actually attributed to "operator error". Reason's Swiss Cheese Model builds on the idea that causation of adverse events is usually multi-factorial — with many factors outside the control of any individual.[4] We must, however, acknowledge the rare situation when harm is due to deliberate intentional acts or gross violations of accepted standards by one or more individuals.

Analysis of adverse incidents will usually reveal weaknesses in the system. This does not mean that our view of adverse events should always be "blame-free". Understanding the relative contribution of the individual and the system to adverse events is sometimes difficult. An "Unsafe Act" algorithm is a method of making such assessments in a fair and just manner. It has been streamlined into to four simple questions by Frankel and Leonard for use by those investigating and analyzing adverse events[14]:

- Did the employee intend to cause harm?
- Did the employee come to work drunk or equally impaired?
- Did the employee knowingly and unreasonably increase risk?
- Would another similarly trained and skilled employee in the same situation act in a similar manner (Reason's substitution test)?

If the first three answers are "No" and the last "Yes" the origin of the unsafe act lies in the organization, not the individual.

A Just Culture is about fair, enlightened, and reasonable assessment of behaviour and produces a working environment that supports high reliability. In such a culture, caregivers feel that they are supported and safe when voicing concerns.[14] Individuals know that they may speak safely on issues regarding their own actions or those of others. They feel able and expected to perform at their best but also feel able to admit weakness and seek assistance when the quality and safety of the care being delivered seems threatened. These workers know that they are accountable for their actions, but will not be blamed for system faults beyond their control. The response to human error or risky behaviour in a fair and just culture is

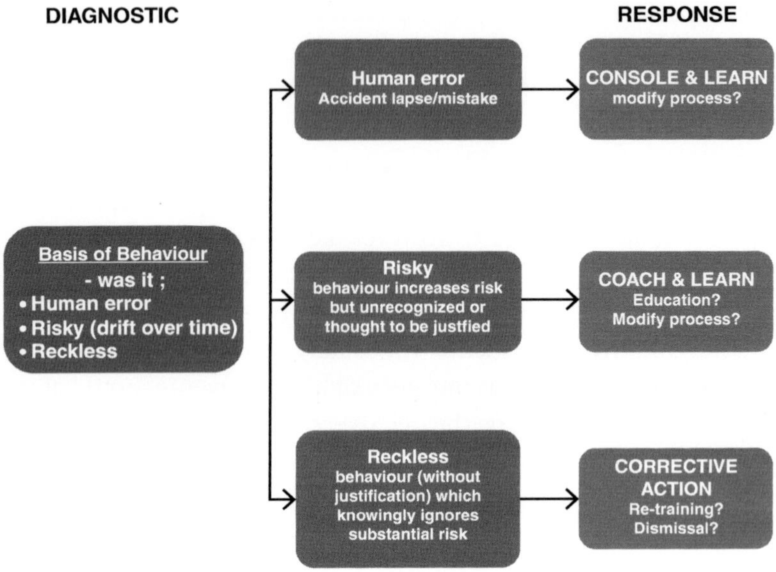

Figure 2. Response to human error, risky, and reckless behaviours (adapted from Mayo Clinic).

learning. Only reckless behaviour provokes corrective action (Figure 2). Near-misses (no harm) and adverse incidents causing harm are treated in the same way since the action is the same; the difference in outcome is merely due to chance.

Frameworks in Patient Safety

Patient Safety is influenced by a multitude of factors: the structures and systems of healthcare, processes, teams, human factors, environment, the quality of staff training, their knowledge, skills, and attitudes and workplace culture. Patient safety can influence by measurement and monitoring, and finally the contribution of patients to their own safety. The terminology used is diverse, ambiguous, and potentially confusing — error, failure, violation, near miss, harm, adverse event, critical incident. The knowledge relevant to patient safety is spread among clinical professions, systems thinkers, engineers, psychologists, data experts and others. To organize our thinking and our strategies, we need frameworks to facilitate reporting and analysis, frameworks to measure culture and cultural change, measurement and monitoring and frameworks that facilitate training and education on safety.

Frameworks to facilitate reporting and analysis

In 2005 Chang *et al.*,[6] published a classification system for near misses and adverse events based on 5 primary classifications; impact, type, domain, cause, prevention and mitigation — each with sub-classifications. The purpose of the resultant Joint Commission on Accreditation of Healthcare Organizations (JCAHO) *Patient Safety Event Taxonomy* was to facilitate a common approach for patient safety information systems. Standardized data would make it easier to file patient safety event reports and to conduct consistent root cause analyses.

In 2009, The WHO World Alliance for Patient Safety devised the conceptual framework for an ICPS.[1] Its aim was to define, harmonize and group patient safety concepts into an agreed classification that facilitated learning and improving patient safety across systems. The ICPS framework helps categorize patient safety information using agreed definitions and preferred terms and is based on 10 high level classes and 48 key concepts which have been defined and assigned preferred terms to facilitate understanding and transfer of information (Figure 3).

Frameworks to facilitate cultural change, measurement, and monitoring safety

In 1998 Vincent *et al.*[5] published a framework for analyzing risk and safety in clinical medicine in order to facilitate a systematic approach to safety and error reduction. The framework described the factors influencing clinical practice and therefore the causes of patient safety incidents. Its purpose was to guide patient safety incident investigations, to generate methods of assessing risk, and to promote and focus research on the causes and prevention of poor clinical outcomes.

The Patient Safety Framework model suggested by Frankel and Leonard[14] summarizes the elements required to ensure organizations,

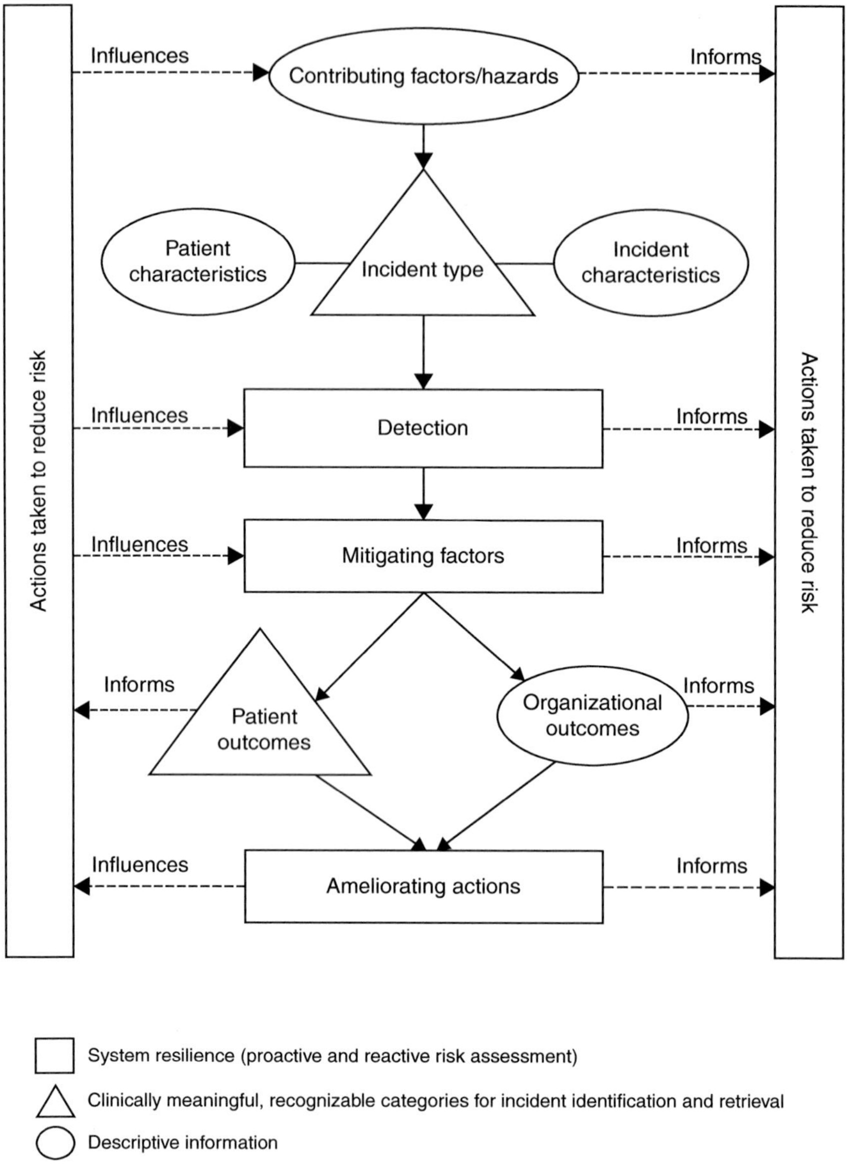

Figure 3. Conceptual framework for the international classification of patient safety.[1]

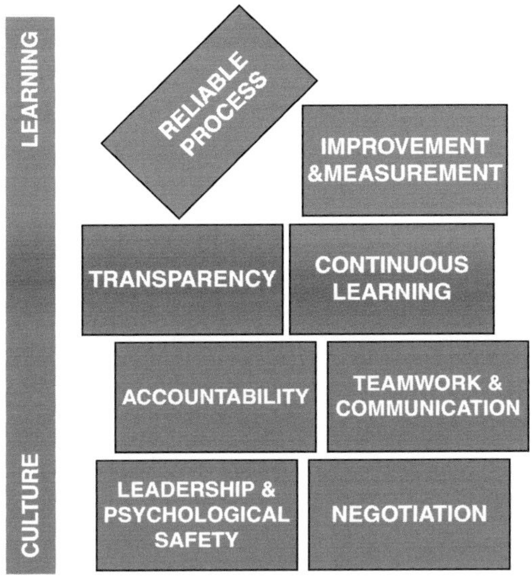

Figure 4. Essential components for a patient safety strategy.[14]

systems and teams are capable of delivering safe, reliable care (Figure 4) and has been adopted by NHS England and others.

The Manchester Patient Safety Framework (MaPSaF) was designed for use within the NHS.[15] It is a tool to help organizations and teams assess their progress in developing a safety culture. MaPSaF uses critical dimensions of patient safety and describes five levels of increasingly mature organizational safety culture. The dimensions relate to areas where attitudes, values and behaviours about patient safety are likely to be reflected in the organization's processes, e.g. investigation of adverse incidents, staff education, and training in risk management. MaPSaF can be used:

- To facilitate reflection on patient safety culture.
- To stimulate discussion about the patient safety culture.
- To reveal differences in perception between staff groups.
- To help understand how a more mature safety culture might look.
- To evaluate intervention(s) needed to change the patient safety culture.

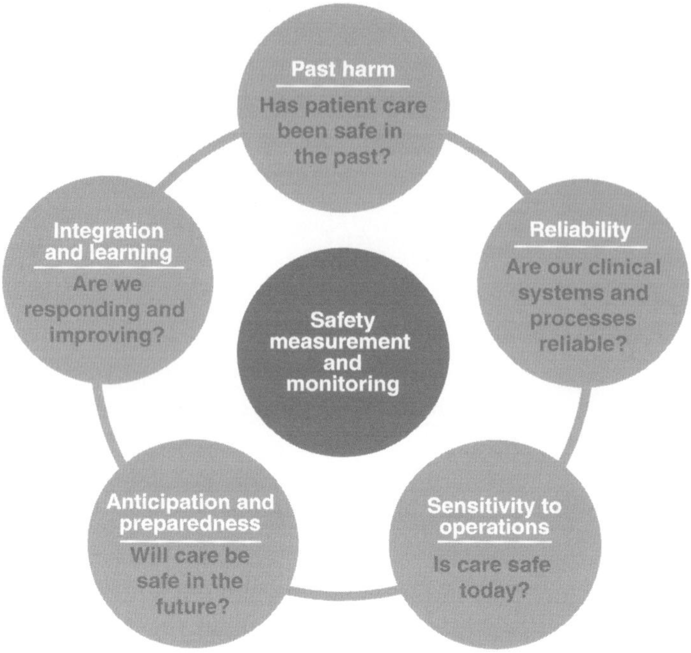

Figure 5. Framework for the measurement and monitoring of safety.[16]

In 2013, work by Charles Vincent led work for the Health Foundation to develop a framework for the measurement and monitoring of safety.[16] The framework (Figure 5) builds on the question "Is our healthcare organization safe? — by posing several (more discriminating) questions:

- Has patient care been safe in the past?
- Are our clinical systems and processes reliable? Is care safe today?
- Will care be safe in the future?
- Are we responding and improving?

Staff safety and fulfillment

While this section will focus on the psychological, (rather than the physical) safety of staff, it would be wrong to overlook the physical dangers posed, to ICU staff in particular, by outbreaks of life-threatening transmissible disease e.g. the 2014/2015 Ebola crisis. In such circumstances, it is important that appropriate personal protective equipment (PPE), training and other guidance is available as early as necessary. During the treatment of repatriated victims of Ebola, the appropriateness and timeliness of supply of PPE, and training of staff was contentious.[17]

Staff need access to designated PPE early enough to receive training and become proficient with its use before there is a significant risk of receiving infected patients. A real-world evaluation of how to use, and how long to work in PPE is also important. Simply issuing guidelines and protocols on PPE and cross-infection precautions and expecting staff to manage is unacceptable. Such behaviour would suggest to staff that they, and their safety, are not valued by their organizations.

Work related stress and burnout are under-recognized threats to the health and safety of ICU staff. Burnout is a colloquial term describing a state of work-related mental exhaustion and may be the antithesis of engagement. Table 1 summarizes the risk factors that have been advanced for burnout. It is more likely to occur in younger members of staff and where staff morale and engagement is poor. Conflict between staff or staff groupings (particularly in the often close-knit community of an ICU) and lack of clear protocols (particularly regarding end-of-life care) generate stress which may damage morale and, in some individuals, lead to burnout.[18,19]

Poorly motivated and engaged staff, working in a poor workplace culture is associated with more patient safety incidents,[20] thus setting up a downward spiral of more incidents, more stress, and decreasing morale. Some have argued that the wellbeing of healthcare staff is a missing quality indicator and healthcare institutions are increasingly recognizing that quality of care and patient safety are partly dependent on the employee wellness

In ICU, failure to provide 'care for the carers' may have unwelcome consequences, not least the risk of adverse events, suboptimal care, and poor outcomes. There is little evidence on which to design interventions, but expert opinion suggests the use of multiple approaches at individual, departmental, and organizational level as summarized in Table 2. Giving staff some control and flexibility and valuing their contributions to the workplace appear to be helpful in preventing burnout. This aligns with the

Table 2. Suggested risk factors for burnout in staff.

Intrinsic factors	Extrinsic factors
• Younger workers	• Workload
• Single status	• Choice and control
• Childlessness	• Recognition and reward
• Neuroticism	• Supportive work community
• Low self-esteem	• Fairness and Justice
	• Conflict in Values (individual organizational

Table 3. Multi-level interventions which may reduce the risk of burnout.

Individual	**Unit**	**Organizational**
		Staff engagement
Stress management	Flexible working/rostering	Resource provision
Involvement in research	Leadership development	Policy development
Assertiveness training	Collaborative decision making	Promoting a learning culture
Time management skills	Employee mentorship	Organizational values
Coping strategies	Teambuilding & social support	Hospital management style
Interpersonal skills	Improved end of life care	

ethos of quality improvement in which front-line staff have a central role in redesigning, testing and improving new, more reliable, ways of working.

References

1. Conceptual Framework for the International Classification of Patient Safety version 1.1 (2009). Available at: http://www.who.int/patientsafety/taxonomy/icps_full_report.pdf.
2. Kohn, LT, Corrigan JM and Donaldson MS (2000). *To Err is Human: building a Safer Health System.* Institute of Medicine, National Academy Press, Washington.
3. Valentin A, Capuzzo M and Guidet B (2006). Patient safety in intensive care: results from the multinational Sentinel Events Evaluation (SEE) study. *Intens. Care Med.*, 32, 1591–1598.
4. Reason J (1990). *Human Error.* Cambridge University Press, Cambridge.
5. Vincent C, Taylor-Adams S and Stanhope N (1998). Framework for analyzing risk and safety in clinical medicine. *BMJ*, 316, 1154–1157.

6. Chang A, Schyve PM and Croteau RJ (2005). The JCAHO patient safety event taxonomy: a standardized terminology and classification schema for near misses and adverse events. *Int. J. Qual. Health Care*, 17, 95–105.
7. Leape L (2002). Reporting of adverse events. *N. Engl. J. Med.*, 347, 1633–1638.
8. Pronovost P, *et al.* (2008). Improving the Value of Patient Safety Reporting Systems. Available at: http://www.ahrq.gov/professionals/quality-patient-safety/patient-safety-resources/resources/advances-in-patient-safety-2/vol1/advances-pronovost_95.pdf.
9. Beckmann U, Baldwin I, Hart GK and Runciman WB (1996). The Australian incident monitoring study in intensive care: AIMS-ICU. An analysis of the first year of reporting. *Anaesth. Intens. Care*, 24, 320–329.
10. Wu AW, Pronovost P and Morlock L (2002). ICU incident reporting systems. *J. Crit. Care*, 17, 86–94.
11. Mahajan RP (2010). Critical incident reporting and learning. *Br. J. Anaesth.*, 105, 69–75.
12. Evans SM, Berry JG and Smith BJ (2006). Attitudes and barriers to incident reporting: a collaborative hospital study. *Qual. Saf. Health Care*, 15, 39–43.
13. Perrow C (1999). *Normal Accidents: Living with High-Technologies*, 2nd Edition. Princeton University Press, Princeton NJ.
14. Frankel A and Leonard M (2008). Essential Components for a patient safety strategy. *Perioper. Nurs. Clin.*, 3, 263–276.
15. Manchester Patient Safety Framework (2006). Available at: http://www.nrls.npsa.nhs.uk/resources/?entryid45=59796.
16. Vincent C, Burnett S and Carthy J (2013). The measurement and monitoring of safety. Health Foundation, London.
17. MacIntyre CR, Chughtai AA and Seale H (2015). Uncertainty, risk analysis and change for Ebola personal protective equipment guidelines. *Int. J. Nur. Stud.*, 52, 899–903.
18. Azoulay E, Timsit E and Sprung CL (2009). Prevalence and risk factors of intensive care unit conflicts: the Conflict Study. *Am. J. Respir. Crit. Care Med.*, 180(9), 853–860.
19. Luce JM (2010). A history of resolving conflicts over end-of-life care in intensive care units in the United States. *Crit. Care Med.*, 38, 1623–1269.
20. Montgomery A, Panagopoulou E, Kehoe I and Valkanos E (2011). Connecting organizational culture and quality of care in the hospital: is job burnout the missing link? *J. Health Organ. Manage.*, 25, 108–123.

Policies and Procedures

Andrew T. Levinson and Mitchell M. Levy
Division of Pulmonary/Critical Care Medicine
Department of Medicine
Alpert Medical School at Brown University
Providence, Rhode Island, USA

Key Points

1. ICU admission, discharge, and triage policies can ensure efficient and equitable transitions of care.
2. Checklists, protocols, bundles, and guidelines are tools that can be used to support implementation of new ICU policies and procedures.
3. ICU policy development should be based on a vigorous quality improvement program.
4. Quality improvement is a formal approach to the analysis of performance and systematic efforts to improve it.
5. Accurately measuring and reporting performance faces a variety of technical and logistical challenges that must continue to be addressed through ongoing feedback and refinement.

Introduction

An efficient highly performing intensive care unit (ICU) requires the development and continuous refinement of policies for the delivery of care. Checklists, protocols, bundles, and guidelines are powerful tools to support implementation of and improve ICU policies. Essential to the improvement of ICU policies and procedures is the ongoing collection and dissemination of both process and outcome measures. The accurate measurement and reporting of quality data is becoming even more important as it is becoming increasingly recognized by the public and policy makers and being linked to financial reimbursement.

Admission and Discharge Policies

All ICUs should have specific policies and processes in place for admitting, discharging, and triaging patients. These policies should be regularly reviewed and modified systematically to meet the specific needs of the hospital and communities that the ICU serves.

The Society for Critical Care Medicine (SCCM) published guidelines for ICU admission, discharge and triage in 1999. They are currently in the process of being updated and revised. It is recommended that healthcare systems tailor admission and discharge guidelines specific for their unique hospital and patient populations.

Admission criteria

Admission criteria should be based on a variety of criteria and factors. Current guidelines utilize several models for ICU admission criteria, including prioritization, diagnosis model, and objective parameters. Most ICUs with admission and discharge criteria utilize a combination of the three approaches, adapting them to their specific community and hospital.

In the prioritization model, patients who are critically ill and hemodynamically unstable who stand to benefit from mechanical ventilation, vasopressors, and other intensive specialized therapies are prioritized for ICU admission. Conversely, patients with no identifiable benefit for critical care, such as patients with stable CHF or who are conscious and with normal vital signs after a drug overdose, are not admitted to the ICU. Similarly, patients who are deemed too sick to benefit from ICU admission as they have no chance of clinical improvement and/or have an irreversible terminal illness are admitted elsewhere.

In the diagnosis model for ICU admission criteria, patients with specific clinical diagnoses, including acute myocardial infarctions with signs end organ dysfunction, respiratory failure with high likelihood of intubation, septic shock with a need for vasopressors, and acute stroke with decreased sensorium, are admitted to the ICU.

Finally, in the objective parameters model patients with specific vital signs such as a mean arterial pressure <60 mmhg or abnormal lab values such as a serum sodium <110 mmol/L or >170 mmol/L are deemed to meet ICU admission criteria.[1]

Discharge criteria

Existing guidelines also recommend that there be clear objective criteria for when a patient is to be discharged from the ICU. These may include when a patient's condition has improved and they no longer require critical care (CC) services. Discharge policies should also address when a patient has clinically worsened and a decision has been made to no longer continue critical care (CC) and to now focus on end of life care. Discharge criteria should be consistent with hospital admission criteria for intermediate and floor level admissions.[1]

Triage

In many healthcare systems the number of potential ICU patients is often significantly greater than the available ICU capacity can accommodate. When the number of potential patients is greater than the number of available beds there must be specific policies and procedures in place. Policies may include empowering the ICU director to make admission and discharge decisions for all critical care and intermediate or step down beds and/or boarding patients in other areas (such as a post-procedure holding area or post-operative care unit), assuming the staff are capable and appropriately trained to care for such patients. Ideally, policies will be identified ahead of time for the early transfer of patients who need ICU admission criteria, assuming they are stable for transfer.[1]

Ethical issues

ICU admission and discharge criteria often expose a variety of controversial ethical issues and societal issues, especially with regards to end of life care and resource allocation. A study of intensivists, ICU nurse managers, and ICU charge nurses in one academic Canadian ICU found that in a third of all admitted patients at least one caregiver considered the care inappropriately aggressive for the end-of-life period.[2] Another study of intensivists and nurse managers from 447 hospitals found that 46% of respondents thought that their patients received too much care "sometimes or frequently".[3] A recent study of five ICUs queried intensivists daily about how many patients on their census had no chance of recovery and correlated the results with daily ICU and ED census data. The study found that intensivists considered 38% of the patients they cared for on days when there were no free ICU beds were thought to have no chance of recovery. Often during these same time periods there were critically ill patients boarding in the emergency departments awaiting ICU admission.[4] As the demand for CC services continues to increase, many of ethical and societal dilemmas related to ICU care must continue to be addressed.

Tools to Implement ICU Policies and Procedures

Checklists, protocols, bundles, and guidelines are tools that can be used to support implementation of new ICU policies and procedures. These tools decrease variability in care and enhance the translation of evidence-based medicine to the bedside.

Checklists are the least complex tools and have been shown to facilitate efficient, high-quality care. Checklists are simple reminders to facilitate routine care patterns, like the provision of deep vein thrombosis (DVT) prophylaxis.

Protocols are precise detailed plans to guide a regimen of therapy and provide a guide to clinicians to a default therapy. Protocols are of varying complexity and drive behaviour towards a common standard. Their prescriptive nature facilitates use in both routine bedside care and clinical research.

Guidelines are systematic statements of policy, rules, or principles, which serve to capture the rules of clinical judgment, but provide little direct assistance in clinical decisions. Often less proscriptive, they serve as general guides for clinical management.

Bundles are a set of interventions, distilled from evidence-based guidelines, which target specific disease states. The assumption underlying the development of bundles is that 'bundling' proven interventions, together should result in better outcomes than when implementing them individually. Monitoring compliance is a key to the successful utilization of care bundles to drive change in behaviour.[5] It is important to emphasize that these tools serve to enhance, not replace the skills of the bedside clinician. They aid in bridging the gap between the discovery and publication of new knowledge with clinical implementation. This path of knowledge translation can help lead to a broad-based application of best practices for appropriate patients.

Two examples of multi-faceted interventions in the ICU to improve care include the Michigan experience with an intervention to reduce catheter-related blood stream infections (CR-BSIs) and the Surviving Sepsis Campaign's (SSC) performance-improvement initiative for sepsis management.[6,7] These projects used local interdisciplinary teams, introduced education, and monitored performance using checklists (CR-BSI) or bundles (SSC). Local commitment allowed for large scale implementation. In Michigan, the median CR-BSI rate dropped from 2.7/1,000 catheter days to 0 at 3 months and was sustained over the next 18 months. In 29,470 patients with severe sepsis and septic shock worldwide over a 7.5 year period, the SSC initiative demonstrated that increased compliance with sepsis performance bundles was associated with a 25% relative risk reduction in mortality rate.

Despite these and other quality metrics successes, not all of the results have been positive. Decreased time from knowledge acquisition to bedside care may lead to unintended consequences. The first example of this is the story of tight glucose control. In 2001, Van den Berghe reported that normalization of glucose in critically ill cardiac patients, i.e. tight glucose control, was associated with decreased mortality. This was rapidly translated into clinical practice in medical and surgical ICUs worldwide. Over the next 9 years, studies suggested these findings may be less pronounced in the medical patients, culminating in the NICE-SUGAR trial, which demonstrated harm to these patients, attributable to much higher rates of severe hypoglycaemia in the intensive insulin group.[8]

A second example of the potential deleterious effects of widespread application of quality metrics is in treatment of community-acquired pneumonia (CAP). The Joint Commission established a 4 hour goal for antibiotic administration in response to two large retrospective studies, demonstrating improved outcomes with earlier antibiotic administration As an unintended consequence, the accuracy of a clinical diagnosis for CAP declined, leading to excessive antimicrobial use and misuse.[9] The Joint Commission has since added a diagnostic category of 'diagnostic uncertainty' and increased the time goal to 6 hours. These stories serve to remind that ongoing evaluation is central to the quality movement. Rapid translation of evidence into clinical practice can sometimes result in unintended consequences. Ongoing evaluation and reassessment is important to recognize and address unanticipated results.

Overview of Policy Development and Establishing a Quality Improvement Program

Hospitals and ICUs worldwide have embraced the field of quality improvement (QI). Policy development should be based on a vigorous quality improvement program.

QI includes four essential phases: development, implementation, evaluation, and maintenance. Each phase has key features. The first step of the development phase is to establish a collaborative interdisciplinary leadership group. This group is central to the success of the QI project and so members need to be selected thoughtfully. Members from all parties affected by the potential intervention should be represented, this may include local experts. This team guides the process and needs to have shared commitment to both QI and a collaborative approach.

Understanding the target environment is important for the initiation of a QI project. Characteristics of the target ICU, size, hospital and ICU type, regional culture, and other factors, are essential in the success of a QI initiative. A mature and high functioning ICU with prior QI experience may perform differently than a QI-naive ICU. Prior experience with successful QI initiatives can help guide what forms data measurement and feedback work best with a specific IUC team. Pre-existing systems for data monitoring and program implementation can decrease the project costs and help ensure sustainability. Goals should be achievable, thus understanding baseline practices is essential. Specific QI efforts should target process issues and clinical outcomes for which the specific ICU is poor performing in. If an ICU is already doing well with regards to a specific process or outcome measure investing significant time and effort in a QI project will likely be very low yield.

Implementation of Policies

After establishing the scope and goals, making a plan for implementation is the next step. Understanding the target environment will aid the process, utilizing existing assets and targeting potential barriers shape implementation. Deborah Cook and colleagues demonstrated that barriers to implementation are not necessarily complex, but easily overlooked.[10] Poor communication between the bedside nurse and physician was one of the main reasons for inconsistent use of semi-recumbence. Through an understanding of process and barriers, solutions may be identified to improve compliance.

Multi-faceted interventions are more effective than single interventions for influencing behavioural change. Guidelines and education alone are unlikely to make substantial changes, so the addition of audit and feedback systems is important. While designing an audit and feedback system, both outcome (long-term) and process (short-term) measures should be considered. There are arguments both for and against the use of either one, so that understanding the benefits of each becomes important. Examples of outcome measures include incidence of Ventilator Associated Conditions (VACs), CR-BSI, ICU length of stay, and mortality. Tracking and reporting outcomes data is usually quite feasible as most institutions collect this data, but demonstrating change may be more difficult. Process measurement, i.e. a marker of 'what we do', such as time to antibiotics, is more difficult to track and may require new systems, personnel and financial investments. However, process measures are more likely to show change and success over a short period of time. Outcomes measures are often better accepted, because they are more obvious measures of patient care. Linking process measures to patient outcomes may facilitate acceptance of specific performance metrics and lead to improved compliance.

The final piece of a QI program is sustaining the effort. Depending on the complexity of the intervention and level of success, sustaining the initial process may require variable work. Balancing cost in terms of manpower and financial resources with value, or impact is essential. Augmenting or a downscaling of the audit and feedback system will depend on success in measured outcomes. Not all achievements will decay at the same rate, so the maintenance phase has to be dynamic, and institution-specific, similar to implementation.

Running a successful QI project requires sustained, but incremental interdisciplinary teamwork. At the heart of its success and maintenance is leadership and perseverance — continuous pursuit of improvement and sufficient resource allocation to allow it to succeed and persist over time. A full review QI implementation is beyond the scope of this chapter, a useful resource is the 'how to' guide published by Curtis *et al.*[11]

Measurement of Performance

Essential to the quality movement is the process of measuring performance. Developing and revising ICU policies and procedures should be based on the ongoing measurement of performance. Audit and feedback are key aspects in any intervention targeting change in clinical practice behaviour.

Often there exists a gap between clinician-reported perception of practice patterns and audit of actual practice. This 'perception/practice gap' is well described, and supports the potential need for measuring and reporting practice performance.

Physicians can have unrealistic expectations around their own competency and performance when compared with external assessments. They also may have inflated views around the adequacy of care they provide. A survey of ICU directors comparing perception of care provided versus actual care delivered demonstrates this gap. Perceived adherence to low tidal volume ventilation and tight glycaemic control was 79.9% and 65%, while actual adherence was 2.6% and 6.2%, respectively.[12]

Physician reporting and clinical experience can play a role in patient care, but evidence suggests that outside evaluation provides a better assessment of practice patterns, and therefore a better basis for informing high quality and reliable care.

There exists significant practice variability that may not be detected unless there is ongoing quality measurement. In a classic study, only 54.9% of 6,712 patients in the USA received care that was compliant with recognized best practices for preventative care.[13] This variability in performance may be due to the complexity of patient care, individual patient physiology, professional values, cost, or other important processes. When deviation is due to knowledge deficits, oversight, or the faulty application of knowledge, it is unacceptable. Variability linked to poor outcomes has been demonstrated in the ICU. Adherence to Infectious Disease Society of America guidelines for the treatment of severe CAP was only 57.8% in a cohort of 529 ICU patients.[14] Mortality was higher in the guideline non-adherent population. Other deviations are frequently linked to worse outcomes.

Limiting variability is central to the quality movement, but has been met with resistance. Standardization of care is seen as an attack on physician and patient autonomy, and a minimization of the importance of physician experience. Some feel that the experience garnered cannot be replaced with quality metrics. Reliance on clinical experience has been called into question. In a systematic analysis of 62 published studies, the majority of these studies suggested a steady decline in both physician competency and patient-centred clinical outcomes after completion of training.[15] Thus, dependence on accrued knowledge, i.e. 'experience', alone may not be in the best interest of patients.

Accurate quality measurements can be logistically and technically challenge. There is the potential for surveillance bias and other confounding and any proposed measure needs to be validated and scrutinized to make sure there are not unintended consequences. For example, hospitals are compared for their venous thromboembolism (VTE) prophylaxis rates and subsequent risk adjusted VTE rates. However, one recent study demonstrated that in hospitals with high rates of VTE prophylaxis, and therefore higher quality scores for VTE prevention, there was also increased use of non-invasive imaging to look for VTE and the result is higher risk adjusted rates of VTE in these hospitals.[16]

Quality measurements are increasingly becoming important for practitioners and hospital systems. In the United States, the National Quality Forum (NQF) is a public–private partnership that endorses consensus standards for performance measurements. Performance measures are selected based on their scientific acceptability, clinical importance, usability, and feasibility. To be endorsed by the NQF, the measures must be evidence based, tested and validated, and supported by key stakeholders as well as community representatives. Endorsed measures are adopted by both public and private funders and healthcare systems. Examples of current NQF measures relevant to critical care practice include appropriate antibiotic selection for CAP, spirometry testing for patients with chronic obstructive pulmonary disease (COPD), and 30-day all-cause mortality following hospital admission for COPD.

Communities with limited resources face particular challenges when it comes to quality measurement. A retrospective study of rural Critical Access Hospitals (CAHs) in the US found that they were less likely to have high scores on key process of care measures. CAHs also had higher 30 day mortality for common ICU diagnoses such as pneumonia, CHF, and acute myocardial infarction.[17] One potential benefit of the increase in widespread quality measurement is the potential for improvements for all patient populations, including those in minority groups with historically decreased access to quality care. Since the introduction in the US of tracking for the adherence to process of care measures for myocardial infarction, pneumonia, and CHF, there has been an improvement in the quality of care delivered to all patient populations and a narrowing of the gap between the quality of care provided to members of minority groups in the United States.

Compliance with Physician Reporting

In the United States, reporting of physician and hospital data on quality measures is becoming increasingly common. More and more it is becoming mandated and tied to the reimbursement of both hospitals and individual providers. One of the factors that makes interpreting quality reporting particularly challenging is that there is significant regional practice variation on Medicare quality indicators.

Even prior to the implementation of the landmark Affordable Care Act (ACA), in the United States there have been significant national efforts to collect and disseminate information on quality measurements. The Deficit Reduction Act in 2004, authorized the Centres for Medicare & Medicaid Services (CMS) to develop data infrastructure and to involve various stakeholders in identifying and validating key performance. The ultimate goal is linking payments to individual physician and hospital performance.

Key components of the ACA Congress mandated in 2010 include identifying quality and performance gaps in the healthcare system, approving and utilizing quality measures developed by independent groups, and then utilizing them for public reporting and linking them to payments. Currently over 76 inpatient quality reporting measures are being reported, including those that relate to management of Acute Myocardial Infarction (AMI), congestive heart failure, and pneumonia. In addition, the CMS recently decided to require hospitals to report adherence to the National Quality Forum's severe sepsis and septic shock management bundle.

The results of mandated reporting of adherence to quality measures have been mixed. Recent demonstration programs funded as part of the ACA showed significant financial savings and improvements in core quality measures when healthcare organizations were given financial incentives and increased flexibility in the delivery of care not tied to fee-for-service payments.

With inpatient quality reporting, significant improvements in rates of achievement for process measures in the management of heart failure and pneumonia have been achieved. For example 93% of patients in 2006 with AMI, received aspirin on arrival to the hospital, but this increased to 99% in 2010. Similarly only 55% of patients with AMI received cardiac catheterization percutaneous intervention (PCI) within 90 minutes of presentation in 2006 but this increased to 91% by 2010.

While there has been significant progress on reported compliance with process measures with the advent of required reporting of quality measures, there has not always been a corresponding improvement in outcomes, including mortality.

A 2015 study evaluating the effect of hospitals participating in the American College of Surgeons National Surgical Quality Improvement

Program (ACS NSQIP) did not yield positive results. The study used propensity score matching to compare mortality data and information on serious post-surgical complications (myocardial infarction, pneumonia, acute renal failure) for over a million patients in 263 participating NSQIP hospitals and 526 non-participating matched hospitals. While there was a trend towards improved outcomes in both the hospitals that participated in the quality reporting program and those that did not, enrollment in the program was not associated with any significantly improved post-operative outcomes or reduced costs.[18]

Quality reporting is now being linked to payments to healthcare systems and for individual practitioners. The Physician Quality Reporting System (PQRS) requires the successful and satisfactory reporting on multiple quality measures in the areas of patient safety, effective clinical care, and cost efficiency, among other areas. Examples include percentage of patients with COPD who are prescribed a bronchodilator and percentage of patients with a diagnosis of CAP who are prescribed appropriate empiric antibiotics.

For physicians in the United States, the PQRS was initially voluntary. However, in 2015, it became a requirement. Physicians now face graduated decreases in Medicare reimbursement if they don't have successful and satisfactory reporting.

Accurately measuring and reporting performance faces a variety of technical and logistical challenges, especially as more and more mandated measures are introduced. One major challenge is that cases may be identified through administrative billing data, which for a variety of both financial and logistical reasons may not accurately reflect clinical conditions and care.

There are also a variety of other potential confounders to public reporting of quality data. A 2015 report by the Institute of Medicine (IOM), *Vital Signs: Core Metrics for Health and Health Care Progress* noted that the current push for quality measures is often haphazard, disorganized, and disjointed and does not take into account confounding by comparing different patient populations.[19] The report proposed focusing efforts and resources on a group of core measures, including an index for the receipt of basic preventative measures, access to care patients need, the delivery of care best supported by current scientific evidence, and life expectancy.

In addition to linking government and private payments to performance measurements, there is a push towards sharing this information not just with payers but also with the public. Public reporting is based on the belief that informing consumers of healthcare will ultimately both improve accountability of healthcare organizations as well as quality of care. For example, in the United States the Consumer Assessment of Healthcare Providers and Systems (CAHPS) database managed by the Agency for Healthcare Research and Quality disseminates patient reported information about topics such as provider communication and accessibility for individual practices as well as healthcare systems.

It remains unclear if the dissemination to the public of quality measurement data changes consumer behaviour and therefore improves care.

A major barrier to improvement is that the public perception of quality healthcare is not always consistent with performance data. A 2009 systematic review of available studies did not find much evidence that consumers provided with information on patient experiences and specific quality measures changed their decision making about the care they selected.[20]

Perhaps, when publicly reported information is more patient friendly and readily available, as well as more validated and risk adjusted, that it will ultimately serve to improve the quality of care delivered system wide.

Conclusion

Developing and maintaining effective policies and procedures is truly of critical importance in ensuring a smoothly operating and efficient ICU. Ongoing quality improvement using quality measurements is becoming increasingly important in caring for the critically ill.

References

1. Task Force of the American College of Critical Care Medicine, Society of Critical Care Medicine (1999). Guidelines for intensive care unit admission, discharge, and triage, *Crit. Care Med.*, 27(3), 633–638.

2. Singal RK, Sibbald R, Morgan B, Quinlan M, Parry N, Radford M and Martin CM (2014). A prospective determination of the incidence of perceived inappropriate care in critically ill patients. *Can. Respir. J.*, 21(3), 165–170.
3. Ward NS, Teno JM, Curtis JT, Rubenfeld GD and Levy MM (2008). Perceptions of cost constraints, resource limitations, and rationing in United States intensive care units: results of a national survey. *Crit. Care Med.*, 36(2), 471–476.
4. Huynh TN, Kleerup EC, Raj PP and Wenger NS (2014). The opportunity cost of futile treatment in the ICU. *Crit. Care Med.*, 42(9), 1977–1982.
5. Ferrer R, Artigas A, Levy MM, *et al.* (2008). Improvement in process of care and outcome after a multicenter severe sepsis educational program in Spain. *JAMA*, 299(19), 2294–2303.
6. Pronovost P, Needham D, Berenholtz S, *et al.* (2006). An intervention to decrease catheter-related bloodstream infections in the ICU. *N. Engl. J. Med.*, 355(26), 2725–2732.
7. Levy MM, Rhodes A, Phillips GS, *et al.* (2015). Surviving Sepsis Campaign: association between performance metrics and outcomes in a 7.5-year study. *Crit. Care Med.*, 43(1), 3–12.
8. The NICE-SUGAR study investigators (2009). Intensive versus conventional glucose control in critically ill patients. *N. Engl. J. Med*,. 360(13): 1283–1297.
9. Kanwar M, Brar N, Khatib R and Fakih MG (2007). Misdiagnosis of community-acquired pneumonia and inappropriate utilization of antibiotics: side effects of the 4-h antibiotic administration rule. *Chest*, 131(6): 1865–1869.
10. Cook DJ, Meade MO, Hand LE and McMullin JP (2002). Toward understanding evidence uptake: semirecumbency for pneumonia prevention. *Crit. Care Med.*, 30(7), 1472–1477.
11. Curtis JR, Cook DJ, Wall RJ, *et al.* (2006). Intensive care unit quality improvement: a "how-to" guide for the interdisciplinary team. *Crit. Care Med.*, 34(1), 211–218.
12. Brunkhorst FM, Engel C, Ragaller M, *et al.* (2008). Practice and perception — a nationwide survey of therapy habits in sepsis. *Crit. Care Med.*, 36(10), 2719–2725.
13. McGlynn EA, Asch Sm, Adams J, *et al.* (2003). The quality of health care delivered to adults in the United States. *N. Engl. J. Med.*, 348(26), 2635–2645.
14. Bodi M, Rodriguez A, Solé-Violán J, *et al.* (2005). Antibiotic prescription for community-acquired pneumonia in the intensive care unit: impact of adherence to Infectious Diseases Society of America guidelines on survival. *Clin. Infect. Dis.*, 41(12), 1709–1716.
15. Choudhry NK, Fletcher RH and Soumerai SB (2005). Systematic review: the relationship between clinical experience and quality of health care. *Ann. Intern Med.*, 142(4), 260–273.

16. Bilimoria KY, Chung J, Ju MH, *et al.* (2013). Evaluation of surveillance bias and the validity of the venous thromboembolism quality measure. *JAMA*, 310(14), 1482–1489.
17. Joynt KE, Harris Y, Orav J and Jha A (2011). Quality of care and patient outcomes in critical access rural hospitals. *JAMA*, 306(1), 45–52.
18. Etzioni DA, Wasif N, Dueck AC, *et al.* (2015). Association of hospital participation in a surgical outcomes monitoring program with inpatient complications and mortality. *JAMA*, 313(5), 505–511.
19. Institute of Medicine (2015). *Vital Signs: CoreMetrics for Health and Health Care Progress.* National Academic Press, Washington, DC.
20. Faber M, Bosch M, Wollersheim H, *et al.* (2009). Public reporting in health care: how do consumers use quality-of-care information? A systematic review. *Med. Care.*, 47(1), 1–8.

Evidence-Based Medicine

Bram Rochwerg and Waleed Alhazzani

Departments of Medicine (Critical Care) and Clinical Epidemiology and Biostatistics, McMaster University, Hamilton, Ontario, Canada

Key Points

1. Clinical practice must be guided by evidence summaries however, these can be cumbersome for individual clinicians to perform.
2. Evidence summaries must be evaluated in the context of the quality or certainty of the data.
3. Factors such as risk of bias, imprecision, inconsistency, publication bias, and indirectness must be considered when evaluating certainty of the evidence summaries.
4. The Grading of Recommendations Assessment, Development and Evaluation working group (GRADE) process for clinical practice guideline development incorporates these important steps to its methodology.
5. GRADE clinical practice guidelines provide clear, systematic and transparent actionable guidance to practicing clinicians.

Introduction

The specialty of critical care medicine (CCM) requires a high level of care to achieve its mission. The field is faced with a need to address the demands of who should be the recipient of such care, and under what circumstances.

Even for standard therapeutic choices for common diseases in the intensive care unit (ICU), critical care (CC) physicians are often challenged with making decisions to help their patients. The complexity of health problems, wide range of diseases, and the rapid development of literature in CCM makes decision-making a challenging and a more complex task to achieve. CC physicians, similar to other clinicians, need to consider the balance between benefits and harm of an intervention compared to alternative interventions, patients' values and preferences, as well as cost when making these decisions. Caring for critically ill patients utilizes a large proportion of healthcare budgets, including caring for patients in the last days of their life. This poses a challenge, not only for CC physicians, but also for administrators and policymakers. In order to deal with these demands, clinicians need to make decisions based on scientific evidence from controlled studies, whenever available, rather than relying solely on clinical experience or physiological studies which may not always be accurate. The concept of evidence-based medicine has become widely accepted and used to tie clinical practice with scientific evidence. Prior to the era of evidence-based medicine, clinical decisions were based on clinical experience or expert opinion, physiological rationale, and sometimes on personal beliefs. Although it is important to take these factors into account, it is now universally accepted that there should be no substitute for evidence based practice. Ideally clinicians should seek the best available evidence at the highest quality. As simple as it may sound, in reality, it is not that simple. The process involves several steps before the successful transition from evidence to practice can occur.

Over the years, the amount of literature in CCM has grown substantially; the diagnostic and therapeutic tools have rapidly developed and continue to expand. This is accompanied by the increasing demands for providing optimal care for critically ill patients in the ICU. Therefore, optimal transition from evidence to practice could be challenging, and tools that help to assess quality of the evidence are of great value.

Principles of Evidence-Based Medicine

Guyatt *et al.* described the three core principles for evidence-based medicine[1]:

1. Detecting and summarizing the best available evidence; high quality systematic reviews and systematic summaries of the evidence are generally the preferred sources.

2. Evidence-based medicine is a guide to help us decide how confident or certain we are about the therapeutic effect of an intervention, the accuracy of a diagnostic test, or a course of a disease.
3. Transition from evidence to practice requires consideration of other factors in addition to certainty of evidence. These factors include the balance between benefit and harm, patients' values and preferences as well as cost.

Summary of the evidence

Narrative (non-systematic) reviews are still commonly published; this approach lacks rigour and is subject to the influence of personal bias. This can delay recognizing beneficial or harmful effects of an intervention, or lead to inaccurate conclusions that could, potentially, be harmful. Historically, it took more than a decade to recognize and recommend an intervention that has been shown to be beneficial, while other interventions recommended by non-systematic reviews have long since been shown to be non-beneficial or even harmful. For example, hydroxyethyl starches were commonly used in resuscitating patients with sepsis and septic shock. Multiple conflicting trials were published over the years; it was not until recently, a systematic review of randomized controlled trials (RCTs) showed that the use of hydroxyethyl starches in this population is associated with increased risk of death and acute kidney injury.[2]

Generally, reviewers start with clear and explicit inclusion criteria that reflect the question of interest, followed by a systematic and comprehensive search strategy to identify the highest quality studies, preferably RCTs, and subsequently, summarizing the effect sizes across relevant studies.

As with other specialties, CC physicians are challenged by the lack of time and methodological skills to conduct high quality systematic reviews. Therefore, it is crucial to identify reliable sources that summarize the evidence such as the Cochrane Collaboration or the American College of Physicians Journal Club.

Quality of the evidence

After identifying the summary of evidence for a specific intervention versus another intervention, we have to determine how certain we are that these estimates approximate the truth, and how confident we are that we can use the results in treating our patients. The degree of confidence in these estimates will vary according to internal and external validity of the evidence.

Historically, the evidence hierarchy relied primarily on the study design. Commonly, RCTs rank first, followed by observational studies with a control arm, non-controlled observational studies, physiological studies, and lastly, expert opinion. Each professional society used different ranking tools to assess the quality of evidence; this can be ambiguous and confusing for practising physicians. For example, clinical practice guidelines have varied in the way they ranked the evidence. The inconsistency in determining the quality of evidence, and the inattention of other elements of the internal validity of studies, was a universal problem. Recently, a more comprehensive framework has been developed by the GRADE. The main purpose of GRADE was to provide an approach for clinical practice guideline development,[3] but it was also designed to facilitate the assessment of the quality of evidence and the confidence in the estimates. The quality of evidence could be rated as high, moderate, low, or very low. As we would expect, estimates from RCTs start as high quality of evidence, although, if the RCTs suffer from issues with design and execution, imprecision, inconsistency (heterogeneity), indirectness, or publication bias, our confidence in the estimates will be lower. The larger the limitations, the less confident we are. Therefore, estimates from RCTs do not necessary imply high quality of evidence. Similarly, observational studies start as low quality of evidence, although, our confidence in the results could increase if, for example, the treatment effect was very large. We can make strong inferences from observational studies that examined early use of antibiotics in patients with sepsis.[4] In this setting, although the study is observational in nature, our confidence in the results is high because of the associated strong treatment effect.

Moving from evidence to decision

Traditionally, medical innovation and uptake of new interventions has been slow and limited by an inability to circulate the information on a large scale to clinicians. Clinical practice guidelines (CPGs) have long provided an outlet for experts to meet, summarize best practices and provide an outlet for knowledge translation through publication and dissemination. Many stakeholders utilize CPGs for their benefit. Clinicians often rely on them as resources to help guide the management of individual patients, hospitals or administrators may use them to help drive organizational policies and patient-care initiatives, and finally, governmental organizations will use them as standards to evaluate health indices and to help make healthcare funding decisions.

The ultimate goal of all guideline developers is to improve patient care and, as such, it becomes important to ensure the guideline development process and recommendation formulation is standardized, systematic, and bias-free. Most importantly, expert CPG developers must properly evaluate the current evidence surrounding a specific recommendation and this evaluation must be included in determining the strength of recommendation. There are many historical examples of guideline committees that made strong recommendations based on 'expert' opinion with low quality or uncertain evidence; such recommendations may have significant deleterious effects on patients. A clear example is the case of hormone replacement therapy (HRT). Organizational guidelines strongly recommended HRT to post-menopausal women based on low quality evidence from observational studies that demonstrated an improvement in terms of cardiovascular outcomes. Once higher quality evidence became available, it was shown that HRT therapy was, in fact, harmful when administered to these patients.[5] This highlights the importance of CPGs and their need to consider the quality of evidence rather than relying on consensus or expert practice.

Since the mid-2000s, the GRADE methodology has gained increasing recognition for use in guideline development. GRADE provides an explicit and systematic approach to recommendation formulation that includes formal evidence evaluation. Subsequently, multiple large international societies have adopted the GRADE approach for use in their CPG documents. Although other guideline systems exist, GRADE has some advantages.[3] GRADE methodology was formulated by an international group of developers from around the world (the GRADE working group) who constantly evaluate the process and look to make improvements. GRADE offers a clear separation between quality of evidence assessment and strength of recommendation. Although the quality of evidence is considered integral when deciding on the strength of recommendation, these processes are separated in time (first the evidence is evaluated, then the recommendation is formulated). Other factors are also considered in the strength of recommendation determination such as cost, feasibility, and the balance of costs and benefits of the specific intervention. GRADE contains explicit instructions for evidence evaluation in terms of when to upgrade or when to downgrade the quality of evidence and which factors to consider. GRADE provides a transparent process of how to move from evidence synthesis to recommendation formulation and acknowledges the variation that is bound to occur at a patient level secondary to individual values and preferences. Finally, clear and pragmatic directions are provided to clinicians and stakeholders on how to respond to either weak or strong recommendations. It is for these reasons that GRADE methodology is gaining international recognition for its approach to CPG development.

Practice Guideline Development

The process of CPG development includes forming a guideline panel, steps necessary to decide on questions, search for and summarize the best available evidence, evaluate the quality of evidence using GRADE methods and producing a clinically relevant and comprehensive list of recommendations using the Evidence to Decision (EtD) framework. Most often guideline panels are formed by international societies or governmental organizations. The first step is usually to form a panel composed of content experts, methodology experts, important stakeholders and administrative personnel. One of the most important considerations in deciding on panel members is to consider potential issues with conflict of interest (COI). COI has the potential to derail the guideline development process and introduce unwelcome bias that may influence the formulation of recommendations. Both financial and intellectual biases should be considered. Multiple approaches to dealing with COI management have been employed by CPG panels but the most important first step is recognition and evaluation of risk.[6] If certain panel members have strong ties to pharmaceutical companies whose products are being evaluated, it may be necessary to exclude them from the guideline development process.

Alternatively, it may be possible to simply exclude them from involvement surrounding recommendations for which they specifically have a COI. Inevitably, this becomes a balancing of priorities, as the potential cost of an overly strict COI procedure is the exclusion of many clinical experts from the guideline panel and a loss of overall credibility. Once the panel has been formed and an approach to COI has been formalized the next step is to decide on relevant topics and clinical questions that the CPG will address. This is often best accomplished via a multi-disciplinary approach involving all potential stakeholders. An increasing number of CPGs have begun including patients in the question prioritization and CPG development process. In effect, this ensures that the final product is patient-centred and relevant to patient care. Patient involvement requires careful explanation to ensure that the patient representative accurately understands the question, and is able to make valid judgements.

Guideline questions should be actionable (i.e. "do this compared to that") and follow the PICO format.[7] This entails specifying in detail the population (P), the intervention being assessed (I), the comparator or alternative intervention (C), and the outcomes of interest (O). This format ensures clarity of recommendations and helps to facilitate the systematic review process. Not all guideline questions are amenable to GRADE review and recommendation formulation. Definitions and descriptive statements (e.g. prognosis, prevalence, statements of fact) are not considered actionable and recommendations should not be made for these statements. Good practice statements are another category of questions for GRADE, in which formal recommendations should not be made.[8] These are specific clinical questions for which there is limited direct evidence, no reasonable alternative and further studies aimed at answering these clinical question are unlikely to be done. The recommendation that physicians should examine their patients on a daily basis is an example of a good practice statement. Although no RCTs exist showing the benefit of this practice, most will agree this recommendation should be followed. It is unlikely that future studies will be done to answer this question, as it is unreasonable for physicians not to examine their patients. There is a potential for guideline panels to apply good practice statements inappropriately in situations where reasonable alternatives exist as *de facto* expert opinion. This practice could sacrifice the integrity of the CPG and should be discouraged.

Once actionable questions are identified for recommendation formulation, relevant outcomes need to be formalized and their importance rated. Guideline developers must assess all outcomes that are potentially important to patients, including harm outcomes. This must be independent of what outcome data are anticipated to be available in the literature. If an outcome is judged to be important (e.g. *Clostridium difficile* infection with stress ulcer prophylaxis), but the evidence is not available, this uncertainty must be acknowledged and considered in recommendation determination. All outcomes are rated by the panel (preferably including a patient representative) in terms of patient-importance on a scale from 1 (limited importance) to 9 (critical).[7] For example, when addressing a question on stress ulcer prophylaxis in critically ill patients, outcomes like gastrointestinal bleeding, pneumonia, and *Clostridium difficile* are patient-important and can be ranked as critical. On the other hand, surrogate outcomes like gastric pH are not patient important, should not be ranked as important and will not contribute to evidence synthesis and final recommendations. This evaluation will become important later during evidence summation.

Once PICO questions have been formalized and outcomes ranked; a systematic review of the literature should be performed. Librarian services may be necessary to help formulate the search strategy and screen titles for relevance. Depending on time and resources available for the specific CPG, a pragmatic search may be adequate. Searches should focus on the best available literature for each question and each outcome of interest. If amenable to pooling, the available literature addressing each question and individual outcome should be meta-analyzed to produce pooled point estimates with corresponding confidence intervals (CI). This is usually the most labor intensive and time consuming component of the guideline development process.

Application of GRADE to Assess Quality of Evidence

Having summarized the evidence, the next step is to apply the GRADE evaluation in order to attach a quality of the evidence for each outcome of each question.[9] This is one of the merits of the GRADE approach; none of the other guideline development tools consider individual outcomes when assessing the quality of evidence.

Quality of evidence is judged on a scale from very low to high depending on specific factors. Quality of evidence can also be considered certainty of evidence. In other words, how certain we are that the estimates approximate the truth. The factors considered as part of the GRADE evaluation include the individual study risk of bias, precision, consistency, publication bias and directness. RCTs usually start as a high quality of evidence and may be reduced to moderate, low or very low quality of evidence if issues exist related to any of these factors. Observational studies traditionally start as a poor quality of evidence and may either be reduced due to these factors or increased if there is a large effect seen, a lack of significant confounders or a clear dose-response gradient is evident.

Risk of bias

Study risk of bias applies to the studies that were included in the evidence summary and pooled estimate of effect. If these studies were poorly done with opportunities for systematic bias we might be less certain in our overall estimate of effect. Factors considered in risk of bias assessment for RCTs include: lack of allocation concealment (those enrolling patients are aware of the group the next patient will be allocated to), lack of blinding (including patients, study personnel, data collectors and analysts), incomplete accounting of patients and outcome events (loss to follow-up, not following an intention to treat analysis plan), selective outcome reporting (not reporting harm outcomes), and stopping early (especially for benefit).[10] Factors considered for observational studies include: failure to develop and apply appropriate eligibility criteria, flawed measurement of exposure and outcome, and a failure to control for potential confounders.[10] Risk of bias, in addition to the other factors, must be assessed individually for each outcome of interest, and if significant issues exist the quality of evidence for that outcome should be lowered.

Imprecision of estimates of effect

Precision is assessed mostly based on the 95% CI around the pooled point estimate of effect.[11] We are more certain regarding our quality of evidence if the point estimate suggests either harm or benefit with tight CI that do not cross unity (a relative risk/odds ratio of 1.0 or a risk difference of 0). This can also be applied to continuous outcomes that are reported as a pooled mean difference or standardized mean difference with CIs. If CIs are wide crossing the point of no effect then it would be reasonable to rate down the quality of evidence for this outcome. If the CIs are very wide for either dichotomous or continuous outcomes then we might rate down two levels for imprecision (e.g. from high to low quality of evidence). Even if CIs appear sufficiently narrow and if sample size and subsequently the number of outcome events are small, one should consider rating down for imprecision.[11]

Inconsistency (heterogeneity)

Inconsistency refers to an assessment of statistical heterogeneity. GRADE suggests rating down the quality of evidence for inconsistency if heterogeneity in results persists even after considering potential *a priori* contributors such as differences in study population, intervention or study methods.[12] Judgement of heterogeneity is based on the similarity of point estimates from included studies, the extent of overlap of their CI based on observation of the Forrest plot and statistical tests such as the Chi-squared and I^2 tests. If significant heterogeneity is found, we would be less certain in our overall estimate of effect and subsequently, the overall quality of evidence would be lowered by one level.

Publication bias

Publication bias may exist as negative trials, especially those funded by industry, may never be published and their results not included in systematic reviews of the literature. Not including these unpublished negative trials will lead to an inflated signal of benefit for an intervention and if publication bias is suspected our quality of evidence should be lowered.[13] Guideline panels should suspect publication bias if studies are uniformly positive and small, especially if industry funded. Formal examination including funnel plots or Eggers statistical test and other regression models may be helpful as well, but requires the presence of at least 10 studies in order to be valid.

Indirectness of evidence

Lastly, directness is assessed based on how closely the individual components of the PICO question of interest for the guideline match the evidence found in the literature search.[14] For example, if we are interested in the effect of a specific intervention in paediatric critically ill patients for our CPG but the data available only examine the intervention in adults, then the overall quality of evidence will likely be reduced for indirectness. The same could be applied if there were significant differences in the intervention, comparator or outcomes studied.

Enhancing the Rating of Quality of Evidence

So far the discussion has been focused on rating down the quality of evidence if specific concerns exist regarding the summation of the evidence available. GRADE also includes three situations, mostly applicable to observational studies, which increase the rating of the quality of evidence if present.[15] If an observed effect in observational studies is large, one might consider increasing the quality of evidence either one or two levels. Similarly, evidence of a strong dose-response gradient or a conclusion that plausible residual confounders would further support inferences regarding the intervention effect are reasons to rate up observational evidence.[15] After considering all of these GRADE factors, the guideline panel will produce an evidence profile. Essentially this consists of a table summarizing the pooled evidence and the GRADE quality of evidence for each outcome of interest.[16,17] The overall quality of evidence for the individual recommendations will be the lowest ranking for any of the outcomes which were deemed of critical importance.[18]

Actionable Recommendations

Now that the evidence has been summarized and evaluated, how do we use this to formulate actionable recommendations? Recommendations are divided into strong or weak and for or against an intervention. The strength of recommendation has important implications for patients, clinicians, and administrators.[19] Strong recommendations mean that most informed patients would choose the recommended intervention. Because of this, strong recommendations are often used to drive hospital and governmental policy. Weak or conditional recommendations mean that individual patient or clinician's choice regarding the intervention will vary depending on individual values and preferences however, still the majority of patients will want this management. Obviously the quality of evidence must be a strong consideration when evaluating the strength of recommendation. For example, in most situations, guidelines panels are discouraged from making strong recommendations in the setting of low or very low quality of evidence. If our certainty in the treatment effect is unclear, we need to temper our enthusiasm for making potentially harmful recommendations (remember the HRT example[5]). However, there are other considerations other than the quality of evidence that GRADE dictates must be included in recommendation formulation and decisions on strength of recommendation.

The EtD framework is a tool developed by the GRADE working group which attempts to formalize these other components and produce a systematic approach to including them in guideline development. The EtD forces guideline panels to look at both the desirable and undesirable anticipated effects of the intervention and decide if they are big or small. Ultimately, a decision must be made regarding the balance of desirable and undesirable effects. In other words, do the benefits of the intervention outweigh any potential harms (e.g. stroke reduction with aspirin compared to bleeding risk). The EtD also focuses on the resources required to rollout the intervention and the costs that could be expected.[20] The strength of a recommendation may be reduced if the intervention is unreasonably expensive with only a small anticipated benefit. These considerations are context-specific and could lead to different recommendations for different regions or countries. Other factors included in the EtD are assessing the impact on health equity, the acceptability of the intervention to relevant stakeholders and the feasibility of implementation. After evaluating all these components of the management question, including but not limited to the quality of the evidence, the guideline panel is then left to decide on the recommendation itself (including the strength and direction). Potentially the biggest strength of the GRADE approach is the explicit description of the process that should accompany any recommendation. A summary of all deliberations and decisions should be included in the recommendation rationale. This ensures transparency and reproducibility. Also, this allows clinicians to better understand the decisions and reasons for individual recommendations and better apply them to their specific patients.

The evolution of evidence-based medicine, the tools available for evidence summary and ultimately CPG development have undergone drastic changes over the last 10–15 years. This has led to systematic, comprehensive and transparent processes that are meant to be patient-oriented and hopefully will improve care. CPGs serve an important role in evidence summary and facilitate the dissemination of good patient care to clinicians worldwide. Although not perfect, GRADE methodology provides a good framework and approach for assessment of quality of evidence and guideline development.

References

1. Guyatt G, Jaeschke R, Wilson MC, *et al.* (2015). What is evidence-based medicine? *User's Guide to Medical Literature*, 3rd Edition. McGraw-Hill Education, USA, pp. 7–14.
2. Zarychanski R, Abou-Setta AM, Turgeon AF, *et al.* (2013). Association of hydroxyethyl starch administration with mortality and acute kidney injury in critically ill patients requiring volume resuscitation: a systematic review and meta-analysis. *JAMA*, 309(7), 678–688.
3. Guyatt GH, Oxman AD, Vist GE, *et al.* (2008). GRADE: an emerging consensus on rating quality of evidence and strength of recommendations. *BMJ*, 336(7650), 924–926.
4. Gaieski DF, Mikkelsen ME, Band RA, *et al.* (2010). Impact of time to antibiotics on survival in patients with severe sepsis or septic shock in whom early goal-directed therapy was initiated in the emergency department. *Crit. Care Med.*, 38(4), 1045–1053.
5. Rossouw JE, Anderson GL, Prentice RL, *et al.* (2002). Risks and benefits of estrogen plus progestin in healthy postmenopausal women: principal results From the Women's Health Initiative randomized controlled trial. *JAMA*, 288(3), 321–333.
6. Guyatt G, Akl EA, Hirsh J, *et al.* (2010). The vexing problem of guidelines and conflict of interest: a potential solution. *Ann. Intern. Med.*, 152(11), 738–741.
7. Guyatt GH, Oxman AD, Kunz R, *et al.* (2011). GRADE guidelines: 2. Framing the question and deciding on important outcomes. *J. Clin. Epidemiol.*, 64(4), 395–400.

8. Guyatt GH, Schunemann HJ, Djulbegovic B and Akl EA (2014). Guideline panels should not GRADE good practice statements. *J. Clin. Epidemiol.*, 68(5), 597–600.
9. Balshem H, Helfand M, Schunemann HJ, *et al.* (2011). GRADE guidelines: 3. Rating the quality of evidence. *J. Clin. Epidemiol.*, 64(4), 401–406.
10. Guyatt GH, Oxman AD, Vist G, *et al.* (2011). GRADE guidelines: 4. Rating the quality of evidence--study limitations (risk of bias). *J. Clin. Epidemiol.*, 64(4), 407–415.
11. Guyatt GH, Oxman AD, Kunz R, *et al.* (2011). GRADE guidelines 6. Rating the quality of evidence — imprecision. *J. Clin. Epidemiol.*, 64(12), 1283–1293.
12. Guyatt GH, Oxman AD, Kunz R, *et al.* (2011). GRADE guidelines: 7. Rating the quality of evidence — inconsistency. *J. Clin. Epidemiol.*, 64(12), 1294–1302.
13. Guyatt GH, Oxman AD, Montori V, *et al.* (2011). GRADE guidelines: 5. Rating the quality of evidence — publication bias. *J. Clin. Epidemiol.*, 64(12), 1277–1282.
14. Guyatt GH, Oxman AD, Kunz R, *et al.* (2011). GRADE guidelines: 8. Rating the quality of evidence — indirectness. *J. Clin. Epidemiol.*, 64(12), 1303–1310.
15. Guyatt GH, Oxman AD, Sultan S, *et al.* (2011). GRADE guidelines: 9. Rating up the quality of evidence. *J. Clin. Epidemiol.*, 64(12), 1311–1316.
16. Guyatt GH, Oxman AD, Santesso N, *et al.* (2013). GRADE guidelines: 12. Preparing summary of findings tables-binary outcomes. *J. Clin. Epidemiol.*, 66(2), 158–172.
17. Guyatt GH, Thorlund K, Oxman AD, *et al.* (2013). GRADE guidelines: 13. Preparing summary of findings tables and evidence profiles-continuous outcomes. *J. Clin. Epidemiol.*, 66(2), 173–183.
18. Guyatt G, Oxman AD, Sultan S, *et al.* (2013). GRADE guidelines: 11. Making an overall rating of confidence in effect estimates for a single outcome and for all outcomes. *J. Clin. Epidemiol.*, 66(2), 151–157.
19. Guyatt GH, Oxman AD, Kunz R, *et al.* (2008). Going from evidence to recommendations. *BMJ*, (*Clin. Res.*), 336(7652), 1049–1051.
20. Guyatt GH, Oxman AD, Kunz R, *et al.* (2008). Incorporating considerations of resources use into grading recommendations. *BMJ*, (*Clin. Res.*), 336(7654), 1170–1173.

Part VI
Financial Management

Funding Systems

Arthur van Zanten
Medical Manager Care Division
Internist-intensivist
Gelderse Vallei Hospital, Ede, The Netherlands

Key Points

1. Critical care (CC) funding varies per country, region, type of hospital (teaching/non-teaching), and type of patient. Costs are substantial estimated at 13–39% of hospital costs and 5–11% of healthcare spending.
2. Diagnosis-related-groups (DRG) funding is commonly used, but may create both underfunding and overfunding related to specific diagnosis categories.
3. Pay-for-performance funding aims to improve quality of care by financial incentives, but has not proved effective in improving outcome.
4. New models of healthcare provision such as Intensive care unit (ICU) regionalization and telemedicine confer new challenges in reimbursement strategies.
5. There is lack of information on ICU research funding, however grants for ICU related science are disproportionally lower related to costs spend on ICU patient care, suggesting underfunding.

Introduction

Treatment of critically ill patients in the setting of an ICU can be considered as one of the most important drivers of the total hospital costs. ICU utilizes expensive medical equipment for monitoring and organ support, costly medications administered mainly via the parenteral route, administration of blood products, extensive use of disposables, and most importantly, the intensity of medical, nursing, and allied healthcare professional staffing. In addition, many other departments and professionals are involved in the multi-disciplinary care of the critically ill patient. Therefore, the total daily costs of CC treatment are substantial.

Inadequate funding of CC may lead to managerial decisions to limit budgets for the ICU department, potentially leading to shortage of ICU bed capacity and/or insufficient staffing levels that may contribute to too early discharge from the ICU to general wards, cancellation of planned surgery for expected post-surgical ICU patients, and/or transfer of critically ill patients to other hospitals. These all indicate serious failure to deliver optimal quality and potentially negatively affect outcome in individual critically ill patients. In contrast, overfunding and low occupancy rates of an ICU may lead to marked financial inefficiency of the hospital and healthcare system.

Costs of CC

It has been estimated in the US that between $121 and $263 billion was spent annually nationwide on patients who required CC. This represents 5.2–11.2% of the total US healthcare spending.[1]

Critically ill patients most optimally are cared for by a multi-disciplinary and integrated team of experts directed by a trained and dedicated critical care physician (an intensivist). The team may comprise intensivists, critical care nurses (CCNs), ICU nurse practitioners, clinical pharmacists, ICU physician assistants, consulting physician specialists, primary care physicians, respiratory therapists, and other healthcare professionals.

A German study dating from 2008 showed that 159 of 407 patients were partially or completely mechanically ventilated. Average costs per ICU day were €1,265 and for ICU days with and without mechanical ventilation €1,426 and €1,145, respectively. Staff costs, comprising 50% of the total costs spend, showed the largest cost share followed by medications (18%) and infrastructure (16%). The need for mechanical ventilation increased the daily costs of resources by approximately 25%.[2]

Variability in Funding Systems

Although funding of CC cannot be separated from the funding of the total hospital system and specific hospital services within the hospital system, several strategies to fund CC treatment are used in the international healthcare setting.

A common system to reimburse hospital costs related to all the aspects of the treatment trajectory ("product") delivered to patients is based on diagnosis-related groups (DRGs) that classify hospital cases into predefined groups based on the International Classification of Diseases (ICD) diagnoses, age, sex, discharge status, procedures, and the presence of complications and/or comorbidities. Funding of CC can be based on DRGs to reimburse hospital care including the ICU period as part of one episode, or using DRGs in combination with surcharges or copayments. In contrast, reimbursement excluding CC from DRG funding with alternative forms of payment, for example per diems or budgets as part of a hospital budget are used in various healthcare systems all over the world.

To make matters more complex, funding is not always sufficient to cover all CC treatment costs. Some systems provide additional insurance coverage for expensive medications that may be reimbursed on top of basic funding. Moreover, in some ICUs all costs incurred from admission to discharge are allocated to the ICU and are part of the budget of the ICU Department; in others, costs for medications, laboratory, radiological, and microbiological diagnostics are part of the budget of those related departments and paid for through hospital budgets or DRGs related to specific activities such as laboratory tests or cultures.

Consultation by other healthcare professionals may be part of the ICU budget, or can be separately reimbursed to the individual healthcare professionals involved. In addition, some systems use integrated funding for hospital and medical costs; in other systems a medical honorarium is separated from hospital costs, potentially leading to divergent incentives, i.e. medical doctors induce higher costs for the hospital, while aiming to earn a higher honorarium.

Given the variety of approaches used in different countries, there is no dominant approach or obvious "best practice" model of funding CC services within DRG systems or outside DRG systems. Every model provides both advantages and disadvantages.

For example, a budget system may lead to better cost containment at a hospital, regional or national level; however, it may also lead to lack of ICU capacity where the need for Critical Care exceeds the available budget. In contrast, a pay-for-performance or DRG system may induce scaling of capacity depending on the availability of patients and related output funding. If the size of the payment reflects the true costs of CC treatment, financial risks for hospitals and healthcare providers are greatly reduced. However, these systems may lead to perverse incentives to increase ICU admission of patients with lower severity of illness, prolong duration of mechanical ventilation and increase the number of interventions (e.g. invasive monitoring). There is limited information in the literature on whether these theoretical considerations on pros and cons in daily ICU practice really play a role. We depend on professional and ethical values of healthcare providers in the ICU, to prevent unwanted effects and exposure to unnecessary CC interventions.

DRG Funding

Diagnosis-related groups funding is based on the assumption that there is small variation in the mean costs of a specific diagnosis treatment combination and that one fee can, on average, cover all the costs involved from the start to the end of the treatment trajectory.

To illustrate pitfalls of the system CC related examples are provided related to the basic principles that are essential for optimal DRG funding performance (Table 1).

Table 1. Basic principles for optimal DRG funding of healthcare systems.

Principle 1	Variations in mean costs should be small among patients within a specific DRG
Principle 2	The number of DRGs produced annually should substantial
Principle 3	The components of costs within the DRG code should be rather similar for different patients

A patient undergoing coronary artery bypass surgery for angina pectoris due to coronary artery stenosis will usually have a pre-operative work-up, hospital admission before surgery, surgery and post-operative ICU admission, ICU discharge, stay in the hospital after ICU discharge, followed by hospital discharge and follow-up in the outpatient department. Nowadays, the number of patients with a complicated course is low, mortality has decreased markedly, and the median ICU stay is limited to 1–2 days. However, where there are pre-existing comorbidities, reopening of the chest, ventricular failure, or infectious complications the length of stay (LOS), the main driver of CC costs, may increase markedly with consequent increase in the total costs of the treatment trajectory. Where a fixed DRG price is paid for the total trajectory in complicated patients funding is not sufficient. When considering the basic principles, there is no problem if most patients (80–90%) have an uneventful trajectory (Pareto rule). From the funding of most uncomplicated patients a small portion of reimbursement budget can be used by hospitals to cover the additional costs of the small group of patients with a complicated trajectory. If many patients are treated annually, as is typical for this diagnosis in cardiac surgery centres, the variation in costs will be limited (principles 1&2), and DRG funding can be considered a feasible and practical funding strategy without major negative side effects. Moreover, hospitals and healthcare providers will aim for low complication rates increasing the quality of care, and will gain financial incentives when the additional costs of complications are low. As all patients within this DRG will typically follow the same trajectory from OR to ICU cost components will be similar with little variations (principle 3).

In contrast, with rarer diagnoses involving lower numbers of patients with large variability in costs and treatment modalities, problems in funding from DRG may arise. Patients admitted to the hospital for urosepsis may be treated with fluids and antibiotics in general wards and discharged after few days of hospital admission without an Critical Care stay. However, some will develop septic shock, necessitating mechanical ventilation, vasopressor therapy, renal replacement therapy, blood transfusions, tracheostomy, and a prolonged stay in the ICU. Consider the situation where a hospital treats 15 patients with urosepsis annually, three more cases with a complicated ICU trajectory may increase the total costs of this DRG group by several hundred thousands of Euros. Typically mean costs will exceed median costs due to skewed distribution. In this case DRG funding may lead to significant underfunding.

CC needs capacity to meet the demand of emergency admissions. If only DRG funding is used there is no coverage of the costs of vacant staffed ICU beds for medical emergencies. This can be circumvented if the price of the DRG is increased with an additional surcharge (e.g. 20%) to aim at an ICU bed occupancy rate of 80%. In this case, a higher actual occupancy rate will lead to better funding at the level of the ICU department and be an incentive to use ICU resources wisely.

In general, DRG funding lacks sensitivity in measuring differences between patients and inaccuracies may result from use of average costs and average prices. More specific appropriate recognition of and payment for teaching hospitals can be an additional problem as staffing patterns may be different and teaching performance may influence efficiency of care processes. In some countries, additional budgets for teaching and academic hospitals may circumvent these specific teaching related financial pitfalls.

In Germany, since the implementation of the diagnosis-related system there has been a continuous lack of finances for the treatment of multiple injured patients. In a study of 442 patients with an average age of 40.5 ± 9.1 years (Injury Severity Score (ISS) 12), the average coverage deficit during an average hospital stay of 13.15 ± 6.3 days was €2,752 per patient. Coverage deficit for patients in group I ($n = 296$, ISS 6.3) was €1,163 with an average hospital stay of 8 ± 4.6 days. In group II ($n = 146$, ISS 23.6), the coverage deficit was €5,973 per patient during an average hospital stay of 23 ± 8.7 days. The ISS, the requirement of blood transfusions and the presence of additional chest trauma were the main drivers of financial coverage deficit.[3]

In another German study in 1631, ICU patients the concept of DRG funding was studied related to patient characteristics and ICU LOS. It was demonstrated that those patients that stayed longer than 20 days more frequently had a sepsis diagnosis (79% versus 33%) and higher in-hospital mortality (23% versus 11%). By stratifying patients in clusters of (Cluster 1: <7 days, Cluster 2: <20 days and Cluster 3:20 days or longer) it seemed possible to design a LOS based reimbursement system. The total costs were markedly different in cluster 1 ($n = 1{,}405$; mean LOS = 2.8; mean cost = €2399), cluster 2 ($n = 190$; mean LOS = 13.4; mean cost = €12,754) and cluster 3 ($n = 36$; mean LOS = 34.9; mean cost = €34,173).[4]

DRG funding can probably be improved by several different methods. Not all basic medical data are recorded optimally, potentially leading to underfunding as some costs go unnoticed. Since the introduction of electronic medical records and Clinical Information Systems workflow and medical documentation can be combined with DRG coding and procedural intervention coding.

Several initiatives address the outliers to develop more rigorous systems. Extended LOS significantly contributes to the total ICU costs. In order to improve DRG systems, identification of the factors that predict prolonged LOS in the ICU could be helpful. Higgins analyzed 12 variables against weighted LOS in 10,862 ICU patients and found that mechanical ventilation and presence of infection on admission prolongs LOS.[5]

Activity-based costing studies in ICUs have shown that time for patient care and costs were poorly associated with diagnosis but better reflected by staffing patterns, ICU levels, and a number of cost drivers, such as admission process, ICU LOS, (non-)invasive mechanical ventilation, haemo(dia)filtration, hospital consultation, and transportation (mobile CC).[6] In the Netherlands an activity-based costing study was performed in order to identify drivers that increase daily costs and workload for intensivists in the ICU. Based on daily SOFA-scores only mechanical ventilation and continuous renal replacement therapy increased workload of intensivists, ICU nurses, and daily costs.[7]

DRG funding of CC will only work if country-specific adjustments are made, depending on the structure of the healthcare system and the CC settings involved. The future demand for CC combined with limited budget for healthcare expenditures will motivate funding bodies to look for the ideal funding of CC and to optimize existing DRG funding systems.

Pay-for-Performance

Pay-for-performance in healthcare was introduced to enhance quality, and provides financial incentives to clinicians or hospitals in order to improve health outcomes. However, clinical outcomes, such as reduced mortality, are not easy to measure. Consequently, most pay-for-performance systems usually are based on process outcomes measurement.

To illustrate the effect of variations in discharge patterns on in-hospital mortality used for pay-for-performance a total of 43,830 patients and 134 non-federal hospitals in Pennsylvania, USA were included in an analysis to calculate hospital-specific risk-adjusted 30-day and in-hospital mortality rates.[8] Mean (SD) risk-adjusted hospital-specific in-hospital and 30-day ICU mortality were 9.6% (1.3) and 12.7% (1.5), respectively. Hospital-specific discharge biases ranged from 1.3% to 6.6%. Large hospitals showed smaller discharge bias compared with small hospitals, making large hospitals appear comparatively worse in benchmarks if in-hospital mortality instead of 30-day mortality was used. Accounting for discharge bias will prevent larger hospitals from being unfairly disadvantaged in public reporting and pay-for-performance.

There is an ongoing debate whether pay-for-performance really improves healthcare outcomes. Even substantial incentives may not change the daily practice of medicine. In some observational studies, incentives were shown to change the practice of medicine, but even when they did, they did not sustainably improve clinical outcomes. Pay-for-performance is criticized since the method is based on corporate management systems where the main relevant outcome is profit. Conversely, the specific demands or outcomes relevant to healthcare may be so different that similar effects may not be expected. To extrapolate and transfer clients, products and product quality to medical processes and outcomes is felt to be difficult. Many important outcomes and processes in healthcare, such as spending time with patients, cannot be easily valued and quantified.

Pay-for-performance is also known as "P4P" or "value-based" purchasing or funding.[9] P4P aims to reward physicians, hospitals, and other healthcare providers when they are able to meet certain performance measures of quality (quality indicators) and measures of efficiency. In contrast, it may penalize healthcare providers in case of suboptimal outcomes, medical errors, or increased costs.

Some studies have shown the magnitude of potential cost savings if preventable ICU complications could be markedly reduced on a national level: ventilator-associated pneumonia (VAP) is a well-known cause of morbidity and mortality in ICU patients. A Canadian study showed the incidence of VAP is 10.6 cases per 1,000 ventilator days (95% CI, 5.1–16.1). VAP increased ICU stay by 4.3 days (95% CI, 1.5–7.0 days) per episode. The attributable mortality of VAP was 5.8% (95% CI, 2.4–14). The number of cases of VAP was estimated to be approximately 4,000 cases per year (95% CI, 1,900–6,100). This resulted in 230 deaths per year with the lower and upper confidence intervals ranging from 0 to 580. VAP accounted for approximately 17,000 ICU days per year or around 2% of all ICU days in Canada. The cost to the healthcare system was $46 million (possible range, $10–82 million) annually.[10]

Most studies fail to demonstrate reductions in financial spend, a pivotal aspect of the basic idea behind P4P. Although scientific medical bodies have approved a limited number of incentive programs, they have expressed marked concerns with respect to the validity of quality indicators, patient and physician autonomy, privacy, and increased administrative burdens.

In an overview of empirical studies in CC narrative, systematic reviews, and commentaries addressing P4P programs[11] the authors concluded that critical care medicine (CCM) would likely become a future target for P4P plans, considering the high cost of care involved, the development of more and better ICU quality of care measures, and the enhanced interest from healthcare regulators and funders. In addition, some implementation barriers to P4P funding in the critical care (CC) setting were provided: selecting evidence based and feasible quality of care measures, motivating the entire interdisciplinary team, integrating multi-faceted behaviour change strategies, and developing informatics infrastructure for timely audit and feedback.

Participation in P4P programs can be considered a potential opportunity for intensivists and ICU teams to improve outcomes for their patients in partnership with regulatory agencies and healthcare funders. However, because many aspects of optimal design of P4P programs in the ICU setting are lacking, high-quality evaluations of their effect on healthcare should be integrated into any P4P strategy and for now should caution widespread uptake before its effects and safety have been proved in the ICU setting.

CC Reimbursement Practices

In Europe, a detailed questionnaire about basic ICU characteristics and ICU reimbursement practices was sent to members of the European

Society of Intensive Care (ESICM) using a comprehensive web-based questionnaire.[12] In total, 447 responses could be analyzed. Of these responding members, 51.5% stated that their ICU received detailed financial information; however, only 15.4% of respondents could identify each cost item for each patient. A majority of respondents (77.6%) stated that their unit's reimbursement system was included in the hospital reimbursement. ICU reimbursement systems were most commonly based on previous year's ICU expenditure (51.0%) and DRG weights (36%).

More recent experts from eight European countries evaluated CC funding by describing their respective ICU reimbursement schemes,[13] clearly demonstrating the variations in systems.

Austria

Austrian ICUs are divided into three categories (1–3), with category 3 ICUs considered to provide the most complex care. Additionally, quality criteria have to be fulfilled (minimal bed number, nurse-to-patient ratio, level of specialization required for physicians in charge of the unit, as well as for coverage during on-call hours). Funding is from a provincial hospital financing system based on the LKF system (Leistungsorientierte Krankenhausfinanzierung performance-based hospital reimbursement), an Austrian performance-related hospital financing system. The basic concept is the combination of main diagnoses derived from the International Statistical Classification of Diseases and Related Health Problems 10th Revision (ICD-10) catalogue and individual medical procedures (e.g. surgery, dialysis), which combine to an overall of 982 case groups. Each of these case groups is reimbursed by a certain number of LKF points. For ICU patients, extra reimbursement is calculated per ICU day, increasing from category 1 to category 3 units by a factor of roughly 1.5 times. Additional reimbursement is generated for each defined medical procedure such as bronchoscopy, ultrasound, and specific antibody treatment. Documentation of ICD-10 diagnoses and daily Therapeutic Intervention Scoring System-28 (TISS-28) scoring, which determines ICU categorization and Simplified Acute Physiology Score (SAPS-II) scoring on admission is mandatory. There are no differences in the reimbursement scheme between teaching and non-teaching hospitals. However, the final conversion for generated LKF points into Euros varies between the nine provinces of Austria and is mainly (politically) determined by provincial governments. Also, the same reimbursement system applies to surgical, medical, neurological, or mixed ICUs. However, reimbursement in surgical ICUs tends to be higher due to more frequent medical procedures provided to surgical patients.

Denmark

The Danish Society of Anaesthesiology and Intensive Care and the Danish National Board of Health developed an ICU–DRG system comprising four groups related to deteriorations in organ failure, and based on a combination of 42 intensive procedure-related codes with specific demands for ICU and duration of mechanical ventilation: ICU–DRG group I: simple organ failure in 1–2 organs — average hospital LOS 10 days, ICU–DRG group II: progressive severe organ failure in 1 organ — average hospital LOS 12 days, ICU–DRG group III: progressive severe organ failure in ≥2 organs — average hospital LOS 14 days, ICU–DRG group IV: severe MODS — average hospital LOS 17 days. The ICU–DRG funding groups are independent of the ICU level (1–3). Short stay patients (LOS <72 hours) are reimbursed using a combination of the main ICD-10 catalogue diagnosis, secondary diagnoses, and procedure-related codes. There are no differences concerning reimbursement of surgical versus medical ICU patients and no differences concerning reimbursement schemes for teaching versus non-teaching hospitals.

Germany

In Germany, ICU funding is based on a DRG system. The basic concept is the combination of a main diagnosis derived from the ICD-10 catalogue and secondary diagnoses as well as procedures listed in the OPS-301 (*Operationen — und Prozedurenschluessel* — operations and procedures classification) catalogue to form a basic DRG code. Patient complexity can modify the DRG code for reimbursement. Several amendments are in place to enhance funding such as length of mechanical ventilation, continuous physician's attendance and minimum stay in the ICU of at least 24 hours.

Complexity is based on a combination of daily assessments incorporating the new SAPS-II (equal to SAPS-II without Glasgow Coma Scale) and an assessment of 10 daily activities from the TISS-28 catalogue. In addition, complex procedures/interventions such as blood products, chemotherapy, central venous catheters, or pacemakers and additional diagnoses, such as severe inflammatory response syndrome, are combined to further increase funding for complex patients. The system incurs relevant administrative burden. There is no difference concerning reimbursement of surgical versus medical ICU patients. There are no differences in reimbursement schemes for teaching versus non-teaching hospitals.

France

In France, hospital DRG funding is now based on four levels of severity mainly relying on comorbidities. Surcharges come from complementary funding based on verified criteria: an official ICU fulfilling the nationwide criteria — board certified intensivist, 24 hours coverage by an ICU physician dedicated to the ICU, nurse-to-patient ratio of 1:2.5 and 1 additional nurse to support every four patients, SAPS-II scores >15 and specific ICU procedures (mechanical ventilation, renal replacement therapy, or vasoactive drugs) used during the ICU stay. In total, these additional funds may account for up to 60% of the total funding of ICUs.

Expensive drugs (antifungal treatment, immunoglobulins, and chemotherapy), are reimbursed independently from the DRG if several criteria are met: medications on a restricted list (<100, updated every year), formal indication approval by health authority, individual prescription, and central preparation by a pharmacist. For teaching hospitals, there is additional funding for students, innovation and research based on the number and quality of publications and participation in on-going trials.

Ireland

In Ireland, healthcare funding is based on a budget system, but also uses DRGs with derived diagnoses from the ICD-10 catalogue. The coding will generate a DRG that is assigned a relative value, which will then provide the average cost of a patient with that diagnosis. This is compared to the actual cost of a patient and a case-mix adjustment is derived. Hospitals are compared to each other nationally, but they are divided into groups with large teaching hospitals in group 1, smaller hospitals in group 2, and stand-alone paediatric hospitals in group 3. Using case-mix adjustment per hospital per group, the fixed budget can be increased or reduced depending on performance as DRG coding is used as a performance indicator and not directly for reimbursement. There are no specific ICU related DRG codes. The actual reimbursement of ICU is not direct, because the ICU also functions as a costing centre. There is no difference between medical and surgical patients with respect to reimbursement nor differences in reimbursement schemes for teaching versus non-teaching hospitals.

Netherlands

In 2005, a DRG based system was introduced. CC costs add up to admission DRGs with specific costing labels for reimbursement (ICU add-ons). During ICU admission, all costs incurred (such as staffing, disposables and equipment, medications, laboratory and diagnostic procedures, and medical consultations by non-ICU physicians) are part of the ICU budget and not related to the hospital admission DRGs. The ICU add-on products are based on three ICU costing groups reflecting ICU complexity levels (low, medium, high). Funding is based on fixed prices per treatment day (a), admission surcharge (only first day) (b), invasive or non-invasive ventilation (c) haemo(dia)filtration (d) surcharge fees applying a normative ratio adding up to the total costs of 20(a): 5(b): 4(c): 3(d), originating from an activity-based costing study.

Healthcare insurance companies can easily validate data from medical records to check hospital claims for reimbursement. There are no differences in reimbursement of medical versus surgical ICU patients, and no differences in reimbursement schemes for teaching versus non-teaching hospitals. The higher volume of ventilated patients in teaching hospitals may increase the ICU budget and circumvent this aspect. Because all costs are in the ICU day price, no additional fees for procedures or medications are available. However, some expensive medications, such as echinocandins, can be reimbursed additionally.

Spain

Healthcare funding is decentralized into autonomous regions (17 plus 2 autonomous cities) having authority on medical issues. All hospitals use the Minimum Basic Data Set (MBDS). The MBDS includes patient variables, episode, diagnosis (ICD-9), and codified procedures. Reference weights of the DRGs are calculated from this dataset, channeled through the autonomous regions to the Ministry of Health, to compare reference and calculated weights at each hospital. In Spain funding for teaching hospitals and non-teaching hospitals is equal.

United Kingdom

In the United Kingdom, hospital reimbursement is based on a system of activity based funding known as Payment by Results. ICU funding is separated from the admission diagnosis funding, which is based on organ support derived healthcare resource groups (HRG). Each patient will have an admission HRG and a separately derived specific CC HRG. Each CC admission episode has a HRG calculated on the basis of the total number of organs supported during the patient's stay. Grouper software is used to derive the HRG from the organ support data supplied. A day rate, which is multiplied by the duration of the ICU admission, is calculated to derive total cost/reimbursement for the episode. There is no difference in the reimbursement between larger and smaller units, medical versus surgical units, or teaching versus non-teaching hospitals. Some treatments, such as haematological drugs, are excluded from the payment by results system and reimbursed separately.

ICU funding in emerging countries

ICU funding is very diverse and multi-layered with wide disparity in distribution of services in many emerging countries. There is information on the Indian ICU reimbursement systems.[14] Marked contrast exists between ICUs in state run hospitals offering near-free services with limited infrastructure and resources and the private sector offering state-of-the-art care to the patient segment with purchasing capacity. In India there is no "one size fits all" formula addressing the reimbursement for intensivists. A fee-for-service model accounts for 82% of overall healthcare expenditure equating to 4.2% of GDP. Private hospitals usually operate on a fee-for-service model with up to 85% patients paying out of pocket and the remaining covered by health insurance.

Appreciation of ICU funding by healthcare providers

Data from the European respondents ($n = 306$) to the ESICM questionnaire on ICU organization and funding showed that supplying detailed financial information makes ICU doctors significantly more satisfied ($p = 0.019$) with their reimbursement system.[12] The most satisfied respondents were those where their ICU reimbursement system used ICU nursing workload scores ($p = 0.018$). ICU physicians would like to be more involved in their unit's financial aspects and would prefer separate funding from the hospital.

Reimbursement imbalances related to actual ICU costs

Several studies have been performed to calculate the actual costs and simultaneous funding of CC in order to study the adequacy of funding. Underfunding or overfunding may be encountered among hospitals as well as among medical specialists involved.

In a teaching hospital from Greece in 2006, an analysis was performed among 312 ICU patients using a macro-costing approach, which focused on the estimation of nominal and actual costs per ICU patient. Data were derived from the annual records of resources consumed in each hospital unit and from hospital balance sheets. Mean actual costs were €16,516, whereas actual reimbursement from social funds was only €1,671. After inflating nominal costs to present values using sensitivity analysis, the reimbursement accounted for 25% of the actual hospitalization costs.[15]

However, in contrast, in Norway, 100% DRG reimbursement did overcompensate observed total hospital costs for open repair of thoracic and thoraco-abdominal aortic disease. The average direct hospital cost for proximal aortic surgery was $15,877 (USD 1=NOK 7.5) while the respective 100% DRG reimbursement including one patient needing a tracheostomy, was $19,803. For patients with distal aortic disease, average direct hospital cost was \$23,005 and DRG reimbursement including patients needing a tracheostomy was \$31,543.[16]

Reimbursement and ICU regionalization

As regionalized ICU care is more common in modern healthcare interhospital transfers (secondary transportation) of critically ill patients may influence costs both at the referring centre as well as at the referral centre. Where there is no surcharge funding for transferred patients referral centres may encounter underfunding as demonstrated by a study performed in such a referral centre among 569 consecutive patients admitted to a tertiary care ICU [17]. Transferred patients had longer ICU LOS (mean 6.0 versus 3.8 days, $p < 0.001$) and hospital LOS (mean 20 versus 15.9 days, $p < 0.001$), and in the group with the lowest predicted mortality of 0–20%, ICU LOS and hospital LOS were significantly higher. In crude cost analysis, costs were \$9,600 higher for transferred patients compared with non-transfer patients (95% confidence interval, \$6,000–13,400). Patients transferred to a tertiary care ICU are generally more severely ill and consume more resources.

Reimbursement and ICU telemedicine

ICU telemedicine programs have now been implemented for 11% of critically ill adults in the USA as a solution for the problem of access to adult critical care services. Implementation of telemedicine is associated with lower ICU (0.79; 95% CI, 0.65–0.96) and hospital mortality (0.83; 95% CI, 0.73–0.94) and shorter ICU (0.62 days; 95% CI, 1.21–0.04 days) and hospital (1.26 days; 95% CI, 2.49–0.03 days) LOS. Furthermore, it was suggested that implementation of ICU telemedicine programs has been associated with lower numbers of malpractice claims and costs.[18] With respect to funding there is lack of information on optimal reimbursement strategies, although the costs of telemedicine have been well studied.

Reimbursement systems and palliative care

Palliative care is considered an integral part of CCM for patients who are critically ill, regardless of prognosis, and is both delivered by intensivists and other physicians in ICU settings. In the context of critical illness, the delivery of palliative care comprises symptom management related to organ failure and family discussions for medical decision about treatment options, such as limiting CC treatments.

In study from Germany in 2009, information on end-of-life decision making and causes of death were obtained for 69 critically ill patients who died in the ICU in order to study how financial incentives may have influenced decision-making.[19] The mean costs were estimated at €1,201,000 for 46 long-stay patients. The revenues were €1,358,000, with an estimated profit of approximately €157,000. If the decision to withdraw or withhold therapy could have occurred three days earlier, the estimated profit reduced to €72,000 (46% of estimated ICU profit). In situations where the decision to withdraw or withhold therapy from patients could have been delayed by three days, the hypothetical profit increased to €217,000 (138% of estimated ICU profit). Although not proved by this study, financial incentives may play a role in clinical decision-making.

Reimbursement and optimization of source documentation

Patient data management systems (PDMS) enable digital documentation in ICUs, and have demonstrated effects on completeness of patient charting and the time spent on documentation. However, these systems are costly and raise the question if such a major investment pays off. Few studies have addressed the effect of PDMS implementation on quality of documentation and funding. In a 25-bed surgical ICU within a German university hospital three years before (2004–2006) and five years after (2007–2011), PDMS implementation only small effects on documentation of reimbursement-relevant parameters were demonstrated, which were too small to offset the total investments in the PDMS.[20]

Research Funding in the ICU

Scientific progress in CCM is essential to further reduce morbidity and mortality of many typical critical illness related syndromes. In general, funding for research in this context is not part of reimbursement of costs for treatment of critically ill patients.

Table 2. Sources of CC research funding.

Commercial	
	Industrial partners and private companies (national and multi-national)
Non-commercial	
	Charities
	Research Councils
	Government departments
	National Institutes of Health, USA
	European Commission
	Internal university schemes

CC research may be funded from various resources depicted in Table 2. The magnitude of research funding and the contributions of commercial and non-commercial funding bodies are not known.

However, there are data from the USA showing that of 19,257 grants funded by the National Institutes of Health, 332 (1.7%) were related to CC and a maximum of 1,212 (6.3%) grants were possibly related to CC, while of 5.2–11.2% of total US healthcare spending is used for CC treatment,[2] suggesting research underfunding related to CCM.

References

1. Coopersmith CM, Wunsch H, Fink MP, *et al.* (2012). A comparison of critical care research funding and the financial burden of critical illness in the United States. *Crit. Care Med.*, 40(4), 1072–1079.
2. Martin J, Neurohr C, Bauer M, *et al.* (2008). Cost of Intensive Care in a German hospital: cost-unit accounting based on the InEK matrix. *Anaesthesist.*, 57(5), 505–512.
3. Garving C, Santosa D, Bley C and Pape HC. (2014). Cost analysis of emergency room patients in the German diagnosis-related groups system. A practice relevant depiction subject to clinical parameters. *Unfallchirurg*, 117(8), 716–722.
4. Neilson AR, Moerer O, Burchardi H and Schneider H. (2004). A new concept for DRG-based reimbursement of services in German Intensive Care units: results of a pilot study. *Intensive Care Med.*, 30(6), 1220–1223.
5. Higgins TL, McGee WT, Steingrub JS, *et al.* (2003). Early indicators of prolonged intensive care unit stay: impact of illness severity, physician staffing, and pre-intensive care unit LOS. *Crit. Care Med.*, 31(1), 45–51.

6. Van Zanten AR, Van der Spoel JI, Ennema J and Zwakkenberg S. (2001). Intensive Care products according to DBC reimbursement: IC financial supportive products. *NVIC Monitor.*, 3, 32–35.
7. Van der Spoel JI, Van Zanten AR, Ennema J, *et al.* (2002). Progress in the pilot study on Intensive Care-products according to DBC reimbursement using SOFA-scores. *Neth. J. Crit. Care.*, 3(2), 26.
8. Reineck LA, Pike F, Le TQ, *et al.* (2014). Hospital factors associated with discharge bias in ICU performance measurement. *Crit. Care Med.*, 42(5), 1055–1064.
9. O'Brien JM Jr1, Kumar A and Metersky ML (2013). Does value-based purchasing enhance quality of care and patient outcomes in the ICU? *Crit. Care Clin.*, 29(1), 91–112.
10. Muscedere JG, Martin CM, Heyland DK (2008). The impact of ventilator-associated pneumonia on the Canadian health care system. *J. Crit. Care.*, 23(1), 5–10.
11. Khanduja K, Scales DC and Adhikari NK (2009). Pay for performance in the Intensive Care unit — opportunity or threat? *Crit. Care Med.*, 37(3), 852–858.
12. Csomos A, Varga S, Bertolini G, *et al.* (2010). Intensive Care reimbursement practices: results from the ICUFUND survey. *Intensive Care Med.*, 36(10), 1759–1764.
13. Bittner MI, Donnelly M, van Zanten AR, *et al.* (2013). How is intensive care reimbursed? A review of eight European countries. *Ann. Intensive Care.*, 3(1), 37.
14. Jayaram R and Ramakrishnan N (2013). Reimbursement for critical care services in India. *Indian J. Crit. Care Med.*, 17(1), 1–9.
15. Geitona M, Androutsou L and Theodoratou D (2010). Cost estimation of patients admitted to the Intensive Care unit: a case study of the Teaching University Hospital of Thessaly. *J. Med. Econ.*, 13(2), 179–184.
16. Mishra V, Geiran O, Krohg-Sørensen K and Andresen S (2008). Thoracic aortic aneurysm repair. Direct hospital cost and Diagnosis Related Group reimbursement. *Scand. Cardiovasc. J.*, 42(1), 77–84.
17. Golestanian E, Scruggs JE, Gangnon RE, *et al.* (2007). Effect of interhospital transfer on resource utilization and outcomes at a tertiary care referral center. *Crit. Care Med.* 35(6), 1470–1476.
18. Lilly CM, Zubrow MT, Kempner KM, *et al.* (2014). Critical care telemedicine: evolution and state of the art. *Crit. Care Med.*, 42(11), 2429–2436.
19. Stachura P, Oberender P, Bundscherer AC and Wiese CH (2015). The possible impact of the German DRGs reimbursement system on end-of-life decision making in a surgical Intensive Care unit. *Wien Klin Wochenschr*, 127(3–4), 109–115.
20. Castellanos I, Ganslandt T, Prokosch HU, *et al.* (2013). Implementation of a patient data management system. Effects on Intensive Care documentation. *Anaesthesist.*, 62(11), 887–890, 892–897.

Cost and Cost-Effectiveness

David J. Wallace
University of Pittsburgh School of Medicine
Department of Critical Care Medicine
Department of Emergency Medicine

Key Points

1. Increasingly constrained budgets place growing emphasis on identifying high value healthcare.
2. Economic evaluations of treatments, protocols and organizational approaches are well suited to critical care medicine (CCM) due to its high morbidity, high mortality, complex interactions, and expensive cost streams.
3. Cost-effectiveness analysis and cost-utility analysis are the most common study designs in stand-alone and nested economic evaluations of intensive care medicine (ICM).
4. Knowledge of the limitations of economic analyses is important to avoid false inference.
5. Recent reporting guidelines should improve transparency and rigor in cost-effectiveness analyses, in turn improving their incorporation into decision-making.

Introduction

Critical care (CC) is expensive and its costs are growing. The Office of the Actuary in the Centres for Medicare and Medicaid Services projects that overall health spending will grow at a rate of 5.7% through 2023 in the United States, which is 1.1% points faster than the growth rate of the Gross Domestic Product. CC accounts for an increasing proportion of these costs, largely attributable to the aging of the population and through the continued expansion of critical care (CC) bed supply.[1] However, despite a substantial financial investment in healthcare, the United States does not report comparable critical care outcomes to similarly resourced countries. The apparent disconnect between the level of spending in the United States and the return on investment has increased interest in methods of determining treatment value and planning resource allocation.

Cost-effectiveness studies are economic evaluations designed to relate healthcare spending to patient outcomes. When there are several approaches to the care of a particular condition, the most cost-effective is the one with the lowest cost per unit of benefit.

Costs

Most generally, cost is defined as the quantity of resources consumed to purchase a good or provide a service. Costs, however, encompass a broad taxonomy of sub-terms, each with a specific meaning in accounting. We will cover the most common cost terms that relate to healthcare economic evaluations in turn: direct costs, indirect costs, intangible costs, marginal costs, fixed costs, opportunity costs, variable costs, and average costs.

Direct costs refer to the part of the price of a good or service that relates to the production of said good or service. This component includes materials, labor and expenses related to production. For medical products and services this means the costs of laboratory tests, radiological exams and administered medications. These costs are related to the quantity of a treatment provided, or in more general terms, the unit of production. Direct costs also cover the economic costs experienced by the families of patients who are critically ill, as well as society at large.

Whereas direct costs are consumed in the process of delivering care, indirect costs represent the cost of lost productivity for the patient, family and informal caregivers. Indirect costs refer to lost productivity in three domains: mortality, absenteeism, and reduced productivity. When a patient dies, lost future earnings represent an indirect cost. For survivors with a new disability, lost productivity is an indirect cost.

Intangible costs are the costs of pain, suffering and other non-financial aspects of disease. Quantifying the value of pain and suffering can be difficult, though their effects are frequently incorporated into quality-adjusted outcome measures.

Marginal cost is the investment required to perform one additional procedure or provide one additional course of therapy. Marginal costs are those costs that vary with production, whereas costs that do not are referred to as fixed (covered below). As a point of clarification, marginal costs are not the full cost of providing the next treatment or the last treatment. If the cost performing the first bronchoscopy is $300 and the total cost of performing two bronchoscopies is $380, the marginal cost is $80. A related concept, incremental cost, refers to the cost of moving from one treatment approach to another mutually exclusive treatment.

Costs that do not vary with the number of patients treated are fixed costs. Examples of fixed costs are the resources required to maintain heating, ventilation, air conditioning, and plumbing to the ICU. Similarly, physician, pharmacist, respiratory therapist, and physical therapist staffing are fixed costs, to the extent that they do not vary within the same day based on admissions and discharges. Nurse staffing is somewhat different, as it can fluctuate based on census and patient acuity within a particular day. In fact, over a longer time frame, other fixed costs can become variable costs — for example, if physician numbers are downsized in response to slowing patient volumes over the course of a year. The majority of hospital costs are fixed costs, consisting of staff, equipment, physical space, and maintenance. For this reason, efforts to reduce hospital costs through a reduction in services will have a negligible effect, unless these efforts are paired with reductions in staff numbers, physical space or fewer capital expenditures.

Opportunity costs are those outcomes that are foregone under the next best alternate allocation of resources, in favor of the therapy in at hand. Logically, given a fixed budget, the resources used to provide a particular therapy can no longer be used for something else. Opportunity cost is an important concept in economics, as it demonstrates the relationship between scarcity and choice. As healthcare resources are not limitless and we must make decisions about which therapies provide the best return on investment.

Variable costs change with changes in production. The cost of disposable goods represents a variable cost. For example, the ICU cost for central lines will be higher in months when more central lines are placed, whereas the cost of electricity will be largely consistent.

Average costs represent the mean cost per unit of treatment. Average costs are separated into two components: short-run average costs and long-run average costs. Short-run average costs vary according to treatment volume. For example, the cost of placing a single patient on an extracorporeal membrane oxygenation circuit includes the costs of reusable equipment and staffing (fixed costs), as well as disposable equipment (variable costs). The next patient placed on the extracorporeal membrane oxygenation circuit will increase overall variable costs (secondary to disposable equipment), but will not increase the overall fixed costs. Therefore, the average cost of care will be lower for the therapy after the second patient is treated. Up to a point, as more patients are treated on the extracorporeal circuit, the average cost of care will be reduced. However, beyond a threshold, the average cost of care will begin to increase. This is because average costs typically have a "U-shape" curve, due to initial fixed costs at one extreme and diminishing productivity at the other. For example, in the case of running an extracorporeal membrane oxygenation circuit, a hospital may begin by employing a single perfusionist. As the number of circuit runs increases, this technician will progressively have less downtime, increasing efficiency. However, once the perfusionist works more than full-time to meet the clinical demand, his or her hourly compensation will increase — and with it increase the overall average cost.

The long-run average cost is a business metric capturing the average cost per output over the long run, accounting for planned changes in the production or delivery process. Hospitals will make decisions about the delivery mechanisms for treatments or procedures that minimize the long-run average cost. Long-run average costs can be lower than short-run average costs by harnessing of economies of scale. In the extracorporeal membrane oxygenation example, the long-run average costs of managing patients with this procedure becomes lower when patient volumes maximize industry, but do not require overtime (overtime costs represent what is known as a diseconomy of scale). Problems related to maximizing efficiency and throughput are certainly not unique to healthcare. Companies such as Netflix, Amazon, and FedEx established market dominance in part through carefully managing long-run average cost and optimizing logistics for efficient delivery of their services (for more on this topic, the reader should explore the related fields of queuing and logistics in operations research.)

For all the terms related to cost, it may be surprising to discover the elusive nature of true costs in healthcare. The more accessible measure for goods and services in healthcare is the charge. Unfortunately, the charge may vary substantially from the cost of a good or service, and the relationship may be higher, lower or equivalent. This is because charges are the amounts billed to individuals, which in turn vary according to discounts, deductibles, copayments and coinsurance. However, billed charges do not always represent all costs for the individual. Furthermore, pricing systems vary between providers, translating into widely different charges at different facilities.[2,3]

Every hospital has a master file of all costs and charges for every hospital service. The ratio between what a day in the hospital costs and what is charged is the cost-to-charge ratio. The closer the ratio is to one, the more narrow the difference between actual costs and the hospitals gross charges. However, even this approach is limited to the known extent of costs.

Determining the full costs of a treatment in a healthcare facility is challenging. Traditionally, hospitals have used the ratio of costs-to-charges (RCC) or relative value units (RVU) to determine the costs for a particular service, intermediate products or procedures.[4] Activity-based costing, a more recent form of cost accounting, offers some advantages to RCC- and RVU-based approaches.

The RCC is calculated by dividing the total costs for a year by the total charges. The resulting ratio is then multiplied by a particular charge and to arrive at the assigned cost. This method of determining costs is more accurate at higher levels of aggregation, such as diagnosis related group (see Ref. 4 for a detailed example of how RCCs can result in different cost estimates for a teaching hospital compared to a community hospital). RCCs also fail to take advantage of modernized inventory and procedural tracking systems. These technological improvements capture more information on overhead, supply, and throughput — facilitating better cost accounting than the RCC summary measure.

The RVU, method of assigning costs uses information from a national database of procedures and weights based on complexity. Unfortunately, the RVU approach to cost can lead to misleading conclusions. While RVUs are associated with procedural complexity, much of manufacturing overhead cost is unrelated to procedural complexity.

Activity-based costing is a form of cost accounting that takes more nuanced approach to allocating production cost and overhead. Under activity-based costing costs are assigned to products and services according to individual consumption of resources. This approach typically assigns more of the total costs to direct costs than in conventional accounting.

RCC, RVU, and activity-based costing are not the only three methods of determining costs in healthcare; however, they are the most prevalent.

Type of Cost Studies

The four most common cost evaluations are cost-minimization studies, cost-benefit analysis, cost-effectiveness analysis, and cost-utility analysis. Each analytic approach has advantages and disadvantages, and provides different outcome metrics; therefore, selection of method should be tailored to the specific question at hand.

Cost-minimization analysis

Cost-minimization studies are used most frequently to compare the overall treatment costs of medications. Cost-minimization studies make the assumption that the medications under consideration are absolutely equivalent — including therapeutic benefit, frequency of adverse reactions and duration of therapy. From the standpoint of study design, when there is no measurable difference between two treatments, a traditional cost-effectiveness analysis approach cannot mathematically be performed (because the denominator of the cost-effectiveness summary statistic would approach zero). This special situation lends itself to cost-minimization analysis. The analysis focuses solely on cost, with the scales tipping in favor of the medication that is less expensive.

While the design of a cost-minimization study is appealing in its simplicity, some question the real world application of the analysis.[5] First, cost-minimization analyses cannot be prospectively planned in conjunction with a clinical research study (in that the design requires clinical equivalence between treatment options, which is not known in advance when evaluating a new therapy). As planned cost evaluations are becoming increasingly common in CCM,[6,7] the inability to build this study design into the analysis is a significant shortcoming. Second, under conditions of uncertainty (which are present in all evaluations), it is difficult to confidently conclude that two therapies have wholly equivalent outcomes (a necessary condition of cost-minimization analysis). Third, with increasingly more specific outcomes and effects, it becomes less likely that two treatments are equivalent across all domains. Collectively, these limitations weaken the case for cost-minimization analyses. An exception to the first limitation is when a clinical trial is explicitly evaluating equivalence or non-inferiority between two treatment options. In that setting, a concurrent cost-minimization study can be planned from the outset. Alternatively, cost-minimization studies may follow negative result or non-inferiority trials as a means of evaluating comparable treatments on cost grounds.

An example of this approach was recently published by the (SEDCOM) (Safety and Efficacy of Dexmedetomidine Compared With Midazolam Study Group. The SEDCOM study evaluated the efficacy and safety of dexmedetomidine compared to midazolam for critically ill patients.[8] The 68-centre trial randomized 366 mechanically ventilated patients to either dexmedetomidine or midazolam over a two-year period. There was no difference in the primary outcome: time at targeted sedation level. However, interest remained in dexmedetomidine, as the intervention group spent fewer days on mechanical ventilation and dexmedetomidine was a non-benzodiazepine class of medication. The investigators performed a nested economic evaluation using the same patient data, to determine the total ICU cost difference between the treatment strategies. As a secondary goal, the investigators evaluated specific cost drivers in each study arm.

Total CC costs comprised the cost of ICU stay, cost of mechanical ventilation, cost of treating adverse drug reactions and finally the cost of the study drug itself. CC stay costs were estimated using a decelerating ramp, with hourly costs on day 1 of $406 per hour, day 2 with $203 per hour and $184 per hour on all subsequent days in the ICU. A decelerating ramp for ICU costs is a potentially reasonable cost-weight strategy, as the majority of costs occur in the beginning of an ICU stay.[9] For adverse events, the cost streams included the costs of diagnostic tests, procedures, consultations and treatments. In an adjusted analysis, the authors determined that dexmedetomidine was associated with higher acquisition costs ($1,826 and $80, respectively). Nevertheless, a dexmedetomidine strategy was less expensive overall in the ICU, primarily through a significant reduction in days on mechanical ventilation (median cost savings: $6,584) and less frequent management of adverse drug reactions (median cost savings: $229).

For ICUs that use continuous infusions of midazolam as a sedative for patients requiring mechanical ventilation, the cost-minimization results provide some new financial insights. High drug acquisition costs may have discouraged hospital pharmacies from purchasing dexmedetomidine considering its efficacy at achieving target sedation is equivalent to midazolam. However, the SEDCOM economic analysis shows that a sedation strategy using dexmedetomidine may have lower overall costs than midazolam from the perspective of the institution.

Important limitations of the study, however, deserve attention. While the authors used a decelerating cost per hour by day in the ICU, adjusted length of stay was not separately reported. Furthermore, the parent SEDCOM study did not report a significant length of stay difference between the treatment strategies. This apparent discrepancy is noted by the study authors, and attributed to risk adjustment differences between the studies. For pharmacies considering adopting dexmedetomidine into their regular practice, the adjusted length of stay numbers would allow local cost calculations to be performed, as well as perform more granular hourly cost estimation.

Long-term outcome effects, and therefore the attendant cost streams, from each sedation strategy are also left unanswered by the study. From the standpoint of achieving target sedation levels, the medications were equivalent. However, if there are long-term cognitive or psychological differences between survivors in the treatment arms, these costs and effects were not captured. The SEDCOM cost-minimization study used the institution for its cost perspective, which simplifies the economic analysis, but may not capture all relevant endpoints (positive or negative).

Overall, there is growing criticism of the cost-minimization approach to economic evaluation.[10] Most recently, cost-minimization was subject to a literature review of publications since 2001.[11] The authors note that the opportunities for appropriate cost-minimization evaluation are becoming vanishingly rare, and furthermore conclude that this method of economic analysis is "not only dead but should also be buried."

Cost-benefit analysis

Cost-benefit analysis, also known as CBA, is the second study methodology covered in this chapter. Cost-benefit analyses date back to the 19th century and work of Jules Dupuit, a civil engineer and economist. At the time Dupuit was interested in the construction of public bridges, and the conditions under which construction could be justified. Cost-benefit analysis as an economic tool, however, did not immediately experience widespread adoption. It was not until the 1950s that the analysis saw more regular use, and even later for its transition into the healthcare space.

Cost-benefit analyses summarize the net benefits and net costs for a particular therapy by converting all benefits and costs into monetary values. Expressed as a ratio, the benefit-to-cost ratio is a measure of the expected return on investment. Cost-benefit analysis draws heavily on the concept of Pareto optimality. When an economy (or part of an economy) is in the state of being Pareto optimality (also called Pareto efficient or Pareto optimum), no resources can be redistributed within the system to achieve a better overall health state. **Pareto optimality** should not be confused with the **Pareto Principle**. The **Pareto Principle** derives from Pareto's observation that 20% of the population in Italy owned eighty percent of the land. This asymmetry is present in many other contexts, to such an extent as to become the 80–20 rule, or the **Pareto Principle**.

Cost-benefit analyses are performed in three stages: (1) measure treatment costs; (2) measure clinical outcomes; and (3) determine if benefit valuation is greater than cost valuation. A downside of cost-benefits analyses is the challenge of financially quantifying health outcomes. Consequently, cost-effectiveness analysis is infrequently used as an economic evaluation in critical care research. A PubMed search performed on 6 May 2015 using the MeSH term "Cost-Benefit Analysis" as a major term without lower hierarchy terms (due to lower term overlap with other economic evaluation types), MeSH term "Intensive Care" and restricted to publications in the last 20 years did not identify any studies employing strict cost-benefit analysis methodology. Two studies used the term cost-benefit analysis in the title and abstract; however, neither was a cost-benefit analysis using strict criteria of cost accounting for outcomes.[12,13]

Cost-effectiveness analysis

Our third cost-effectiveness study design is called cost-effectiveness analysis or CEA. CEA compares the relative costs and outcomes for two more treatment strategies. The difference between two treatments is expressed as a ratio of the change in health state (denominator) to the cost of the treatment (numerator). CEA and cost-utility analysis are used increasingly in CC research, both as stand-alone evaluations[14,15] and bundled prospectively with clinical investigations.[6,7]

CEA uses the incremental cost-effectiveness ratio (ICER) to measure a proposed therapy against a comparator. The ICER is the difference between the cost-effectiveness ratio of the proposed therapy and the cost-effectiveness ratio of a comparator therapy. As a formula the ICER is expressed as:

$$(\text{Costs}_{\text{proposed}} - \text{Costs}_{\text{comparator}}) \div (\text{Outcomes}_{\text{proposed}} - \text{Outcomes}_{\text{comparator}})$$

or

$$\text{Cost-Effectiveness Ratio}_{\text{proposed}} - \text{Cost-effectiveness Ratio}_{\text{comparator}}.$$

The ICER is a simplification intended to facilitate summarizing the change in health state associated with the proposed treatment. The intention of the ICER is to provide a means of balancing potentially competing priorities: an individual patient's treatment preference and society's willingness to pay for that preference.

CEAs are often shown in a cost-effectiveness plane (Figure 1). Cost-effectiveness planes are divided into four quadrants, representing the

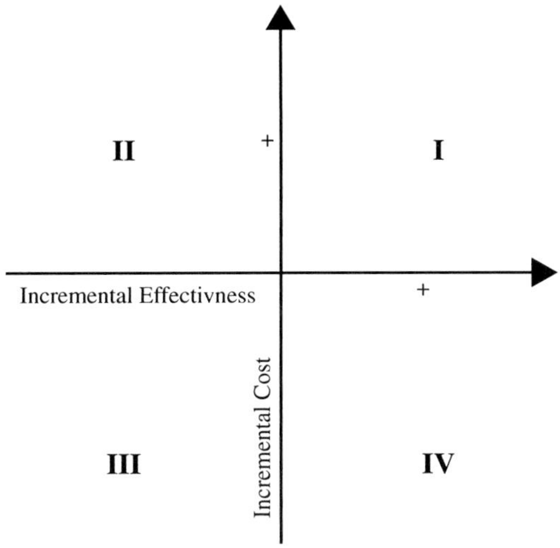

Figure 1. Cost-effectiveness plane.

incremental difference between proposed therapy and comparator therapy. Therapies in quadrant I are both more effective and more costly. These interventions may be adopted, depending on societies' willingness to pay threshold. Therapies in quadrant II are more expensive and less effective that current therapy, thereby classified as "dominated." These therapies should not be adopted. Therapies in quadrant III are cost reducing and quality reducing, but may nevertheless be attractive to a healthcare system. With a constrained budget, therapies in quadrant III have the potential to free up resources for other healthcare interventions with higher yield on the investment. Like therapies in quadrant I, this decision will be based on a willingness to pay threshold. Therapies in quadrant IV are both less expensive and more effective, and are thereby classified as "dominant." These therapies should be adopted.

Some are critical of the ICER as an overly simplistic measure of appraising a treatment value.[16] The argument stands that neither a ratio nor a difference in ratios can answer how many patients will benefit, how much the therapy will cost and how the healthcare system plans on paying for the new therapy. While these criticisms have merit, the ICER is a generally accepted representation of the two components required to assign value. More concerning, however, is evidence of publication bias in the healthcare economic literature.[17] In a 2006 systematic review of published cost-effectiveness studies, study authors identified a bias towards publication of more and less favorable ICERs, with fewer reports in the intermediate range. Furthermore, studies conducted with industry support were more likely to publish results with ICERs below the societal willingness to pay threshold. The authors conclude with an appeal for a more transparent reporting process and greater methodological rigor in healthcare economic evaluations.

In 2013, recognizing growing problems with economic evaluations of healthcare, 10 academic journals simultaneously published reporting guidelines for health economic evaluations.[18] The Consolidated Health Economic Evaluation Reporting Standards (CHEERS) guideline is a checklist designed to standardize reporting and facilitate presentation consistency for editors, reviewers, and researchers. The framework was developed using a modified Delphi process, comprised of experts in health economics, clinical epidemiology, decision-making, and technology assessment. The panel also included physicians in clinical practice and members with experience in guidelines development. Though the development of the guidelines was a sponsored event, the final recommendations were entirely the work of the task force. The framework has 24 individual points, separated into six manuscript categories: (1) title and abstract; (2) introduction; (3) methods; (4) results; (5) discussion; and (6) other. The full task force recommendations are contained in a separate publication.[19]

Cost-utility analysis

The final economic evaluation covered in this chapter is the cost-utility analysis. The cost-utility analysis is a special case of CEA where outcome measures are adjusted for life quality. Fittingly, a frequent outcome measure in cost-utility assessment is the Quality Adjusted Life Year (QALY). A QALY is based on the number of years of life that would be extended from a particular therapy. QALYs weigh the duration of health gains against the quality of the time, from 1.0 for perfect health to zero for being dead (1 QALY = 1 year of life × 1 utility value). Any disability can factor into QALY adjustment. For example, a year of life complicated by the systemic effects of chemotherapy might be valued at 0.7 QALYs. Some methods of quality adjustment, such as the EuroQol-5D, allow for negative health states (indicating there are conditions regarded as worse than death). Perhaps surprisingly, some disease states are associated with higher quality of life scores for patient than before their diagnosis.

Complicating matters further, patients may not experience all costs or benefits from a therapy at the time it is applied. Recognizing that benefits and costs experienced in the future are less valuable than immediate costs and benefits, cost-utility analyses discount future costs and health states. The discount is based on uncertainty, anticipated economic inflation and patient's general preference for immediate gains over those in the future. Similarly, the benefit of one patient living five additional years is not equivalent to ten patients each living six additional months.

Failure to discount both costs and benefits creates an economic and policy scenario called the Keeler–Cretin procrastination paradox. Under conditions without discounting, we would forever favor healthcare programs that take place sometime in the future, rather than investing in programs today. Based on worldwide economic growth, future costs and benefits should be discounted at 3% per annum.

In 2006, the Institutes of Medicine's Committee to Evaluate Measures of Health Benefits for Environmental, Health, and Safety Regulation produced *Valuing Health for Regulatory CEA,* a general set of recommendations on the conduct of CEA.[20] The report highlights that no single quality measure is clearly superior others, and that researchers, analysts and decision makers must use judgment in selecting a particular approach. The report notes that recommendations based on QALYs will bias towards therapies that benefit the young (who have greater potential for increased QALYs), whereas analyses targeting total lives saved will assign the same impact value whether the recipient is middle aged or elderly. Rather than endorsing a single economic metric, *Valuing Health for Regulatory CEA* recommended regulatory agencies report four measures of cost-effectiveness: cost of life saved, cost of year per life saved, cost of quality-adjusted year of life saved, net cost of quality-adjusted year of life saved.

Decision analysis is a type of economic analysis that combines information on costs, outcomes and probabilities for competing management strategies, and produces summary measures to facilitate selections. Decision analyses are often useful for untangling complex cost streams where intuition alone reliably leads to poor strategy selection. At their core, decision analyses rely on the decision trees and Markov models.

Decision trees expand from individual nodes representing individual decisions, subsequently branching to next level decisions. At any particular decision point, the cumulative probability of choices is equal to one (all possible decisions are accounted for). As you move through a particular branch of a decision tree into progressively smaller limbs, cumulative costs and consequences are accumulated. Conventionally, the decision tree is drawn extending from left to right, with decisions drawn as squares and chance nodes drawn as circles. Outcomes are usually drawn as boxes or triangles. A simplistic decision tree is shown in Figure 2, illustrating the management and outcomes of a patient with respiratory insufficiency. Conceivably, the full accounting of cost streams for management of respiratory insufficiency could produce a fuller set of branches and greater arborization in the tree.

Knowledge of the accuracy and range of plausible values for each node is paramount in a decision tree. The researcher should use the best possible evidence for each value, advisably with a systematic review or

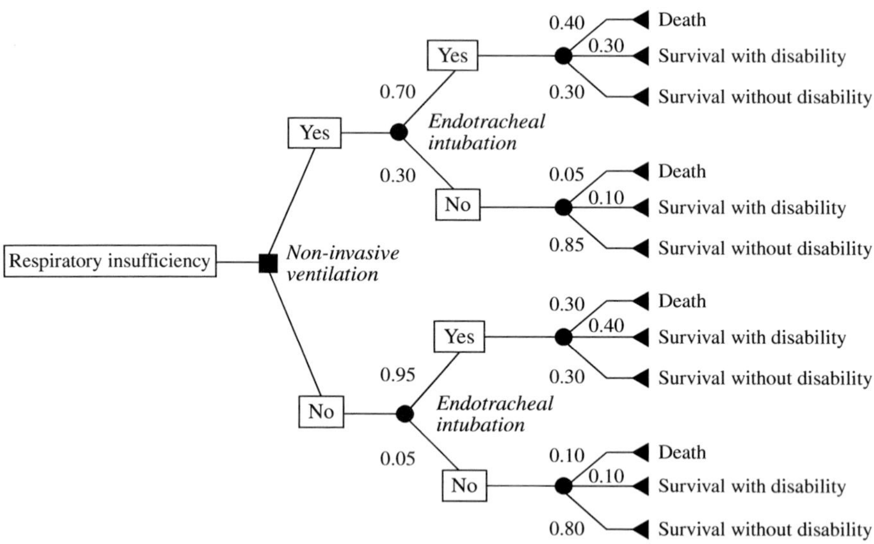

Figure 2. Decision tree for the management of respiratory insufficiency showing a probability for each branch.

meta-analysis. In all cases, a range of values should be explored with a sensitivity analysis. As values for cost and probability are changed in the sensitivity analysis, thereby evaluating the stability of the conclusion of the analysis. When small changes to a particular variable result in large changes in the conclusion, the analysis is said to be sensitive to that variable. Sensitive variables are compelling candidates for further research, as tighter value ranges would result in more stable conclusions. On the other hand, variables that do not have much effect on the conclusion are either more firmly established (narrower range of plausible values) or the variable simply does not have a large an effect in the entirety of the clinical pathway.

Markov models are another method of performing a decision analysis. Unlike decision trees, which are linear, Markov models include recursive relationships between health states. Figure 3 shows a simplistic Markov model linking volume overload to renal failure and two health states.

An individual can remain in any given state, or cycle between states. The only terminal state in the model is death. Markov models also include the effect of time, thereby isolating where events take place during the simulation. Finally, Markov models are capable of evaluating more complex interactions between health states.

The standard method of analysis with a Markov model involves a hypothetical cohort of patients. Patients enter the model in varying health states. Then the model cycles and patients are redistributed to other health

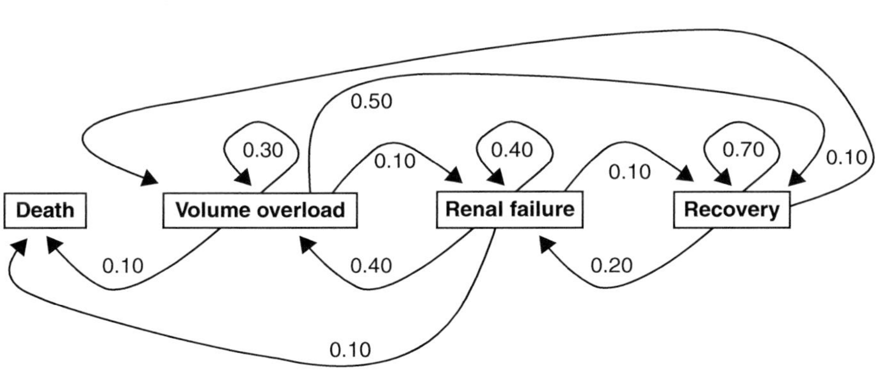

Figure 3. Markov model for renal failure, volume overload, recovery, and death showing a probability for each branch.

states based on the underlying probability of each transition. Once all transitions between health states are complete, outcomes are re-assigned and then summed to produce totals. Markov models are also run using a multi-way sensitivity analysis called Monte Carlo simulation. In a Monte Carlo simulation, values for any or all variables in the model are changed simultaneously. Additionally, starting values for each variable are picked randomly from pre-specified distributions of the variables. The model is run repeatedly, producing both outcomes and 95% confidence intervals.

League tables are aggregated lists of therapies and cost-effectiveness measures. The motivation for creating league tables is to inform healthcare policy and promote high value spending. An example of one large online league table is the CEA Registry, a comprehensive database of over 4,300 cost-utility studies across a range of conditions published through 2013. The registry represents an ongoing effort by Tufts University to compile available evidence on the value of healthcare interventions and promote standardized methodologies.

While league tables have the potential to both inform policy and spending decisions, league tables are also subject to misinterpretation or false inference. For fair comparison, studies listed in a league table should be methodologically similar, occur during the same time frame and generally the same setting. Furthermore, the user of the league table should evaluate to what extent the conditions of the league match the candidate environment. Hopefully the CHEERS guidelines will improve consistency and transparency in cost-effectiveness reporting which in turn will facilitate comparisons of effectiveness and cost across interventions.

Conclusions

CC is a major driver of overall healthcare spending. CEA complement efforts to identify winning therapies by identifying the best approaches for a given price. With high morbidity, high mortality, complex interactions and expensive cost streams, CCM is a natural home of these types of analysis. However, cautious interpretation of cost-effectiveness remains extremely important, as misuse and misunderstanding regarding cost-effectiveness is common.

References

1. Wallace DJ, Angus DC, Seymour CW, *et al.* (2015). Critical care bed growth in the United States. A comparison of regional and national trends. *American J. Respir. Crit. Care Med.*, 191(4), 410–416.
2. Rosenthal JA, Lu X and Cram P. (2013). Availability of consumer prices from US hospitals for a common surgical procedure. *JAMA Intern. Med.*, 173(6), 427–432.
3. Aliferis L. (2015). Variation in prices for common medical tests and procedures. *JAMA Intern. Med.*, 175(1), 11–12.
4. Young DW. (2007). The folly of using RCCs and RVUs for intermediate product costing. *Healthc Financ Manage.*, 61(4), 100–108.
5. West TD, Balas EA and West DA (1996). Contrasting RCC, RVU, and ABC for managed care decisions. A case study compares three widely used costing methods and finds one superior. *Healthc. Financ. Manage.*, 50(8), 54–61.
6. Peek GJ, Mugford M, Tiruvoipati R, *et al.* (2009). Efficacy and economic assessment of conventional ventilatory support versus extracorporeal membrane oxygenation for severe adult respiratory failure (CESAR): a multicentre randomised controlled trial. *Lancet*, 374(9698), 1351–1163.
7. Mouncey PR, Osborn TM, Power GS, *et al.* (2015). Trial of early, goal-directed resuscitation for septic shock. *N. Engl. J. Med.* 372(14), 1301–1311.
8. Riker RR, Shehabi Y, Bokesch PM, *et al.* (2009). Dexmedetomidine vs Midazolam for Sedation of Critically Ill Patients: A Randomized Trial. *JAMA*, 301(5), 489–499.
9. Kahn JM, Rubenfeld GD, Rohrbach J, and Fuchs BD (2008). Cost savings attributable to reductions in ICU length of stay for mechanically ventilated patients. *Med. Care*, 46(12), 1226–1233.
10. Briggs AH and O'Brien BJ (2001). The death of cost-minimization analysis? *Health Econ.* 10(2), 179–184.
11. Dakin H and Wordsworth S (2013). Cost-minimisation analysis versus cost-effectiveness analysis, revisited. *Health Econ*, 22(1), 22–34.
12. Beauregard CL and Friedman WA (2003). Routine use of postoperative ICU care for elective craniotomy: a cost-benefit analysis. Surgical Neurology [Internet]. Available at: http://www.sciencedirect.com/science/article/pii/S0090301903005172.
13. Branch-Elliman W, Wright SB, and Howell MD (2015). Determining the ideal strategy for ventilator-associated pneumonia prevention: Cost-benefit analysis. *American J. Respir. and Crit. Care Med.*, 2015, 192(1), 57–63.
14. Fowler RA, Mittmann N, Geerts W, *et al.* (2014). Cost-effectiveness of dalteparin vs unfractionated heparin for the prevention of venous thromboembolism in critically ill patients. *JAMA*, 312(20):2135–2145.

15. Angus DC, Clermont G, Watson RS, Lindu-Zwirbie WT, Clark RH and Roberts MS (2003). Cost-effectiveness of inhaled nitric oxide in the treatment of neonatal respiratory failure in the United States. *Pediatrics*, 112(6 Pt 1), 1351–1360.
16. Diamond GA and Kaul S (2009). Cost, effectiveness, and cost-effectiveness. *Circ. Cardiovasc. Qual.* Outcomes, 2(1), 49–54.
17. Bell CM, Urbach DR, Ray JG, *et al.* (2006). Bias in published cost effectiveness studies: systematic review. *BMJ*, 332(7543), 699–703.
18. Husereau D, Drummond M, Petrou S, *et al.* (2013). Consolidated Health Economic Evaluation Reporting Standards (CHEERS) statement. *BMC Med.*, 11(1), 1–1.
19. Husereau D, Drummond M, Petrou S, *et al.* (2013). Consolidated Health Economic Evaluation Reporting Standards (CHEERS) — Explanation and Elaboration: A Report of the ISPOR Health Economic Evaluation Publication Guidelines Good Reporting Practices Task Force. 16(2), 231–250.
20. Committee to Evaluate Measures of Health Benefits for Environmental HASR, Services BOHC, Institute of Medicine (2006). Valuing Health for Regulatory Cost-Effectiveness Analysis. National Academic Press, Washington, DC.

Budget Management

Andrew Webb
Clinical Professor, Faculty of Medicine, University of British Columbia, Vancouver, Canada

Key Points

1. Budgets are numerical expressions of plans and are control standards against which results can be compared. The critical care (CC) budget describes expenses required to achieve annual objectives.
2. A revenue budget describes revenue generation from patient care, education and research. An operating expense budget includes costs of day-to-day CC operations, including wages, equipment, and supplies but there is no fixed relationship between cost and price charged.
3. The budget should be reviewed and developed in consultation with other services to ensure the annual plans for the CC unit and its role in providing services to others can be accomplished financially.
4. The performance of the CC department is monitored against agreed activity, quality and financial targets. Variances are discussed and explained and actions put in place to correct the variance.
5. Cost improvement programs focus on innovative methods of care delivery that streamline processes and reduced wasteful steps and their consequent cost.

Introduction

Budgeting is a fundamental part of managing CC: it involves allocating resources deliberately and prudently to achieve program objectives. This includes planning approved goals into specific projects and activities, staffing, and procurement of resources. Budgeting aims to optimize resource use in the short-, medium-, and long-term. Short-term budgeting focuses on planning operations, whereas medium- and long-term budgeting should have a strategic perspective.

The budgeting context for CC

CC is regarded as a high resource consumer with increasing demand for all aspects of CC. A simplistic view sees CC as a service that is difficult to deliver and requires significant resources. Hospital funding methods do not usually separate CC from other specialties; CC is funded mostly as an overhead to these specialties' costs. This important conceptual point mirrors the way many non-intensivists view the service. Prospective payment systems for hospital care may not cover the cost of the CC component (explicit rationing). Regardless of the funding system used, the same basic information is necessary to estimate the required resources or what can be done within the available resources.

CC financing and funding has many possible sources, mostly determined by the hospital's reimbursement mechanisms. Budgeting and financing systems of CC vary widely.[1,2] The use of CC resources also varies widely between countries of comparable wealth and similar population death rates. In the USA, almost half of all hospital deaths involve an ICU stay, whereas in the United Kingdom, CC is involved in one out of five hospital deaths.[3] The different examples of how the hospital and its CC units can be financed include for-profit, not-for-profit, and government-funded.

For-profit

In this example, the payer is usually the commercial insurance industry whose primary responsibility is to their shareholders. Like business, a for-profit hospital cannot survive unless costs are lower than charges. In this model, the CC manager focuses his/her efforts on maximizing the unit's revenue and minimizing its costs.

Not-for-profit

In a not-for-profit organization, revenue that exceeds costs is reinvested to support growth and development. Not-for-profit hospitals receive operating funds from two sources — consumers and philanthropy. In this situation, the CC manager needs to ensure costs are lower than revenue income (which is approved by the hospital's senior management team during the annual budget building process).

Government-funded

In hospitals funded by government, the CC manager needs to ensure providing care is accomplished within a pre-defined budget. In some government-funded systems, maintaining efficiency (ensuring costs are below revenue) leads to reinvestment for growth and development. Some organizations limit access to CC by limiting the number of funded beds (implicit rationing) with a fixed budget for a financial year irrespective of demand changes. Others have increased CC capacity on the back of activity based funding systems where additional capacity provides additional income to increase CC budgets.

Defining the Budget

Budgets serve a dual purpose. They are numerical expressions of plans and they are control standards against which results can be compared. The CC budget describes expenses required to achieve annual objectives, such as a given case volumes. This means a CC budget is a statement of expected revenues and expected expenses over a defined time period. The objective of the CC budget are to:

- describe its annual plan numerically,
- create a basis for evaluating its financial performance,

- create control standards against which results can be compared,
- create cost awareness by the ICU staff.

Each service within the hospital may be a 'cost centre' or a 'profit (revenue) centre'. Cost centres typically produce services that are not directly charged to third-party payers e.g. housekeeping. Some clinical services, e.g. radiology and laboratory, can be regarded as cost centres. The profit centres (e.g. surgical departments) have their costs attributed in charges to third-party payers directly, and their charges also include the costs of the cost centres. CC can function either as a cost centre, trading internally, or a profit centre charging third-party payers directly, or as a mix of the two. In the latter case, some are charged directly, e.g. patients admitted primarily for CC and/or discharged directly to other institutions.

Types of budgets

Revenue

A revenue budget describes revenue generation from patient care (revenue from patient billings and government funding), education (revenue for teaching students) and research (revenue from research agencies and industry). There is no fixed relationship between costs of a service and the price charged for the service.[4] In for profit systems, the price includes the profit. In government funded healthcare systems, the price can be distorted by many factors including political policies, accounting policies, and cross-subsidization within the hospital. Cross-subsidization may reduce the effective cost of low volume, expensive therapies by assigning part of their cost to the price of high volume, less expensive interventions.

Operating expense

An operating expense budget includes costs of day-to-day CC operations, for example wages, equipment, and supplies. The budget may be fixed or variable. A fixed budget means resources are committed to a specific cost centre for the budget period and are based on planned workload. In this model expenditure control is the only way of managing the budget. A variable budget means resources change with volume, workload or service demand. In this model, the revenue budget flexes with activity and allows the budget to keep pace with activity. There is also the possibility of volume efficiency as more activity achieves a lower unit cost.

Hospitals sometimes attempt to associate costs with particular patient cases which is called case-mix accounting. In this approach, a complete financial picture of all costs is developed for treating individual patients grouped into similar classes on the basis of resource use.

Expenses in CC operating budgets can be direct (for example, staffing expenses, disposable expenses, pharmaceutical costs) or indirect (costs of services provided by others to the CC department). Indirect costs may be attributable to activity, e.g. the costs of physiotherapy, laboratory, radiology, housekeeping, etc., or may be considered as an overhead, for example the cost of utilities. Indirect costs may not appear in the CC operating expense budget. They may be considered as direct costs of the service providing department, a 'central expense' for all patient care units in the hospital or shared between service-receiving and service-providing departments, or internally traded as an expense to the service-receiving department.

Where indirect costs are considered to be direct costs of the service-providing department they carry the risk of fluctuation in demand and changes in costs of delivering the service. If demand increases, their budget may not be sufficient. If the demand decreases, the resulting overcapacity causes inefficiency and unnecessary hospital costs.

Indirect costs considered as a central expense of provided from a fixed budget of the service-providing department deviations from the agreed service level will have budgetary or operational consequences for both the service-receiving and service-providing departments. The absence of a direct financial link makes mitigation of the risk of significant budget variance particularly difficult.

Where indirect costs are internally traded internal prices are defined for the services provided to the CC department from other departments. The budget contains both the direct and the indirect costs. The risk of increased service demand is borne by the service-receiving department.

Capital budget

A capital budget includes a schedule equipment acquisitions planned in the budget year. Capital expenditure may be depreciated over the lifetime of the equipment and shown as a depreciation expense in the operating expense budget.

Costing Models

CC costing methodology

Many attempts have been made to measure the resources used in CC. However, as noted in a review by Gyldmark,[5] comparisons between studies are difficult as different studies have included different elements of resource use.

'Critical to Success'[6] reported large variations in CC practice and subsequently costs. Resource data collected in a standardized manner is an essential component of modern CC practice. Approximately 50–60% of the total CC costs are direct costs. Up to 90% of these are staff costs. Some costs are fixed and independent of activity level (e.g. cost of space) while others vary according to the volume and content of care (e.g. costs of materials and pharmaceuticals). Staff costs are often considered as fixed costs; however, if staffing is flexible according to patient numbers, some of the staff costs are variable costs.

Assessment of the costs of CC may follow a 'top-down' approach or a 'bottom-up' approach. The 'top down' approach to costing allocates total hospital costs, collected retrospectively, to a departmental level using some allocation statistics.[5] Often, total CC costs are derived from the hospital budget and apportioned by the number of patients to produce an average cost per patient. While this approach avoids laborious costing of individual patients it is not capable of comparing the costs of individual patients or groups of patients as it assumes that individual patients consume an identical amount of resource on a daily basis.

The bottom-up approach necessitates the accurate, prospective measurement of resources at a unit level that are ascribed to individual patients.[7,8] For example, delivering an analgesic would be costed by measuring the numbers of syringes used, the analgesic itself and the amount of nursing time required to prepare and deliver the drug. Against these values, unit costs are assigned. While this approach facilitates costing of individual patients and groups of patients it is laborious, complex, and expensive to operate.

Various hybrid costing methodologies have been used in CC. Defining patients according to a dependency measure (in its simplest form high dependency care or critical care) attempts to overcome the assumption that resources are distributed evenly between patients in the 'top-down' approach. A period of 'bottom-up' calculation may be used to define the costs of the high dependency patient assuming remaining costs are distributed amongst the CC patients.

Assigning costs

Assigning costs to individual patients or groups of patients help in both budget and assessing changes in CC activities. Costs may be assigned based on time in the CC unit (usually by day) or by using a weighted procedure method.[4]

Using time as a proxy for costs assumes all patients require roughly similar therapeutic interventions and procedures. Weighted procedure methods assign a relative weight for resource consumption of common procedures and therapeutic interventions, considering materials, pharmaceuticals, equipment, and staff. The total costs, including those from the use of other services, are divided according to the number and relative weight of the procedures and interventions performed.

Costs may be apportioned according to CC intervention.[9–11] The earliest was the Therapeutic Intervention Scoring System (TISS).[9,12] The original TISS assessed 76 therapeutic interventions and monitoring tasks summarized to a single sum score that provides a proxy measure of cost, including both the material and labor costs. A shorter version with 28 items was developed subsequently.[10] The weighted procedure method using the TISS or other similar instruments does not measure all CC activities so will inflate costs of those activities measured by an amount to cover those that are not.

Some studies found a significant relationship between daily TISS scores and individual patient costs[13] while others do not support this hypothesis.[10] TISS was originally described as a method for quantifying therapeutic interventions and has been adapted extensively in individual ICUs to reflect local practice. This clearly affects comparison between different ICUs.

The Medical Economics and Research Centre in Sheffield, UK developed their own method of CC costing, starting with the identification of budgetary components associated with resource use. The selection of the most important components was based on relevance, data availability and ease of collection. The validity of the data was considered. This process led to the definition and grouping of components as 'cost blocks' (Table 1).[8]

The UK Intensive Care National Cost Block Programme launched in 1999, as a standard method of costing for CC overcoming the complexity of existing systems and the heterogeneity of accounting practices employed by individual UK NHS trusts.[14] It was developed with the principle aim of facilitating meaningful comparisons between individual CC units.

A number of factors influence the varying degrees of expenditure on CC in different hospitals. Technological developments, differences in unit characteristics and differences in methods of costing are thought to be three such factors.[5] Heterogeneous case-mix is another problem. A study of the cost of individual patients admitted to a Canadian ICU found that the 8% of their patients who consumed the highest costs equated to the same amount of resources as the 92% of patients with the lowest costs.[15] The cost block method overcomes the problem associated with different methods of costing, insofar as more accurate study of the costs and consequences of CC can prevail.

Managing the Budget

Assessing resource requirement

In most healthcare systems budgets are reviewed annually. The budget should be reviewed and developed in consultation with other services to ensure the annual plans for the CC unit and its role in providing services to others can be accomplished financially. One of the most important

Table 1. Cost components collected within each cost block.[8]

Cost block	Cost components
1. Capital Equipment	Linear standard depreciation
	Maintenance
	Annual lease and hire charges
2. Estates	Water, sewerage, waste and energy
	Building and engineering
	Maintenance and decoration
	Rates
	Building depreciation
3. Non-Clinical Support Services	Administration
	Management
	Cleaning
4. Clinical Support Services	Radiology
	Laboratory services
	Physiotherapy
5. Consumables	Drugs and fluids
	Top 10 drugs and fluids
	Disposables
	Nutritional products
	Blood and blood products
6. Staff	Consultant medical staff
	Other medical staff
	Technical staff
	Nursing staff
	Bank and agency nursing staff
	Administrative staff

determinants of budget need is the number and type of cases that will be treated. This will be informed by historical trends and consultation with other services using CC services. The consultation should focus on changes in service provision of departments using CC services to identify if their needs may change, e.g. appointment of staff that perform procedures that depend on CC. As the annual budget is developed cost pressures need to be identified such as:

- Salary increases;
- Drug and material price increases;
- Changes in reimbursement processes or policies;
- Investment in new technologies;
- Service contract price increases.

All systems for financial management within the CC unit have to operate within the resource constraints of the overall health system. The demand for CC services continues to increase and is not matched by a commensurate increase in healthcare resources. The reasons for the increase in demand are multi-factorial but include:

- Aging population.
- Increased public expectation.
- Technological advance.
- Changes in disease demography.

Strategies for dealing with the imbalance between resource and demand include reducing demand, limiting supply (implicit rationing), and improving efficiency. CC budget management systems must seek to rationalize expenditure since the only other alternative in a resource limited healthcare system is rationing of the service.

Budget monitoring

Hospital organizations usually establish a process by which necessary data are collected, distributed and evaluated by all patient care unit managers. The hospital generally identifies what it considers to be performance indicators and measures variance (actual performance versus what was planned).

- Financial, e.g. cost per unit of service.
- Staffing, e.g. cost per unit of service or staff paid hours as a percentage of total paid hours.

- Workload.
- Productivity, e.g. staff productivity index.
- Utilization, e.g. workload per patient or activity.

The CC manager is required, following review of the data, to identify reasons for variance and the activities that will be instituted to bring the budget back in line with what was predicted in its initial development. An example of the types of data and the processes used for this type of analysis is shown in Table 2. When an area of significant change is identified, the CC manager should examine and identify potential reasons for the variance. These may include increases or decreases in service activity and/or workload. Effective budget management requires an action plan to manage the variance to zero.

The fixed budget model

This model focuses on the use of expenditure budgets as the overall control mechanism (as opposed to a financial reconciliation of income and expenditure budgets). In this model, hospital revenue is redistributed to cost centres as an allowance, or expenditure budget. The CC cost centre is expected to deliver a service to support other departments. Targets are set and must be delivered within the scope of the budget allocated.

As the hospital sets budgets there is an opportunity to negotiate an adjustment to the expenditure budget based on known or projected changes in activity, demand or performance. This would normally occur on an annual basis, with *ad hoc* review during the year as necessary. The CC budget is negotiated in the context of the previous year's performance and an estimate of CC activity required to support the hospital's performance targets for the next year.

The budget for a CC unit should, as a general principle, reflect the actual make-up of the department. Each component of the service should be represented in the budget just as it is represented in the actual delivery of service (Table 3). In a fixed budget, overhead and indirect costs (e.g. cost of maintaining buildings, costs of support by other departments) are not attributed to the ICU and are treated as a hospital overhead or as part of another department's budget. Indeed some costs (e.g. sterile supplies,

Table 2. A typical monthly variance analysis report.

Portfolio/department	Critical Care
Report for period ended	XX/XX/XXXX
Responsible manager	XXXXXXXX

	Period			Year to date			Reason for variance	Action required/taken
	Budget	Actual	Variance	Budget	Actual	Variance		
Contract income								
Other income								
Revenue								
Salaries								
Benefits								
Contract labor								
Medical/surgical supplies								
Drugs								
Sundry expenses								
Expenses								
Net before amortization								

Table 3. A general model for a fixed ICU expense budget.

Staff	ICU managerial staff
	Medical staff
	Nursing staff
	Administrative support staff
	Technical support staff
	Educational staff
	Research staff
Equipment	Replacement
	Maintenance
Supplies	Pharmacy
	Blood and blood products
	Disposables
	Sterile supplies
	Administrative supplies
	Catering supplies
Diagnostics	Laboratory
	Radiology
Support services	Operating room
	Allied Healthcare Professionals
	Religious support services
	Mortuary services

laundry of sheets) are often not attributed to the ICU budget. Thus many ICUs are not expected to budget or manage expenditure on many of the items in Table 3.

Throughout the year, the performance of the CC department is monitored against agreed activity, quality and financial targets. Variances are discussed and explained and actions put in place to correct the variance.

With a fixed budget there is relatively little bureaucracy. Once the budget is set financial management is focused on containing expenditure. A fixed budget helps to focus attention on hospital objectives (rather than departmental agendas). It can work extremely well in smaller hospitals, where close liaison across cost centres is possible and staff can work together towards common shared goals. However, the CC department is exposed to the risk of increased demand, due to a change in another department's activity. It can be difficult to make significant service changes, or to develop new services, as there is no direct link between externally negotiated funding and the budget.

The variable budget model

This model recognizes that CC activity is determined by the activity of user departments. A trading account allows the CC department to recoup costs related to patient activity (variable costs) from user departments thus maximizing flexibility. User departments gain access to CC beds that may otherwise be closed to contain expenditure within a fixed budget. A small fixed budget is usually maintained to cover costs that are not related to patient activity (fixed costs).

A central theme of the trading account is the direct relationship between income and expenditure. It seeks to factor in relevant aspects of providing CC services: availability of staff, resources for equipment, consumables and drugs and the relationship between referring clinicians and the unit. The model attempts to match the flexible use of capacity with a parallel flexibility in funding. For CC units this principle has the added advantage of minimizing the financial risk through uncontrolled demand. Generally, the fixed costs are determined by the number of beds expected to be available or the predicted activity. In this respect the fixed costs budget is exactly the same as it would be in a fixed budget model.

Conversely the variable costs are those directly associated with activity. These are the costs that will change as a result of one more or less bed day of activity (Table 4). The trading account generates an income that is directly related to patient activity and expenditure is managed according to this income. Because the fixed budget devolved to the CC department is a fraction of the total expenditure, each user department is given a budget from which they can purchase their ICU service.

Service-receiving departments have a budget for their use of CC, shifting the financial responsibility for referral to the referrer. The financial risk of CC activity is moved to the source of such activity and budget

Table 4. A general model for a variable ICU budget.

Revenue	Income per patient day
Staff expenses	Bedside nursing staff
Supplies expenses	Pharmacy
	Blood and blood products
	Disposables
	Sterile supplies
	Administrative supplies
	Catering supplies
Diagnostics expenses	Laboratory
	Radiology
Support service expenses	Operating room
	Allied Healthcare Professionals
	Religious support services
	Mortuary services

management is focused on balancing income and expenditure rather than simply containing expenditure. In larger hospitals where close liaison between cost centres may be difficult, interaction is made more explicit. Developments in all interacting cost centres are forced to take account of the implications for CC.

A well-run trading account requires accurate and timely activity monitoring. Clearly the overall financial risk to the hospital does not disappear but it makes explicit the requirement to think through at a proper strategic level the impact and cost of CC services.

Managing Cost Efficiency

Resource limitation in the healthcare system as a whole must be matched by a reduction in expenditure. This can be achieved by increased efficiency (reduced cost per patient treated) or by reducing demand. Increasing efficiency is difficult as technological advance (in this context technology includes pharmaceuticals) will, in the majority of cases, increase costs. However, some technological developments may be cost beneficial.

Although the trading account model allows the CC unit to increase its income according to demand that leaves a reduction in resource somewhere else in the healthcare system. This may be appropriate if the priorities of the healthcare system can tolerate that reduction and wider use of trading accounts is one way of matching resource consumption to whole system priorities. A simple example may be the choice between two equally effective antibiotics: one is expensive to purchase but does not require laboratory measurement of levels, while the other is cheap but does require laboratory levels. Using the trading account model the first antibiotic may be the best choice.

The fixed budget model leaves expenditure control as the only way of managing the budget and cost efficiency, i.e. providing more activity for the same cost or providing the same activity at a lower cost. If the budget was based on system-wide priorities this would not matter, although there is little scope for accommodation of changing priorities. Furthermore, using the antibiotic example from above, most would select the second antibiotic since the costs of the laboratory measurements come out of another department's budget.

Cost improvement programs focus on innovative methods of care delivery that streamline processes and reduced wasteful steps and their consequent cost. Staff costs make up the major part of all CC expenditure such that the most effective way of reducing expenditure is to reduce staff costs. Increased efficiency can be achieved by reducing the average numbers of nurses per patient. Alternatively, efficiency in terms of cost per patient may be achieved by reducing the numbers of skilled nurses per patient and supporting them with unskilled assistants. Flexibility in staff rosters may reduce costs by reducing dependency on temporary or casual staff that are usually more expensive than permanent staff. Non-staff costs may be controlled by formulating agreed policies for admission and treatment taking into account real cost benefits where alternative treatments are associated with differing costs. This approach can most obviously be applied to formularies for drug choice and stock lists for disposables. For materials and disposables bulk purchase policies between departments or hospitals will usually reduce unit costs.

Costs of CC vary between units and are, in part, dependent on the organization of the unit. An open unit may have little in the way of treatment or admission policies with little control of expenditure. A closed unit will usually have well developed policies and uniformity of treatment leading to better expenditure control.

Since the fixed cost element is not related to patient activity a large ICU will have lower average costs than a small ICU. This is because treatment of a larger number of patients means the fixed costs represent a smaller proportion of the total. Thus a larger unit is more efficient than a smaller unit in economic terms.

Capital Expenditure Budgets

Capital assets

A capital asset is a tangible productive resource with an expected life in excess of one year. Capital assets are typically either land, buildings or equipment. Capital assets usually require repair and maintenance and have a cost that is amortized over the expected life of the asset. Many healthcare systems provide a separate funding stream for the purchase of major capital assets. Some healthcare systems consider the capital assets as an overhead to the system with central budgeting of resources to provide the assets. In some healthcare systems, the payer makes revenue charges for capital assets to increase awareness of the costs of using assets, to provide incentive to use them efficiently and to promote the forward planning of asset replacement. In these systems, assets are brought into the balance sheet at their purchase cost and subsequently revalued as a result of either periodic assessment (land and buildings) or annual indexation (equipment). Each asset is given an asset life and a calculation is made resulting in a charge to the hospital's revenue account. For example, a ventilator with a 10 year life would be written down to a zero book value by 10 revenue account charges over a 10-year period (assuming zero inflation). This charge to revenue is termed depreciation.

Alternative funding of capital equipment

In a variable budget, CC department surplus revenues may be used to fund or part-fund capital purchases. Where hospitals have trust funds then equipment purchases may be possible from them. Each hospital will have its own arrangement. Funds are often left to CC by grateful relatives and these are often restricted in use to improving the CC environment.

Another alternative is leasing. While leasing is often less cost efficient than straight purchase it is a way of financing a purchase without using scarce capital funds. Accounting rules distinguish between two types of lease: the finance lease and the operating lease.

The finance lease is regarded as a simple finance arrangement entered into in order to get something for which funds are not immediately available. In such an arrangement, leasing charges are typically the total purchase costs plus finance charge with the ownership passing to the lessee from the lessor after the final payment has been made. A finance lease is accounted for as though the asset were purchased from capital funds.

An operating lease should be seen as a type of rental agreement. Key features of an operating lease are that ownership does not automatically pass to the lessee at the end of the lease. It is also required that the total paid over the life of the lease (after deducting sums for inflation and for the inherent finance charge) does not exceed 90% of the original purchase price. This is known as the 90% rule.

Generally speaking, for best value to be obtained, a lease with the longest period that is also consistent with the 90% rule is most competitive. The life of a lease should reflect the expected life of the equipment, which is often nearer 10 years than 5, and leasing quotes should be obtained for a number of lease periods, e.g. five, seven, and nine years.

Because it is like a rental agreement an operating lease payment is charged in full to the operating expense account. Any lease deal needs provision to have been made in the revenue budget. Rolling forward equipment provision from lease to lease is, therefore, a lot less difficult than obtaining new equipment where the costs of the lease need to be provided in full. However, before re-leasing replacement equipment consideration should always be given to purchasing (or renting for an extended period) the old equipment from the leasing company. It may, after all, not need replacing!

References

1. Vincent JL, Takala J and Flaaten H (2012). Impact of reimbursement schemes on quality of care: a European perspective. *Am. J. Respir. Crit. Care. Med.*, 185, 119–123.
2. Bekes CE, Dellinger RP, Brooks D, *et al.* (2004). Critical care medicine as a distinct product line with substantial financial profitability: the role of business planning. *Crit. Care Med.*, 32, 1207–1214.
3. Wunsch H, Linde-Zwirble WT, Harrison DA, *et al.* (2009). Use of intensive care services during terminal hospitalizations in England and the United States. *Am. J. Respir. Crit. Care Med.*, 180, 875–880.
4. Finkler SA (1982). The distinction between cost and charges. *Ann. Intern. Med.*, 96, 102–109.
5. Gyldmark M (1995). A review of cost studies of intensive care units: problems with the cost concept. *Crit. Care Med.*, 23, 964–972.
6. Audit Commission (1999). Critical to Success: the place of efficient and effective critical care services within the acute hospital. HMSO Publications Centre, London.
7. Edbrooke D, Stevens V, Hibbert C, *et al.* (1997). A new method of accurately identifying costs of individual patients in intensive care: the initial results. *Intensive Care Med.*, 23, 645–650.
8. Noseworthy T, Konopad E, Shustack A, *et al.* (1996). Cost accounting of adult intensive care: methods and human and capital inputs. *Crit. Care Med.*, 24, 1168–1173.
9. Cullen DJ, Civetta JM, Briggs BA and Ferrara LC (1979). Therapeutic intervention scoring system: a method for quantitative comparison of patient care. *Crit. Care Med.*, 2, 57–60.
10. Miranda DR, de Rijk A and Schaufeli W (1996). Simplified therapeutic intervention scoring system: the TISS-28 items — results from a multicenter study. *Crit. Care Med.*, 24, 64–73.
11. Sznajder M, Leleu G, Buonamico G, *et al.* (1998). Estimation of direct cost and resource allocation in intensive care: correlation with Omega system. *Intensive Care Med.*, 24, 582–589.
12. Keene R, and Cullen DJ (1983). Therapeutic intervention scoring system. Update. *Crit. Care Med.*, 11, 1–3.
13. Havill J, Caspari M, McConnell H, *et al.* (1997). Charging for intensive care using direct nursing hours as the cost marker. *Anaesth. Intensive Care*, 25, 372–377.
14. Edbrooke D, Hibbert C, Ridley S, *et al.* (1999). The development of a method for comparative costing of individual intensive care units. *Anaesth.*, 54, 110–120.
15. Noseworthy T and Jacobs P (1995). Cost control in the ICU. *Curr. Opin. Crit. Care*, 1, 324–328.

Part VII

Emergency Preparedness

Disaster Response

Morgan McMonangle
Consultant Vascular and Trauma Surgeon
St Mary's Hospital,
Imperial College Hospitals NHS Trust, London

Francesca Rubulotta
Consultant and Senior Clinical Lecturer,
Anaesthesia and Intensive Care Medicine
Imperial College Hospitals NHS Trust
Imperial College School of Medicine
University of London, London

Key Points

1. A disaster may be defined as any large-scale regional incident, natural or manmade, typically occurring unexpectedly, leading to major disruption.
2. The four phases of emergency management of disaster are mitigation, preparedness, response, and recovery.
3. A successful disaster response is dependent on being well resourced with a well trained and rehearsed emergency response system. Very small changes or "errors" in the initial phases of a disaster management plan can have large organizational consequences.
4. The mantra of disaster triage is to perform the greatest good for the greatest number.

5. An individual's perception and orientation to a crisis is case specific and depends on whether or not victims are optimistic about the future. Second victims are healthcare providers who are involved in an adverse patient event, or medical error and become victims because they are traumatized by the event.

Introduction

Although major disasters have a low probability of occurring, they have devastating consequences when they do. Designing a response structure around each event is difficult, especially when public resources are low.[1–3] The response to a disaster involves many different teams and organizations in the provision of the broad range of resources required. For example, although the emergency medical service (EMS) responds to the majority of day-to-day emergencies, this service is severely disrupted after a disaster. Instead of an immediate response, the accepted window for action may be longer. For example, after an earthquake, most survivors are rescued within the first 24–72 hours; hence, a 48 hour time-period is a commonly defined performance window. Thereafter, mortality & morbidity increases with each passing hour.[1] The quicker a disaster response is provided the better the outcomes. It is often the lack of effective disaster management and leadership in the early stages that propagates problems. Initial issues include a lack of prior planning & training, poor financial backing, poor resource provision, difficulties associated with handling complex situations and adapting to an ever changing challenging environment.[2,3]

What is a Disaster?

A disaster may be defined as any large-scale regional incident, natural or man-made, typically occurring unexpectedly, leading to major disruption of the normal infrastructure and affecting the inhabitants directly. An extraordinary emergency response is required in its aftermath, due to the normally available resources being overwhelmed. A Multiple Casualty Event exists whenever normal healthcare resources are strained beyond the normal surge capacity, but are not yet overwhelmed. Once overwhelmed, this escalates into a Mass Casualty Event.[3]

When should a "Disaster" be declared?

A disaster is declared when the number of casualties in need of treatment (either pre-hospital or in-hospital) overwhelms the normal system beyond the point where effective or safe care can be delivered. This may be due to the presence of:

- Multiple patients needing treatment or rescue
- Environment which is challenging

Although the absolute number of patients is relative to the healthcare system, the normal emergency system (rescue or healthcare) within the region cannot adequately cope because of limiting factors. These may include resources, which may not be available (e.g. pre-hospital) or capacity surge, where the hospital system is overwhelmed. Additionally, the geographical spread must be considered. The containment of the incident may be Closed or Open:

- Closed disaster — a single event in a specific location (e.g. building collapse), typically occurring over a finite time and location. The strain on resources is predictable.
- Open disaster — occurs over a much wider geographical area or time (ongoing disaster). Examples include; armed conflict, earthquake, pandemic, heat wave, radiation fallout, others.

Expectations after a disaster

A Major incident may be classified according to its size and effect (burden) on the infrastructure. Further classification includes:

- Simple versus compound
- Size subdivided into minor, moderate, or severe
- Compensated versus uncompensated

Simple versus Compound

A disaster is deemed simple when the infrastructure (e.g. roads, health service) remains intact. A disaster is compound when it has lost its effective infrastructure. For example, a multi-vehicle collision is classified as a simple disaster because the normal access infrastructure for rescue and delivery remain intact. If, however, the same incident occurs due to a motorway collapse with destruction of the normal rescue pathways, it becomes compound.

Size

This describes the magnitude of the number of casualties that have overwhelmed the system, which is relative to the system itself. Typical descriptions based purely on numbers are labelled minor (25–100 casualties), moderate (100–1,000 casualties) or severe (>1,000 casualties). Typically, 10–20% of the total number affected by the disaster (including the dead) will present to hospital, with a mixture of injuries. This figure appears to be constant across a whole variety of mass disasters.

Compensated versus uncompensated

All major incidents will require mobilization of additional resources. If these ensure adequate support then the disaster is described as compensated. An uncompensated disaster is one where the normal system can no longer cope, despite additional resources. This may result from massive absolute numbers of casualties, unavailability of specialist care or equipment (e.g. chemical, biological, radiation (CBR)) or the incident has occurred in a remote region where access and delivery of care is too difficult.

Resource Management

All hazard approach

This describes a system, typical in most western countries, which is capable of dealing with all types of major disasters, including special circumstances (i.e. those requiring specific specialized skills or equipment such as large scale burns, large numbers of children or specialized decontamination facilities for CBR).[3]

Resource capability and limitations

A successful disaster response is dependent on being well resourced with a well trained and rehearsed emergency response system. This includes frontline teams in addition to disaster management, command, and transportation. Even with a highly trained and resourced response team, the speed and efficiency of the response is limited by the infrastructure, which may have been destroyed, the availability of medical personnel and their experience in dealing with the specifics of the incident. Other limitations include the psychological burden of human loss and other environmental disruption.

Infrastructure limitations

Necessity provisions include; adequate, safe food and water, electricity, lighting, shelter, transportation (both in & out of the danger zone) and communications. An open disaster may have a number of casualties in need of evacuation but with loss of access roads, or air access. The challenge is timely access to reach the disaster zone and provide secure evacuation of injured patients. Planning this action requires both response team and patient safety. Predicting the extent of environmental damage is almost impossible and even the most experienced response plan may need to be adjusted as the specific infrastructure limitations come to light.

The team involved may be multi-disciplinary including healthcare specialists in addition to the fire service, police or other security bodies. Suitable transport platforms may be different or specialized, requiring additional planning. The best trained and rehearsed teams are efficient at a speedy response without compromising service or safety of either the teams or patients. However, most teams do not deal with major disasters on a regular basis and the biggest challenges remain the variability of conditions, recourse and skill availability, with developing countries being hit hardest due to their lack of good rescue infrastructure.

Medical limitations

This includes available personnel and their skill level, especially in dealing with disasters, diagnostic technology (e.g. CBR), drugs, fluids or blood availability. Disaster triage is a unique algorithm not normally used in day-to-day practice, but may be a rate-limiting factor for an effective response. Poorly performed triage will contribute to an inefficient response thereby quickly overwhelming the system.

The Disaster Response

Broadly speaking, the response to a disaster may be divided into the acute response phase and the external response phase. The acute response phase is generally short, ranging from 24 to 72 hours or until external assistance (e.g. governmental, non-governmental or international aid agencies) can be dispatched. During the acute phase, local health facilities are easily overwhelmed. In the 1992 earthquake in Turkey, first aid given by lay survivors significantly improved survival of entrapped victims. As part of an action plan, local facilities and health providers or even lay persons should be integrated into the initial disaster response. This training should ideally be provided during the preparation and mitigation phases of disaster preparedness. Risk knowledge, regional vulnerabilities and the likely type of disaster that may occur, with its associated injury patterns, will help assist the local and acute response in the immediate aftermath.

A response takes time and the majority of deaths or casualty burden have already occurred prior to response mobilization (or even knowledge that a response is necessary!). However, three different levels of response are recognized:

- Level One Response — typically involves the escalation of the normal emergency services available at local level only. It may include the use of non-emergency services and vehicles for rapid transportation out of the disaster zone or to hospital. An escalation of the normal hospital services is also expected, including immediate discharge of patients where possible and cancellation of non-essential surgeries and investigations to free-up room for the expected casualty surge.
- Level Two Response — the regional or state-wide response that typically involves the mobilization of out-of-area resources from neighboring regions into the disaster zone, including supplies and personnel. Disaster command is usually regional working in close conjunction with other local command systems.

- Level Three Response — aid from outside agencies at national, governmental or even international level. This is typically reserved for large scale disasters. Often the numbers affected exceed 1,000 with an even greater population displaced over time.

It is the Level One (i.e. immediate local) response that has the potential to be most effective in the immediate aftermath on both mortality and morbidity. The immediate role of the other response levels is to support the Level One teams, in particular to replenish supplies or provide additional networks (e.g. personnel, food, water, equipment, etc.). A typical Level One response includes frontline medical teams at the incident site, a medical Coordinator on site, who works on triage and in parallel with the Incident Commander (command and control unit). Level One should work as a team. A team is "a small number of people with complementary skills who are committed to a common purpose, performance goals, and approach for which they hold themselves mutually accountable".[4] Teamwork may be deficient in several ways, especially during acute care, and these flaws can interact and impair patient outcomes.

There is good evidence for the value of realistic patient simulation (RPS) in the training of trauma team members.[5,6] RPS is demonstrating potential in improving Level One response outcomes.

It is interesting to note that the military are often the first on the scene after a large-scale disaster, because they may be mobilized in large and well-equipped teams. The hierarchical command structure allows most military systems to respond to a major disaster in a rapid and coordinated fashion. They have ready access to resources and are equipped to perform vital functions such as resource distribution, security, search and rescue, logistics assistance, field hospital staffing and transportation to otherwise unreachable communities.

A Command and Control unit should be initiated contemporaneously with level One response and this should incorporate other responsible units (typically 5–7 units) including; safety officer, medical officer, press officer, etc. The Command and Control unit must have an effective and robust communications network to receive information and distribute instructions to all teams involved along the command chain. This unit is also responsible for audit and governance. One good example of this is the response seen after the 2013 Boston Marathon bombings, where effective outcomes were the product of repeated team drills including simulation and communication amongst disciplines providing initial care, including EMS and trauma surgeons.[7]

The four phases of emergency disaster management

Since the turn of the 21st century, and especially the 9-11 attacks in New York City in September 2001, disaster preparedness has taken a more prominent role in modern healthcare. Current expert consensus defines four phases of emergency management: mitigation, preparedness, response, and recovery (Figure 1).

- Mitigation — the prevention of future emergencies by minimizing the effects of a disaster. This activity occurs both prior to and after an event. An example is buying life or home insurance.
- Preparedness — the preparation for managing the emergency directly. Examples include; evacuation plans, water and food supplies or fuel consumption. Preparedness is planned before the emergency occurs.
- Response — the safe and effective response to an emergency. This takes place during or in the immediate aftermath of an emergency and is the actual application of the plan. Examples include; disconnecting gas supplies after an earthquake.
- Recovery — the rebuilding phase after the emergency has subsided aimed at restoring a normal or preferably improved situation or environment. This might require a considerable financial assistance.

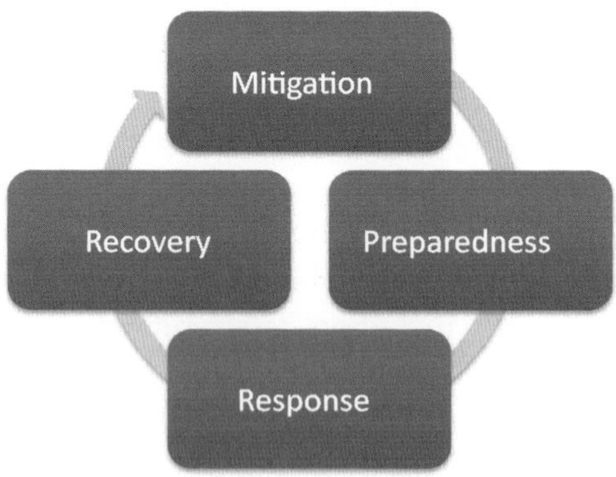

Figure 1. A four-phase model of disaster response.

Adequate preparedness at a local level must address vulnerability. Emergency disaster management plans must be designed looking at the balance between capacity and susceptibility to hazards. At a community level, potential hazards are identified and prioritized in a vulnerability assessment. In addition, an evaluation should focus on the community's capacity to manage a situation based on the resources and how these may be utilized. Preparedness includes the training and education of public health officials and community responders with respect to the disaster plan. Training must provide skills and knowledge. In a large-scale incident, disaster outcomes can be variable. The affected population is most vulnerable during early stages and before basic public health measures (water, sanitation, shelter) are implemented.

Prevention is therefore part of preparedness and it is divided into three phases:

- Primary prevention — the goal is to prevent the transmission of diseases. Action plans in this phase include promoting healthy practices (e.g. water treatment, basic hygiene as well as mosquito nets, etc.).
- Secondary prevention — the aim is to identify and treat any disease in the population and to prevent progression to a more serious stage. Actions include alleviating symptoms of disease (e.g. oral rehydration solution) and early detection and treatment of TB or dysentery, for instance.
- Tertiary prevention — the aim is to reduce permanent damage from diseases. Examples include rehabilitation after trauma injuries.

Any systematic analysis must look at all components of the preparedness program to identify weaknesses. All changes recommended after assessment must be aimed at outcome improvement. Interventions must be prioritized according to significance; for example, an expected disease with a high mortality must be addressed before a less frequent condition.

The Hajj is a "mega-gathering" event attended yearly by millions of Muslims from across the world. Planning, communications and logistical support are the foundations of its success. Current studies predict that by 2020, there will be more than 10 million pilgrims in attendance for the event. New construction and supportive infrastructures are already underway to meet the ever-growing needs of the pilgrims. With the improvement of systems and design, there is already a steady decrease in the number of accidents and requests for help. Continuous monitoring of emerging health situations ensures that a simple case of the flu does not become a worldwide epidemic. There will always be a need for emergent care during the Hajj and the Saudi Red Crescent Authority and supportive agencies will be ready to serve those who come to participate. Nearly 200,000 pilgrims that performed the Hajj in 2008 originated from the world's most resource-limited countries, where access to H1N1 vaccine and capacity to detect and respond to H1N1 in returning pilgrims are extremely limited. International efforts may be needed to assist resource-limited countries that are vulnerable to the impact of H1N1 during the 2009–2010 influenza season.[8]

Triage

Medical interventions must be kept to a minimum at the scene (Ground Zero) of a disaster, except for immediate rescue. Ideally, healthcare providers should limit any medical treatment to Triage, Treatment (simple) and Transport (to an appropriate medical facility).

The mantra of disaster triage is to perform the greatest good for the greatest number. This alters the normal standard hospital care, which treats everyone with the same level of care and expectations. Instead, disaster triage revolves around the population ("best for most") rather than the individual ("everything for everyone"), aiming to provide care for the majority of people with the least amount of resources available. Over triage must be avoided as this places an unnecessary strain on resources, potentially leading to failure of the system. Disaster triage has a dynamic equilibrium between the needs of the population and the resources available and is directly dependent upon:

- Number of wounded casualties and their needs (injury burden).
- Number of competent personnel available to provide for the injured.

Triage algorithm

This does not follow the normal triage pathway of emergency hospital or pre-hospital practice because neither resources nor time available will allow for individualized care. The triage algorithm is simple to use, effective and easily understood by all personnel involved. It is also dynamic, as reassessment may become necessary as the incident evolves or resources change. Documentation and labelling are also important and although simple and rudimentary, must be performed accurately. Finally, triage decisions, as authorized by the medical command, must be considered final and be respected.

30-second sieve

Patients are rapidly examined and categorized simultaneously. The unconscious patient is approached following a very simplified, yet effective format, by applying the A–B–C approach.

- Airway — perform chin-lift and a check if patient is breathing. If yes, move on to B. If not, pronounce dead.
- Breathing — if breathing is present or restored, check the respiratory rate. If it is severely abnormal (i.e. <10 or >29 breaths min^{-1}) then categorize it as ***Priority P1*** (immediate life-saving care required). If respiratory rate is within normal limits, then move on to **C**.
- Circulation — Measure the capillary refill time (normal <2s) and pulse rate. If capillary refill time >2s or pulse rate >120 bpm, then categorize the patient as ***Priority P1***. If these parameters are normal, categorize as ***Priority P2*** (urgent care (within 4–6 hours) required).

Patients are categorized according to the likelihood of salvage, which in turn dictates the urgency and rapidity of the treatment required, if any (see Table 1).

- Category One (Red) — These are also Priority P1 patients. Patients have injuries requiring immediate intervention or emergency surgery with a good chance of recovery. These should only receive "minimal acceptable care" in the field and during the early phase of resuscitation, before retriaging and treating appropriately. This typically constitutes about 10–20% of the total casualty load (including deaths) after a disaster. Examples include laparotomy for haemorrhage, thoracotomy, etc.

Table 1. Categorization of trauma.

Category	Description		Colour	Priority	Treatment
1.	**Immediate**	Require immediate life-saving treatment	Red	P1	T1
2.	**Urgent**	Require treatment within 4–6 hours	Yellow	P2	T2
3.	**Delayed**	Require treatment but no defined set time	Green	P3	T3
4.	**Expectant**	1. Unlikely to survive treatment 2. Circumstances dictate that their treatment may compromise the care of others	Blue		T4
5.	**Dead**	Dead	White	Dead	Dead

- Category Two (Yellow) — These are also Priority P2 patients. Patients have injuries requiring surgery, typically within 4–6 hours, but not as an immediate priority. Examples include limb revascularization, burr hole, etc.
- Category Three (Green) — These are also Priority P3 patients. Treatment for injuries is required but there is no set defined time (e.g. limb fracture stabilization, soft tissue suturing, etc.).
- Category Four (Blue) — Severe wounds and unlikely to survive, especially given the current demand on resources as patients may become a drain on resources, where outcomes are likely to be futile. These patients are managed expectantly with analgesia and sedation.
- Category Five (White) — These are patient's pronounced dead at the time of triage. They should be removed to an appropriate location when it is safe to do so and other priorities have been attended to.

Adequate training is required for the safe and prompt use of the triage sieve. Simulation is beneficial at acquiring these competencies and should include training of nurses, paramedics and even non-medical personnel, who may be called upon as part of a disaster response.

In the event of a Mass Casualty Incident (MCI) an Incident Command System (ICS) should be established for triage. A MCI may range from a few patients injured in a bus accident overwhelming a local hospital, to a natural disaster or conflict where hundreds or thousands of victims incapacitate the entire health system of the affected area.

Resources, transportation, access and physical environments are often disrupted. Such austere conditions place huge constraints on the emergency medical care needed by the affected population. The ICS (a large command and control unit) is a hierarchical structure designed to command, control and coordinate the effective emergency response among all agencies and organizations involved in a disaster. This system was developed in the United States (1970) after previous problems identified with MCI, including inadequate planning, poor communications, and lack of appropriate triage. Hospitals can adapt a structure similar to ICS, which is the Hospital Emergency Incident Command System (HEICS). Both ICS and HEICS disaster management are not widespread, and might be absent, especially in developing countries. ICS and HEICS serve as useful tools in basic MCI management as those offer a series of steps that, taken together meet the immediate health needs of disaster victims. The triage team works under the authority of the Triage Officer, with responsibilities for tagging and immediate treatment before releasing patients according to medical priority. On-site care is limited to emergency care only. Teams may need to be rotated where resources or staff are limited, but it is important that decisions made are timely so that the facilities are not overwhelmed.

The function of the search and rescue team is the safe location and evacuation of victims from the impact zone, preferably with transfer to the medical post after triage. The medical post is established as close as is safely possible to the impact zone within a sheltered domain to reduce transfer distances and shorten time to care.

The evacuation team is responsible for the safe transfer of victims to the designated healthcare facility using appropriate transportation with escorts. The walking wounded are often transferred by non-medical transport, but only after all acute victims have been evacuated. Upon arrival at the designated hospital, each patient is retriaged and assessed and more definitive care given.

Triage must be 'absolute' rather than 'relative' with each patient's needs judged as either urgent or not urgent. Categorization is based on:

- The nature or immediate threat to life of the patient's present condition. It is not based on the order of arrival!

- The potential for survival. This is a delicate balance between the prognosis counter-balanced by the availability of resources, which may be a dynamic process as either the patient condition, the environment or the resources available change. This concept is critical and can greatly influence the overall survival rate after a disaster.

The most commonly recognized triage systems, internationally, in MCI are:

- The Simple Triage and Rapid Treatment (START) color coding system.
- The Secondary Assessment of Victim Endpoint (SAVE) secondary triage for more in-depth assessment.

Triage is both an ongoing and dynamic process beginning in the field and repeated at the medical camp or hospital as the patient's condition evolves. Triage is not confined to any one area and may be performed in the field, during transportation or at hospital. Simultaneous triage of multiple victims, together or in different locations, can take place.

The general principles of disaster triage include:

- In borderline survival cases, triage as urgent.
- With injured children, prioritize over adults within the same triage class.
- Give basic stabilization measures to all patients before giving further or more definitive individual care.
- Definitive simple care (e.g. debridement and suturing, antibiotics, plastering of fractures, etc.) is only performed once no more casualties arrive and all urgent injuries have been managed.

To avoid overwhelming the facilities, the most senior clinician oversees the patient flow and triage. A recent systematic review of strategies to manage and allocate scarce resources during Mass Casualty Events found 74 studies, which met inclusion criteria.[3] However, the evidence was sufficient to form conclusions only on two strategies, although the strength of evidence was rated as low. One of these two strategies was looking at optimizing use of existing resources. Unfortunately, commonly used field triage systems do not perform consistently during actual mass casualty events according to this systematic review. The number of high-quality studies addressing other strategies was insufficient to support conclusions about their effectiveness because of differences in study context, comparison groups, and outcome measures. The current evidence base is inadequate to inform providers and policymakers about the most effective strategies for managing or allocating scarce resources during mass casualty events. The author of this review found that a consensus on methodological standards is needed to guide future research. Standards have not been developed to promote consensus interpretations of the evidence supporting individual strategies.

Chaos theory and Disaster Response

Chaos theory has been recently indicated as a useful way to understand a disaster response given how unpredictable it is. "Chaos is the irregular, uncertain, discontinuous aspect of change within the confines of a patterned whole."[2,9] Disaster workers are in constant motion at various locations through space and time as they apply the Command & Control unit or other management systems' tactics. Generally, disaster workers are using "workplace rules" within a "field of action." Workplace rules are interorganizational principles dictated by the Command and Control unit. The field of action can be highly complex and it is defined by the physical workplace plus the external environment. Disaster response organizations and response systems are dynamic systems. Some dynamic systems evolve in exceedingly complex ways, initially appearing to defy any rule. Chaos theory is a way to analyze such systems. In mathematical theory a single law governs the change from order and predictability into unpredictability or chaos for dynamic systems. According to Pietgen *et al.* "there are abrupt qualitative changes — called bifurcations — which mark the transition from order into chaos like a schedule, and 'universal' meaning that these bifurcations can be found in many natural systems both qualitatively and quantitatively".[10] Chaos is a type of nonlinear behaviour emerging along a universal route. At a certain point along this route organizations become highly sensitive to initial conditions and may change abruptly. The form a disaster takes is highly influenced by the initial conditions. During the first 24 hours after an event, disaster organizations appear to exist at the edge of chaos, a position that allows maximum adaptability. Very small changes or "errors" can have large organizational consequences. The accumulation of errors could lead to a second-order phase transition characterized by a period of disconnected organizational fragments that eventually come together to form the new system. More complex, and adaptive structures may emerge from a phase transition. New structures are not necessarily more efficient compared to previous structures or response systems. These are very important findings because these seem to map the essential information about how systems become disorganized or evolve. The challenge at the edge of chaos is how to interpret the options creatively and choose among a multitude of possibilities. Kiel tells us that "Most importantly, during times of high instability such as disasters and occasions when emergency services reach peak levels of activity, it is essential to recognize that stability can only be regained by developing strategies that are themselves unstable. In short, we must match the instability of these environments with management practices and organizational strategies that are dynamic and fluid".[11] All levels of the disaster response should be flexible and adaptive. Managers should look for the unusual. This suggests that it necessary to be open to learning and therefore adapting to what is necessary for the new system. This style of decision making relies on rapid and adequately networked communications, and an exploratory, experimental process based on intuition and reasoning by analogy. Employees should be rewarded for risk taking, and experimentation that creates different options and for making such shifts. This involves top level managers dealing with the politics of coordination and consensus building across organizational and political jurisdictions. The application of chaos theory to disaster management has a number of significant limitations. The question of how helpful chaos theory is for disaster response needs further empirical investigation. Significant resources are needed to maintain the capacity to act in different ways on short notice. An over commitment to flexibility can result in rigidity, particularly when decisive action in a single direction is required. Such organizations can also be indecisive and not be able to make critical decisions quickly.

The Role of Critical Care in Disaster Management

Engagement and education of Intensive Care Unit (ICU) clinicians in disaster preparedness is fragmented by time constraints, institutional barriers, often only being attended to after the disaster has occurred.[12]

A systematic review from 2007 to 2013, was used to formulate a consensus statement by the American College of Chest Physicians on the management of large-scale disasters or pandemics with multiple critically ill or injured.[13] The recommendations are relevant to all front line clinicians, hospital administrators, and public health or government officials working in disaster planning and grouped under the following themes:

- Situational awareness.
- Clinician roles and responsibilities.
- Education.
- Community engagement.

The role of critical care (CC) physicians after a disaster is most likely to be hospital-based where their skills are best used. Involvement includes up-staffing within the unit, expansion of CC beds (including ventilated) to other suitable areas of the hospital (e.g. some HDUs of trauma wards may have capabilities to transform a certain number of beds into ICU-level care). The ICU physician must identify which patients may also be safely stepped-down from a CC environment to allow the bed be used for victims of the disaster, especially post-operative support. This may also include identifying beds within the coronary care unit or acute surgical wards. Many ICU physicians may be called upon to aid in the retriaging of patients once admitted to the resuscitation bay and give expert advice on whether a patient is suitable for ICU-level care including full ventilation, or whether survival is unlikely and comfort-measures only should be applied. As CC is the most expensive aspect of healthcare, the ICU physician has an important role in resource allocation, which also maximizes survival for the most victims while minimizing futile care during a resource-challenging situation.

It is important to secure empty beds when a major disaster occurs due to the resulting large numbers of trauma patients. In the Great East Japan Earthquake on 11 March 2011 air quality monitoring was also required due to the risk of environmental radioactive pollution from the nuclear disaster causing problems with artificial respiration management involving atmospheric air. The variability in damage arising during different disasters thus requires a flexible response from ICUs that handle seriously ill patients.

The role of telemedicine

In 2012 in the United States of America, 8% of non-federally funded ICU beds used telemedicine programs, including installations from overseas, in part driven by the shortage in board certified CC physicians. This technology offers an important input in patient care, which is enhanced by a change in the culture of care and the interfacility, interstate and even intercountry collaboration used to improve care.[14] Smartphone applications are fast becoming essential to emergency responders and the lay public. Currently, 683 applications were identified existing in various price ranges and quality. The Community Emergency Response Teams and the federal Emergency Management Agency (FEMA) had the best apps for National Disaster Medical System responders. The National Library of Medicine's Wireless Information System for Emergency Responders (WISER) app was an excellent app for HazMat responders. The Centres for Disease Control and Prevention (CDC) had high-quality apps for emergency responders in various fields. The American Red Cross had the most useful apps for natural disasters.[14] Best published evidence has demonstrated improved ICU outcomes with telemedicine implementation including ICU and hospital mortality, in addition to cost savings in the form of decreased length of stay and compliance with ICU best practice care. This level of care could be used to enhance remote care and advice in a disaster zone, especially in the event of staff shortages. Between January 1980 and September 2013, 17,565 disasters recorded. During this study period, 878 articles, chapters, books, and presentations were reported. Of these, only six articles described the effectiveness of telemedicine in mock simulations and disaster drills, and 19 articles provided examples of effective use of telemedicine in disaster response. However, these studies demonstrated telemedicine as a valuable tool for communication between frontline humanitarian aid workers and expert physicians at remote locations.[15] Future reports of disaster response should emphasize population-based outcomes as well as logistical details. Response and planning should be based on the projected number of critically ill or injured patients resulting from specific scenarios. Standard ICU management forms and patient data forms to assess ICU surge capacity impacts should be created and utilized in disaster events.[14]

Post-Disaster Effects on Healthcare Staff

How responders and victims are affected by or adapt following a disaster and the disruption of their future perspective is not fully known.[16] An individual's perception and orientation to a crisis is case specific and depends on whether or not they are optimistic about the future and actively involved in unfolding events. A person's ability to act may depend on their belief in whether or not they have a future. The sudden occurrence of a disaster severely qualifies prior concepts of the present and the future.[17] The sudden onset of a disaster "brings one crashing to the present." One of three possible temporal positions can result:

- "Restoration of flexibility" is when the victim resolves the immediate problems and attempts to restore their lives to normal.
- "Permanent loss of flexibility" occurs when an irrevocable change occurs in the social or economic fabric requiring people to redefine these relationships.
- "Presentism" refers to a condition where the need to deal with the necessities of life is so overwhelming that no wider perspective is possible.

Similarly, healthcare professionals can suffer traumatic experiences working in the area of a major disaster. Healthcare professionals can suffer post-traumatic stress disorders or they could become second victims.

Second victims are healthcare providers who are involved in an adverse patient event, or medical error and become victims because they are traumatized by the event. Despite this term being first coined in 2000 in relation to medical error,[17] it is only in recent years that those responsible for training and managing doctors have actively established processes to support staff involved in critical incidents that cause harm to their patients.[18] The second victim is frequently distracted from immediate patient care demands by becoming engrossed in self-reflection, replaying the activities preceding event awareness. Some providers may be unwilling to discuss the event, compounding their anxiety and ability to work. The second victim tends to self-isolate in an attempt to concentrate and focus on precisely what happened.[18] Over time, clinicians move from these worries to an intense fear they will no longer be viewed as trusted colleagues. Ultimately, second victims desperately want to know post-event details so they can make a positive difference in future outcomes.' Managers and senior supervisors should be aware of common high risk situations likely to evoke a second victim response so that clinicians at the epicentre of such events can be deliberately identified, monitored and supported in a timely manner. It is important to touch base with potential victims more than once, as there may be cases in which an emotional impact is delayed or cases in which the victim is unable to talk about the emotional trauma immediately after the event. Well after the chaos of the event has settled and after the second victim has had time to personally process what happened, interviewees expressed that, given a choice, they would welcome conversations about their emotional response with a trusted peer. Peers, especially those who have experienced this phenomenon, can offer powerful healing words and special support based on their personal experience. If the colleague has experience as a second victim, sharing personal stories can be powerful. Even without personal experience, the colleague can still be supportive while anticipating common second victim needs, free from judgment and blame. Ultimately, ongoing reassurance that the clinician remains a respected and trusted member of the clinical team is essential. In the event of team management, appropriate debrief is crucial. During these emotionally charged discussions a facilitator skilled in team dynamics and critical incident stress management (CISM) should coordinate and lead the team discussion. CISM has been used effectively for years in the emergency medical community and was developed to help prevent potentially disabling stress responses among emergency responders to traumatic community disasters such as the Columbine shootings, the Oklahoma City bombing, and the Twin Towers attack. Clinicians should not have to seek support on their own. Key principles should serve as a guide for institutions formalizing a peer support infrastructure keeping in mind that affected staff should always be treated with respect, compassion and administrative support immediately following adverse clinical events.

References

1. Koehler GA, Foley D and Jones M (1992). Computer simulation of a california casualty collection point used to respond to a major earthquake. *Prehosp. and Disaster Med.*, 7(4), 339–347.

2. Adam B (1998). Chernobyl: Implicate order of socio-environmental Chaos. In *Time and Chaos*, CT, Fraser J and soulsby M (eds.), International Universities Press, Madison, pp. 109–124.
3. Timbie JW, Ringel JS, Steven Fox D, *et al.* (2013). Systematic review of strategies to manage and allocate scarce resources during mass casualty events. *Ann. Emerg. Med.*, 61, 677–689.
4. Katzenbach J and Smith D (1993). *The Wisdom of Teams: Creating the High Performance Organization.* Harvard Business School Press, Cambridge, MA.
5. Hammond J, Bermann M, Chen B and Kushins L (2002). Incorporation of a computerized human patient simulator in critical care training: a preliminary report. *J. Trauma.*, 53, 1064–1067.
6. Lee SK, Pardo M, Gaba DM, *et al.* (2003). Trauma assessment training with a patient simulator: a prospective, randomized study. *J. Trauma.*, 55, 651–657.
7. Walls RM and Zinner MJ (2013). The Boston Marathon response: why did it work so well? *JAMA*, 309, 2441–2442.
8. Memish ZA, and the Jeddah Hajj Consultancy Group (2009). Establishment of public health security in Saudi Arabia for the 2009 Hajj in response to pandemic influenza A H1N1. *Lancet.*, 374, 1786–1791.
9. Scott LA, Swartzentruber DA, Davis CA, Maddux PT, Schnellman J and Wahlquist AE (2013). Competency in chaos: lifesaving performance of care providers utilizing a competency-based, multi-actor emergency preparedness training curriculum. *Prehosp Disaster Med.*, 28(4), 322–333.
10. Peitgen H, Jurgens H, and Saupe D (1992). *Chaos and Fractals.* Springer-Verlag, New York, pp. 584–586
11. Kiel L (1995). Chaos theory and disaster response management: lessons for managing periods of extreme instability. In *What Disaster Response Management Can Learn From Chaos Theory.* Conference Proceedings, May 18–19, 1995 Available at: https://www.library.ca.gov/CRB/96/05/over_12.html (Accessed 16 April 2016).
12. Timbie JW RJ, Fox DS, Waxman DA, *et al.* (2003). Allocation of Scarce Resources During Mass Casualty Events. Evidence Report No. 207. Prepared by the Southern California Evidence-based Practice Center under Contract No. 290-2007-10062-I. AHRQ Publication No. 12-E006-EF. 2012:84.
13. Task Force for Mass Critical Care (2014). Care of the critically ill and injured during pandemics and disasters: chest consensus statement. *Chest*, 146(4), 1–41.
14. Bachmann DJ, Jamison NK, Martin A, Delgado J and Kman NE (2015). Emergency preparedness and disaster response: there's an app for that. *Prehosp. Disaster Med.*, Sep 15, 1–5.

15. Latifi R and Tilley EH (2014). Telemedicine for disaster management: can it transform chaos into an organized, structured care from the distance? *Am. J. Disaster Med.*, 9(1), 25–37.
16. Call JA, Pfefferbaum B, Jenuwine MJ and Flynn BW (2012). Practical legal and ethical considerations for the provision of acute disaster mental health services. *Psychiatry.* 75(4), 305–322.
17. Schreiber MD (2015). Toward the way forward: building an emergency mental health system for Israel. *Isr. J. Health Policy Res.* Sep 15, 4, 47.
18. Wu A (2000). Medical error: the second victim. *BMJ.*, 320, 726.

Pandemic Planning

Michelle Murti
Medical Health Officer, Fraser Health, Surrey, Canada
Steve Reynolds
Regional Medical Director, Critical Care, Fraser Health, New Westminster, Canada

Key Points

1. Critical Care Pandemic Planning requires a 'whole-of-society' approach, overall system coordination and planning to maximize preparedness.
2. Pandemic planning scenarios should be broadened from traditional influenza risks to incorporate risks from organisms with a range of pathogenicity and transmissibility.
3. Planning should consider both surge capacity and surge capability for determining infrastructure and human resource requirements.
4. Organizational, regulatory, legal, and ethical frameworks are required for decision making during pandemics.
5. A research agenda for addressing the evidence needs before, during and after a pandemic should be incorporated into planning.

Introduction

"*In preparing for battle, I have always found that plans are useless, but planning is indispensable.*" — Dwight D. Eisenhower (1890–1969)

The last major influenza pandemic prior to H1N1 virus in 2009 was over 40 years earlier, in 1968, when a reassortment of the haemagglutinin yielded a H3N2 variant which replaced the H2N2 strain that had been circulating since 1957. In the past century, there have only been four influenza pandemics (1918, 1957, 1968, 2009) from which to draw our experience and understanding for planning for the next pandemic. The 2009 pandemic was the first one where substantial planning and preparations were in place prior to its onset. However, with limited and out-of-date experiences on which to base planning, many of the assumptions that went into pandemic planning prior to 2009 were based on estimates of severity from a different era. The estimated case-fatality rate of the 1918 pandemic was 1–3%, which was the basis of modeling assumptions for many pandemic plans pre-2009. However, case-fatality rates for symptomatic illness in 2009 were estimated to be between 0.03% and 0.05%.[1] While there were significant levels of morbidity and mortality associated with the H1N1 pandemic, there has been a shift in consideration for planning assumptions to have a scalable response that is adapted to the actual risk, which is likely to be unknown at the start of the pandemic.

In 2010, the World Health Organization's (WHO) Regional Office for Europe assessed pandemic planning activities at the regional and national levels in Europe to identify common elements of successful planning.[2] The essential elements that emerged were communication, coordination, capacity, adaptability/flexibility, leadership, and mutual support. It was also identified that planning should be multi-sectoral, have political support and dedicated funding. Areas identified for further planning included vaccine logistics, use of diagnostic tests and real-time surveillance, as well as improvements to communications and flexibility of response. Despite these statements, an international review of the WHO response to the 2009 pandemic stated that "the world is ill prepared to respond to a severe influenza pandemic or to any similarly global, sustained and threatening public health emergency."[3] The review committee identified structural impediments, operational deficiencies as well as limitations of scientific understanding and technical capacity. These are often the same issues that encumber local hospital and regional planning groups, and need to be considered in planning for the next pandemic.

In addition to the shift in planning, assumptions that will be required to prepare for a novel influenza virus with efficient and sustained human-to-human transmission, there have also been new non-influenza threats emerging such as Severe Acute Respiratory Syndrome (SARS), Middle Eastern Respiratory Syndrome (MERS), and Ebola virus disease (EVD), that demand a different approach to pandemic planning for the healthcare system. Global surveillance and local preparedness to sporadic, but inevitable, international spread necessitate ongoing vigilance to emerging pathogens that may or may not lead to sustained transmission in new locales, but pose a perpetual threat. Pandemic planning is necessary to provide appropriate surge capacity and capability for critical care (CC) preparedness.

Definitions and Descriptions of Pandemics

A pandemic is defined as an epidemic disease of widespread prevalence around the globe.[4] Epidemics such as MERS and EVD that have been localized to specific geographic regions but have had evidence of global spread with more limited ongoing transmission, do not meet the definition of a pandemic without widespread global prevalence. However, planning principles from influenza pandemic preparedness as well as emergency management broadly can be applied to these types of epidemics. The WHO uses a four-phase continuum for assessing influenza pandemics: (i) interpandemic phase (the period between influenza pandemics); (ii) alert phase (a new sub-type of influenza has been identified); (iii) pandemic phase (period of global spread); and (iv) transition phase (de-escalation of pandemic activities).[5] There is continuous risk assessment throughout, and shifts in activity from preparedness to response to recovery and back to preparedness.

Emergency response frameworks used internationally for all-hazards approaches to emergencies typically include a five-phase planning cycle: (i) prevention (planning to avoid/prevent a threat); (ii) protection (ensuring capabilities for security against a threat); (iii) mitigation (reducing impacts from a threat); (iv) response; and (v) recovery.[6] Explicitly considering what can be done in the interpandemic phase to prevent, protect and mitigate the threat of a pandemic should be, and more recently, has been incorporated into planning activities for infectious disease threats. The outbreak of EVD in West Africa has demonstrated how ongoing activities in these three domains can assist in preparedness and lack of activity can propagate an epidemic. Failure to identify the initial spread of the outbreak in Guinea in early 2014 due to deficiencies in global situational awareness and surveillance show the international lack of planning to identify such threats. Ongoing prevention from this type of threat would require an investment of public health and health service resources in impoverished countries to identify and respond to emerging infections. An early coordinated international response, once the threat was identified, would have been far less resource intensive than the sustained and widespread efforts required to manage an epidemic. However, most countries around the world began to protect their own borders from the threat of importation through border screening, monitoring activities and local infrastructure development, instead of investing more heavily in source control efforts to manage the risk of spread.[7] This has resulted in significant mitigation activity within developed countries in terms of increasing capacity at the frontline level for all facilities, development of Ebola assessment hospitals, and the increasing number of Ebola treatment centres capable of managing patients infected with Ebola and other biosafety level four pathogens.[8]

Expansion of the realm of preparedness activities to consider what types of prevention, protection and mitigation are needed requires a framework to consider the types of epidemic or pandemic scenarios to plan for. Early iterations of influenza pandemic plans used single scenario models, based on the high morbidity and mortality estimates from pandemics during the 20th century. The better outcomes from the 2009 H1N1 pandemic, led to development of 'mild', 'moderate', and 'severe' planning scenarios considering increasing case fatality, and impact on the entire population. More recent models have accounted for variability in the risk of transmission (low versus high) of infection as measured by the cumulative attack rate and the basic reproductive number and clinical severity of outcomes (low versus high) as a measure of case fatality rate to develop four planning scenarios.[9] Consideration of the transmissibility and clinical severity of a pathogen is more applicable to planning for non-influenza epidemics and pandemics. For example, MERS has very high clinical severity (case fatality rate estimated at 36%), but typically low transmissibility, where spread has been contained amongst household contacts or within nosocomial transmission settings.

This shift in planning scenarios and range of preparedness activities has also spawned a shift in approach to planning requiring the multi-sectoral, 'whole-of-community' planning. In 2010, just as the world was dealing with H1N1, the European Society of Intensive Care Medicine (ICM) released a series of articles from their Task Force for Intensive Care Unit Triage.[10] The Task Force convened in 2007 to review the literature and confer with experts in the field (critical care (CC), infectious disease, nursing, epidemiology, public health, medical engineering and ethics) to develop Standard Operating Procedures (SOP) for how to operate an intensive care unit (ICU) in two scenarios: (i) during an influenza epidemic and (ii) mass disaster. The intention of the SOP was to provide medical personnel in a hospital direction on how to manage the emergency through guidelines and protocols, and provide the legal basis, authority and organizational relationships during emergency situations. The findings of the Task Force provided important planning recommendations across a range of activities. While the SOP does address the need for coordination and collaboration with 'interface units' within the hospital and regionally through principles of an Incident Management System to organize the overall response, the SOP is primarily designed from the perspective of the ICU as the central planning unit. In 2012, the American College of Chest Physicians' Task Force on Mass CC began updating their recommendations for disaster planning, published in 2014.[11] The primary audience for the findings from this Task Force included clinicians, hospital administrators, public health/ government and medical societies, recognizing that disaster and pandemic planning requires a broad multi-sectoral approach. A dedicated chapter on systems-level planning, coordination, and communication reflects the importance of political leadership to the planning process and the development of a planning and preparedness infrastructure.

In 2012, the Institute of Medicine released their *Crisis Standards of Care, a systems framework for catastrophic disaster response*, in recognition of the "substantial change in healthcare operations and level of care that can be delivered in a public health emergency."[12] Figure 1 shows the framework with key pillars of service delivery of medical care that operate under local, regional and national governments, and are based on ethical and legal bases, and supported by operations, education and information sharing. While all emergencies start local, the framework sets out the roles

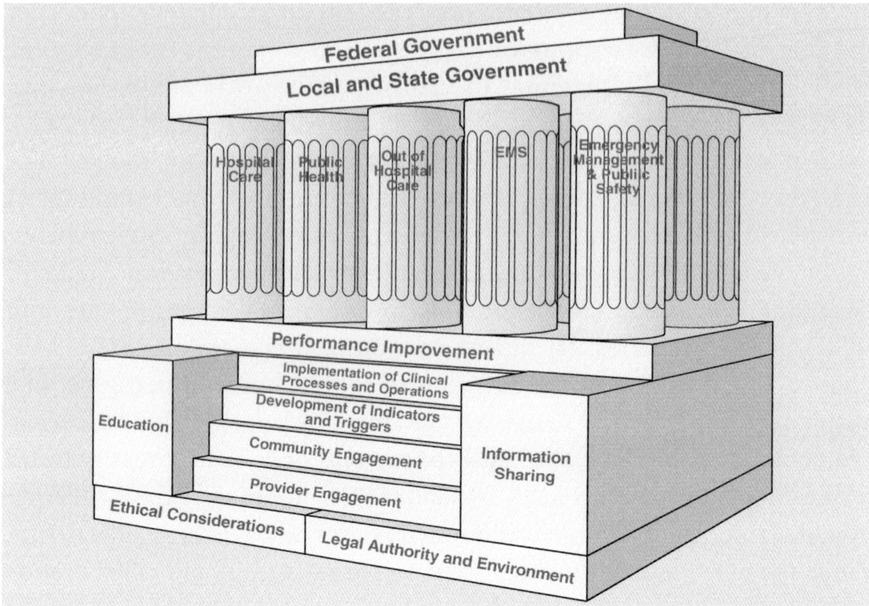

Figure 1. A systems framework for catastrophic disaster response[12] (with permission from the Institute of Medicine).

and relationships from which to build a coordinated, scalable response to an emergency event that overwhelms local resources.

Surge Capacity

The American College of Emergency Physicians (ACEP) defines surge capacity as a measurable representation of ability to manage a sudden influx of patients.[13] This includes both contingency capacity, where existing resources are used to provide functionally equivalent care, and crisis capacity where usual level of care is impossible. Hick *et al.* described this continuum from 'conventional' to 'contingency' to 'crisis' care for disaster events based on levels of increasing demands, and across the areas of space, staff, supplies, standards of care, ICU expansion goals, and level of resources required at the local, regional or national level.[14] Whereas there is often only a limited space to expand capacity within the walls of an ICU, contingency plans include expansion of ICU level care to repurposed areas within the hospital with existing staff managing larger numbers of patients to accommodate the increase in capacity. Crisis operations accommodate an even greater increase in capacity where decisions have to be made on allocation of resources and acceptable alternate levels of care. In addition to total demand on service, the expected duration of surge requirements is important for determining continuity of operations and the alternate levels of care provided within the rest of the healthcare system. Tools for identifying what indicators and triggers can be used by health systems to determine activation of surge capacity plants have been put forward by the IOM Crisis Standards of Care.[12]

Levels of surge used to trigger changes in response can vary based on the jurisdiction, typical operating capacity and by scenario. For example, when short-term surge capacity is anticipated from a mass event, higher levels of surge may be used to trigger contingency or crisis plans. Slower, ongoing high demand scenarios such as an influenza pandemic may use lower cut-offs of overcapacity to trigger implementation of contingency and crisis scenarios. In British Columbia, Canada, ICU overcapacity levels of 15%, 25%, and 40% have been used to define low, medium and high surge levels, and levels above 40% trigger initiation of Emergency Triage Status with provincial coordination of mechanical ventilator allocation through triage teams.

Types of specialty CC provided within a facility may also influence surge capacity planning, such as trauma centres or paediatric units. While not all hospitals with CC services specialize in this level of care, all facilities should be prepared to receive, stabilize and treat these populations for the first 48 hours.[11] This premise of care has also been applied to planning for higher levels of care requiring biocontainment, as in the tiered hospital response to EVD patients and use of Ebola Assessment hospitals that can manage a person under investigation, and Ebola Treatment hospitals with sufficient resources for definitive care.[8] In order to operationalize the coordination of care between holding and specialized facilities, regional plans should include: (i) triage and transfer criteria for specialty patients; (ii) regionally set expectations for non-specialty hospitals level of preparedness; (iii) coordination through a regional triage officer to ensure best available specialty care; (iv) transportation coordination for optimizing site usage; and (v) the legal and human resources agreements to share subject matter expertise where needed across a region. Most facilities have measures for ongoing situational awareness of CC resource utilization due to the daily strain on healthcare systems. However, daily collection and sharing of this type of information for regional decision makers to make coordinated decisions based on accurate and timely information is essential, and preparedness plans should incorporate a Joint Information System for managing measures of utilization and resources during a pandemic. For example, daily assessments at the regional and national level were necessary during H1N1 to ensure equitable access and maximum utilization of ventilation support.

Surge capacity preparedness to meet contingency and crisis demands requires coordinated logistical planning that includes the expansion needs of CC.[11] The Task Force identified a 12 step planning process to achieve the necessary objectives and critical tasks within a facility setting. The aim of the plan would be to identify how within existing hospital resources, those who are the least sick patients could be discharged to community settings, those in intermediate level of care units could be stepped down to general wards, making way for expanded capacity for those who are critically ill. The first step in this process is to identify the team and their organizational authority to conduct the planning process. The team would then need to assess the current capacity and identify the gaps and opportunities where resources are needed to meet surge capacity. Medical leadership within the team is critical during this planning process. This allows pre-set criteria to be developed with clinician input that can be implemented during a pandemic by administration allowing clinical staff to focus on patient care duties. However, due to the impacts on ongoing operations to the rest of the hospital, dissemination of plans requires change management leadership and inclusion of all relevant stakeholders.

In a large pandemic with high clinical severity and resource needs, every area of the hospital will be impacted and needs to agree to and be involved with establishing and practising the plans for their alternative use in a pandemic. Areas that will be expected to deliver higher levels of care than usual require easily moved supplies and equipment, as well as training for staff on their use. Staff training should be based on an inventory of existing skills and training requirements to provide enhanced care.

An assessment of usual services that have impacts on CC will influence contingency plans, and the decision-making process for de-escalation of non-essential services required to shift to surge capacity. A process for continuous improvement, exercises and reassessment should be part of planning and implementation.

Typical facility supply logistics focus on 'just-in-time' inventory management from one or more suppliers to avoid overstocking and expiry of product. Immediate access to stockpiles of essential supplies during a pandemic is required to manage immediate demands while additional supply chains can be established. Most developed countries maintain a national emergency stockpile that can be used to assist local and regional with a 24 hour response through strategically located supply centres. However, local and regional access to these supplies to ensure delivery to the appropriate facilities requires planning and coordination. These plans should also demonstrate that local facilities have plans for how they will best make use of supplies in demand by substituting, conserving, reusing, or reallocating existing and received resources. Local plans will need to address issues of inappropriate sequestering of resources that may occur when a steady supply is not guaranteed, e.g. staff concerns about the lack of sufficient personal protective equipment (PPE) resources to manage their safety. The two main areas of supply chain management in a pandemic plan are PPE and mechanical ventilation support.

Staff safety through the appropriate and knowledgeable use of PPE is critical to maintaining adequate staffing during a pandemic. For new and emerging pathogens, the level of PPE measures may not be well established, as was the case in SARS and the question of need for airborne precautions. Clinical research during pandemics evolves over time, and recommendations on the most appropriate measures may change necessitating corresponding changes to supply chain management and change management with staff. Iterative training and retraining for staff on the use and indications of PPE often need to be developed and disseminated quickly to ensure all staff are adequately prepared for the level of risk they might encounter. Where possible, pre-planning for fit testing, training and assessment of competence in PPE should be initiated and maintained prior to a pandemic because locating and training a competent workforce takes significant time and resource. The duration of PPE supplies for various scenarios will also depend on the level of care expected of the facility. Where all facilities are typically required to manage patients for 48 hours pending transport, higher-level facilities will require longer duration of supplies.[15]

Supply chain management should anticipate pandemics where cases suffer rapid and severe respiratory failure requiring prolonged mechanical ventilation. During H1N1, some countries estimated a 15 times increase in the volume of ICU admissions compared to other seasons, and those most impacted included populations that would require specialized respiratory support, including young children, pregnant women and those who are morbidly obese.[15] Pandemic plans need to include an inventory of existing ventilator supports for both general and specialized populations. If national or regional plans include stockpiled ventilators, plans should ensure they have the mandatory operational, performance, safety and maintenance features to make them immediately available upon deployment, along with the additional operational, communication, training, administration, and other supporting resources required.[11] Supply chain management for ventilation should consider[15]:

- Ventilator Allocation Plans including the full range of ventilation options available and current capacities within the hospital and with the region for coordination with other facilities.
- How additional ventilation support can be increased through reallocation of anaesthesia and recovery room services and the cancellation of elective procedures.
- Where crisis capacity is required, and the regional pandemic coordination team has sanctioned alternate standards of care as part of appropriate crisis standard to meet demands, the use of non-mechanical respiratory support despite mechanical ventilation requirements.

The recent wide spread preparations for EVD patients have highlighted the importance of PPE measures and training, as well as additional facility level logistical requirements. Most facilities do not routinely stockpile PPE for biosafety level 4 pathogens, and do not provide training on the associated infection control practices and procedures of properly donning and doffing such PPE. One of the key findings emerging from the work around preventing EVD nosocomial transmission was the use of a trained observer to supervise donning and doffing procedures to ensure proper completion without breaches. It rapidly became apparent that the physical layouts of ICUs require planning for creation of a special anteroom where supervised donning and doffing could occur, and staffing levels need to accommodate extra personnel for this role. ICU planning also needs to include management of medical waste (solid and liquid) and the associated training required to appropriately store and dispose of waste contaminated with a biosafety level 4 pathogen. This level of biocontainment will also impact the level of ancillary support directly available to the patient through laboratory procedures/protocols for specimen handling, portable imaging services, and other specialty services that require access to the rest of the facility.

For all pandemic planning, management of patient transportation that will be available to support critically ill patients under strict infection prevention and control precautions and/or mechanical ventilation should be considered as part of supply chain logistics. Regional coordination of capacity across facilities has to take into account what type of patient transportation options are available, how quickly they can be available and operating capacity. These plans need to account for staffing and training of transport personnel, and the geography and weather patterns of a region.

Central organization for regional surge capacity requires a Central Triage Committee (CTC) to oversee and coordinate regional ICU usage during a pandemic. Within each facility, an interdisciplinary triage team, led by a CC Leader who has both clinical and administrative expertise and control, is necessary to manage local decision making. While each facility maintains local autonomy of day to day triage and operations, consistent data flow and communication from facilities to the CTC allows for situational awareness to ensure resources are being directed in an appropriate and coordinated way. The CTC oversees the logistical and operational needs, such as PPE ordering and mechanical ventilation usage, monitors and evaluates outcomes, and communicates to facilities to ensure consistency. The CTC may operate as an Emergency Operations Centre (EOC) under an Incident Management System (IMS) to interface with the facilities' EOCs for effective and efficient decision making. Difficult decisions will require rapid assessments from accurate information, ethical and legal input, and potentially additional research to guide oversight and implementation. The CTC also needs to be linked to higher-level jurisdictional (national/international) bodies for coordination beyond the region. Because this infrastructure is infrequently used, regular planning and exercise of the coordination under a CTC is needed to refine the function and communication flow in an emergency situation such as a pandemic.[10,11]

An important role for the CTC is to communicate to facilities and staff on the current level of emergency because of the pandemic and why triage is required. Shifting healthcare teams familiar with a universal access system towards a utilitarian ethic of triage requires clear direction on the need for this type of decision making. Pandemic planning should familiarize staff to this concept, and plan for the appropriate psychosocial supports to assist healthcare providers. Involving staff in the development of clinical decision support systems for triage is necessary to anticipate these types of needs.

Clinical prioritization processes should include: (i) rapid evaluation measures of evidence based prognostic factors, (ii) inclusion and exclusion criteria for ICU admission, (iii) priority level assignment, (iv) frequent reassessment intervals, and (v) appeal/reevaluation processes. Readily available clinical assessment tools should be used to maximize the field locations that can identify the need for ICU care. In general, the need for CC is based on the need for mechanical ventilation and/or vasopressor support. Exclusion criteria are based on:

- prognostic factors for low probability of survival, such as severe and irreversible neurologic events or severe prematurity;
- factors predicting short life expectancy (less than one year).

Prognostic scoring tools, such as the Sequential Organ Failure Assessment (SOFA), have been proposed as additional considerations for inclusion criteria; however, limitations in their validation or predictive ability across all patient population groups prevent their routine use. Other factors, such as potential years of life lost, may also influence assessments of prognostic and life expectancy factors. Based on assessments, patients are either deemed high or medium priority and await ICU admission based on bed availability, or are diverted to other clinical resources for more appropriate care. Reassessments by the local CC triage team at intervals of 48–72 hours are recommended. Assessments require a process for appeals to be considered and managed without undue burden on the care team and adequate support for all involved. Coordination with the rest of facility and other regional services to provide appropriate non-critical care (supportive medical care, community care or palliative care) is required for rapid allocation after triage.[11]

Where pandemic response requires tiered levels of acute care and ICU care, such as specialized EVD treatment units, triage of who is likely to require the highest level of care may mean reviewing individual patients within a central regional committee. This may be feasible when the expected number of total cases is very small, but the impact from any one case is large. In influenza pandemics, the CTC should focus on broader decisions about the type of care provided as the number of patients requiring ICU level care is expected to be high. Individual level care decisions under review by the facility triage team may be escalated during a pandemic based on need for specialized care, or precedent-setting decisions about allocation of care.

Surge Capability

The US Department of Health and Human Services defines 'surge capability' as the *ability to manage patients requiring unusual or very specialized medical evaluation and care.*[16] Where surge capacity focuses on the infrastructure requirements for CC responses to pandemics, surge capability considers the human resources, continuity of operations, and specialized populations that define what type of surge capability exists.

SARS, H1N1, and EVD have all highlighted the extreme importance of staff resource management during pandemics. At a time when increased staffing is required to manage the surge demand, it is likely that there will be significant reductions in available staff due to staff illness/family illness/fear of illness, concerns about personal safety, and poor morale.[15] Unlike surge for a mass event that impacts a specific area and typically for a shorter duration, a global pandemic will result in widespread and cumulative shortages. There will be no unaffected areas for redeployment, and over the course of the pandemic, staff illness, burn-out, and other attrition will further deplete available staffing. Therefore, planning should take into account the predicted increase in staffing demand based on surge level while anticipating a reduction in actual available staff. Modeling tools can assist in estimating staffing requirements based on surge level.[17]

In general, increased staff time for CC can come from increasing hours of existing staff and reallocating staff from other areas to CC. Existing staff may be expected to work longer hours and decrease work hours related to non-CC activities (e.g. administration, elective procedures). Regional coordination should also address the administrative, legal and other barriers to cross-facility redeployment of CC staff through Memoranda of Understanding to maximize allocation to areas with highest need. Reassignment of non-CC staff will require CC staff to take on supervisory roles instead of or in addition to direct care roles to maintain the necessary level of CC expertise for all patients. Regional planning should have mechanisms to allow expedited expanded scope of practice/privileges for staff and students under the emergency provisions of a pandemic. Engagement with the broad range of workforce stakeholders during inter-pandemic periods allows for discussion and the development of the necessary infrastructure to support CC staffing.[10,15]

Planning for expanding staff roles requires coordination between Workplace Health and Safety and administrative databases to review available staff and monitor and maintain the necessary training and skill level of those staff to be ready in case of a pandemic. Fit-testing and training for use of PPE can be time-consuming and best maintained on an ongoing basis. Similarly, preparation and dissemination of infection control and exposure control plans need continuous updating, while recognizing specific needs associated a novel pathogen may emerge over time. In the case of pandemics that impact specific populations, such as a high burden of paediatric patients, staffing requirements will need to adjust for expertise and capacity. For pandemics where cohorting of staff and patients is recommended to prevent spread of infection within the facility, staff rotation restrictions may also impede flexibility of staff allocation.[10]

Those managing healthcare facilities have a duty to provide a safe work environment for their staff, as well as a supportive environment that addresses their psychosocial needs. Strict adherence to infection prevention and control measures are necessary to prevent staff transmission and illness. However, maintenance of these measures may be impeded by the mental and physical tolerability of the PPE, and changing/inconsistent information received about requirements. Facility and regional coordination is needed to provide oversight of infection control practices and a single source of information about required measures that is presented by an expert in risk communication. As well, for the development of consistent practices on how staff accommodations will be addressed to support personal and family needs, stressful conditions, and work refusals.[15] In the development of specialized units for EVD treatment, use of staff who volunteered for the unit facilitated high levels of staff engagement; however, high volumes from a pandemic will demand all available staff who will have a wide spectrum of needs to feel it is a safe and supportive work environment. Placement of social support staff within CC and other settings to monitor, anticipate and be readily available to respond to psychosocial needs of staff is recommended.

A 'whole-of-community' approach is also needed when considering plans for CC surge, as pandemics will put a strain on the entire continuum of the health system with a need for increased capacity and capability within primary care, emergency care and other sectors. Continuity of operations at all levels will be impacted by a widespread pandemic due to reduced staffing and increased demand. Efficient and accessible primary care/public health that provides preventive measures, such as immunization and antiviral prophylaxis, and early triage assessment and treatment is essential to reducing the escalation of need for CC. Other measures, such as mobile assessment units, increased home care support, and opening residential care capacity, may enable increased capacity within facilities and expansion of CC services. Most facility continuity of operations plans should address various levels of reduced staffing scenarios and what are the non-essential services that will be stopped; however, these plans should also incorporate the duration of reduced services and the surrounding health and community services outside of the facility that support those temporary reductions. Regular monitoring and assessment at a local and regional level of facility and community indicators is needed to communicate needs and plan across the health system.

Other specialized resources that contribute to surge capability may depend on the populations impacted by the pandemic. Paediatric CC resource management requires its own planning given the complexity of needs and potential for even further limited capacity compared to available resources. High burden of illness in obese and pregnant populations from H1N1 may demand planning for specialized infrastructure and staff. Transportation plans should anticipate an increased demand for transfers from remote and rural locations to CC facilities where populations may be more vulnerable due to lack of prevention and primary care services and the underlying health status of the population. All of the planning scenarios should also consider the broader context of support required to manage these patients beyond their CC needs. This may include: supportive care and accommodation for family members attending paediatric patients and those transferred from remote locations, cultural and language services, and grief and religious services. Technological resources may facilitate care scenarios, such as the use of dedicated tablets for those under prolonged isolation to communicate with facility care providers as well as their support networks, while reducing the need to expose additional staff to infectious patients.

Ethics of Pandemic Planning

An ethical framework is needed to guide the difficult decision making associated with pandemic planning and the ongoing urgent questions and issues that arise during a pandemic. The process of ethics-based planning should be pragmatic and transparent and enable the planning team to come to a common consensus of the core ethical values underlying decision making, and develop planning principles to guide future decisions. Ethical issues will arise at all levels of care, but a common framework for local and regional coordination provides a more fair and equitable approach for consistent decision making across facilities.[11] These processes require time for reflection and discussion and must be undertaken in the inter-pandemic years. As discussed in this chapter, where triage allocations will be required based on surge demands, there will be a shift towards a utilitarian ethic of healthcare decision making. However, allocation is only one component for planning CC services, and ethical principles of respect, minimizing harm, fairness, autonomy, and reciprocity are key considerations for managing staffing and patient care decisions.

Along with an ethical framework, pandemic planning should be based in legal, regulatory, and risk-management frameworks to guide decision making. Regional, national and international laws must be upheld during a pandemic. For example, countries must comply with the World Health Organization's International Health Regulations on disease notification and sharing of information. Regional laws on the public health provision of emergency powers during a pandemic may allow for expansion of resources available that assist in surge capacity. Development of MOUs and other mechanisms that facilitate movement of staff and infrastructure are also critical preparations.

Research in pandemics

High demand for information needs during a pandemic necessitate active research agenda planning and preparation as part of pandemic preparedness. Early in the course of the outbreak, particularly for novel pathogens, there will be urgent questions to guide the identification, treatment, control and prevention of the infection. International coordination of such research, particularly clinical trials, maximizes efforts in acute and CC settings. Understanding burden of illness, reproduction rate, and vulnerable populations are also key inputs at a global and local level to determining what level of surge capacity may be anticipated for implementation of plans. Protocols for the observational and clinical trial study designs to address anticipated research questions should be developed and approved ahead of time for immediate implementation. Data collection tools that can be used on an ongoing basis with minor revision for adaptation to a pandemic establish ongoing baseline data, avoid introduction during a pandemic, and allow regional, national and international comparison. Ethical review initiated during a pandemic may also restrict the timeliness of research, and pre-approval is recommended. Where pre-approval is not available, a centralized and expedited ethical review process should be used to balance benefits and harms.[18]

Summary

Pandemic planning for CC is an ongoing process. It requires coordination of efforts using a whole-of-society approach to involve the appropriate stakeholders during inter-pandemic periods. While the 'what' and the 'when' of the next pandemic cannot be predicted, planning efforts should develop the necessary basis to address the needs that arise.

"*O happy posterity, who will not experience such abysmal woe and will look upon our testimony as a fable.*" — Petrarch (1304–1374) regarding the Bubonic plague.

References

1. Low DE and McGeer A (2010). Pandemic (H1N1) 2009: assessing the response. *CMAJ,* 182(17), 1874–1878.
2. World Health Organization Regional Office for Europe (2010). Recommendations for good practice in pandemic preparedness. 2010. Available at: http://www.euro.who.int/__data/assets/pdf_file/0017/128060/e94534.pdf (Accessed 16 April 2016).
3. Fineberg HV (2014). Pandemic preparedness and response-lessons learned from the H1N1 influenza of 2009. *NEJM,* 370, 1335–1342.
4. Public Health Agency of Canada (2011). The Canadian pandemic influenza plan for the health care sector. 13 September, 2011. Available at: http://www.phac-aspc.gc.ca/cpip-pclcpi/ (Accessed 16 April 2016).
5. World Health Organization (2013). Pandemic influenza risk management: WHO interim guidance. Available at: http://www.who.int/influenza/preparedness/pandemic/influenza_risk_management/en/ (Accessed 16 April 2016).
6. Federal Emergency Management Agency (2015). Mission Areas. 19 March, 2015. Available at: http://www.fema.gov/mission-areas (Accessed 16 April 2016).
7. Gates B (2015). The Next Epidemic — Lessons from Ebola. *New Engl. J. Med.,* 372, 1381–1384.
8. Centers for Disease Control and Prevention (2015). Interim guidance for U.S. hospital preparedness for patients under investigation (PUIs) or with confirmed Ebola Virus Disease (EVD): a framework for a tiered approach. Available at: http://www.cdc.gov/vhf/ebola/healthcare-us/preparing/hospitals.html (Accessed 16 April 2013).
9. Ministry of Health and Long-Term Care (2013). Ontario health plan for an influenza pandemic 2013. Avaiable at: http://www.health.gov.on.ca/en/pro/programs/emb/pan_flu/pan_flu_plan.aspx (Accessed 16 April 2013).
10. European Society of Intensive Care Medicine's Task Force for Intensive Care Unit Triage during an Influenza Epidemic or Mass Disaster. *Intensive Care Med.,* 36 (1), 1–79.

11. Sandrock CE (2014). Care of the critically ill and injured during pandemics and disasters: Groundbreaking Results from the Task Force on Mass Critical Care. *Chest,* 146(4), 1–41.
12. Institute of Medicine (2012). Report. Crisis standards of care: a systems framework for catastrophic disaster response. Available at: http://iom.nationalacademies.org/Reports/2012/Crisis-Standards-of-Care-A-Systems-Framework-for-Catastrophic-Disaster-Response.aspx (Accessed 21 March 2012).
13. American College of Emergency Physicians (2010). Health care system surge capacity recognition, preparedness, and response. Available at: http://www.acep.org/Clinical — Practice-Management/Health-Care-System-Surge-Capacity-Recognition,-Preparedness,-and-Response/ (Accessed October 2011).
14. Hick JL, Barbera JA and Kelen GD (2009). Refining surge capacity: conventional, contingency, and crisis capacity. *Disaster Med. Public Health Prep.* 3(2), 59–67.
15. Manuell ME, Co MDT and Ellison RT (2011). Pandemic influenza: implications for preparedness and delivery of critical care services. *J. of Intensive Care Med.* 26(6), 347–367.
16. US Department of Health and Human Services (2012). Public Health Emergency, Medical Surge Capacity Handbook. Available at: http://www.phe.gov/Preparedness/planning/mscc/handbook/Pages/appendixd.aspx (Accessed 14 February 2013).
17. Nap RE, Andriessen PHM, Meessen NEL, Miranda DDR and Van Der Werf TS (2008). Pandemic influenza and excess intensive-care workload. *Emerging Infectious Disease,* 14(10), 1518–1525.
18. Gabriel LEK and Webb SAR (2013). Preparing ICUs for pandemics. *Curr. Opin. Crit. Care,* 19, 467–473.

Index

D

E

F

G

H

I

J

K

L

Q

R

U

V

W

Y